I0034876

Biostatistical Methods and Applications in Health Research

Supported by real-world case studies, this essential textbook provides a detailed overview of the use of biostatistical tools and methods, enabling students and researchers to undertake their own research with confidence and understanding.

After a general introduction to the field, the book provides a step-by-step description of the essential statistical methods that are foundational to analysing data from clinical trials, epidemiological studies and other health-related research. From basic concepts such as probability and distribution through to hypothesis testing, regression analysis, survival analysis, meta-analysis and systematic reviews, each chapter is designed with a clear pedagogical approach featuring explanatory diagrams, real-life examples and sample problems. Later sections of the book cover clinical trial design and analysis, diagnostic testing, Bayesian methods and machine learning. Through this detailed, comprehensive treatment of the key tools and methods, the book encourages readers to develop their own critical thinking skills, recognising good or bad pieces of research when they see them, asking questions about where evidence and assumptions come from or choosing the most appropriate biostatistical methodologies in their own research.

Written by a team of experts with extensive teaching experience in this field, this is the ideal textbook for graduate students and researchers across the biomedical sciences, from public health to epidemiology to clinical medicine.

Vivek Verma, Assistant Professor, Department of Statistics, Assam University Silchar, Assam, India.

Hafiz T.A. Khan, Professor of Public Health and Statistics at the University of West London and a Professorial Fellow at the Oxford Institute of Population Ageing, University of Oxford, UK. For the last three decades, he has been involved in teaching applied statistics, public health, demography, health economics and research methods. He has published more than 260 research articles in various international journals.

Dilip C. Nath, Former Vice-Chancellor of Assam University and Professor of Statistics at Gauhati University, India. He has published more than 200 research papers in reputed national and international journals. His current research interests are in biostatistics, medical statistics, demography and actuarial statistics.

Kenneth C. Land, John Franklin Crowell Professor Emeritus of Sociology at Duke University, where he is also a research professor at the Social Science Research Institute. He worked as faculty in the University of Illinois at Urbana-Champaign and the University of Texas at Austin and has published more than 450 research papers in various international journals.

Biostatistical Methods and Applications in Health Research

A Case Study Approach

Edited by Vivek Verma, Hafiz T.A. Khan, Dilip C. Nath, and Kenneth C. Land

Routledge
Taylor & Francis Group

LONDON AND NEW YORK

Designed cover image: Getty Images

First published 2026
by Routledge
4 Park Square, Milton Park, Abingdon, Oxon OX14 4RN

and by Routledge
605 Third Avenue, New York, NY 10158

Routledge is an imprint of the Taylor & Francis Group, an informa business

© 2026 selection and editorial matter, Vivek Verma, Hafiz T.A. Khan, Dilip C. Nath, and Kenneth C. Land; individual chapters, the contributors

The right of Vivek Verma, Hafiz T.A. Khan, Dilip C. Nath, and Kenneth C. Land to be identified as the authors of the editorial material, and of the authors for their individual chapters, has been asserted in accordance with sections 77 and 78 of the Copyright, Designs and Patents Act 1988.

All rights reserved. No part of this book may be reprinted or reproduced or utilised in any form or by any electronic, mechanical, or other means, now known or hereafter invented, including photocopying and recording, or in any information storage or retrieval system, without permission in writing from the publishers.

Trademark notice: Product or corporate names may be trademarks or registered trademarks, and are used only for identification and explanation without intent to infringe.

British Library Cataloguing-in-Publication Data
A catalogue record for this book is available from the British Library

ISBN: 978-1-032-70097-7 (hbk)
ISBN: 978-1-032-70099-1 (pbk)
ISBN: 978-1-032-70100-4 (ebk)

DOI: 10.4324/9781032701004

Typeset in Sabon
by Apex CoVantage, LLC

Contents

Figures

Tables

Contributors

Abdulsalam Ahmed, Senior Researcher Department of Community Health, Ibrahim Badamasi Babangida University Nigeria, Nigeria

Dibyojyoti Bhattacharjee, Professor in Statistics, Department of Statistics, Assam University, Silchar, India

Prativa Choudhury, Research Associate, Department of Paediatric Surgery, All India Institute of Medical Sciences, India

Robert Cook, Senior Research Fellow, School of Health, Education, Policing and Sciences, University of Staffordshire, United Kingdom

Kishore Kumar Das, Professor in Statistics, Department of Statistics, Gauhati University, India

Anjan Kumar Dhua, Professor of Paediatric Surgery, Department of Paediatric Surgery, All India Institute of Medical Sciences, India

Prabudh Goel, Professor in Paediatric, Department of Paediatric Surgery, All India Institute of Medical Sciences, India

Gagan Gunjan, Assistant Professor in Medicine, Department of Medicine, Rajendra Institute of Medical Sciences, India

Ahmed Hossain, Associate Professor of Biostatistics, College of Health Sciences, University of Sharjah, United Arab Emirates

Nazim Husain, Research Officer (Unani), Regional Research Institute of Unani Medicine, India

Nuha Ibrahim, Research Officer, Evidence Centre, Health Research Board (HRB), Dublin, Ireland

Divya Jain, Associate Professor in Ophthalmology, Department of Ophthalmology, Post Graduate Institute of Child Health, India

Amirhossein Jalali, Associate Professor in Biostatistics, School of Medicine, University of Limerick, Limerick, Ireland

Denny John, Professor of Health Economics, MS Ramaiah University of Applied Sciences, India

Hafiz T.A. Khan, Professor of Public Health and Statistics, College of Nursing Midwifery and Healthcare, University of West London, United Kingdom, and Professorial Fellow, Oxford Institute of Population Ageing, University of Oxford, United Kingdom

Masuma Khanam, Research Scholar, Department of Statistics, Assam University, India

Anoop Kumar, Assistant Professor in Pharmaceutical, Delhi Pharmaceutical Science and Research University, India

Mukesh Kumar, Assistant Professor in Statistics, Department of Statistics, MMV, Banaras Hindu University, India

Dilip C. Nath, Professor Emeritus, School of Applied and Pure Sciences, The Assam Royal Global University, Guwahati, Assam, India

Gholamreza Oskrochi, Professor of Statistics, College of Engineering and Technology, American University of the Middle East, Kuwait

Kamalesh Kumar Patel, Scientist II, Clinical Research Unit, All India Institute of Medical Sciences, India

Pratibha Prasad, Assistant Professor in Neurology, Department of Neurology, All India Institute of Medical Sciences Patna, India

Shafiqur Rahman, Associate Professor of Statistics, School of Natural and Physical Sciences, University of Papua New Guinea, Papua New Guinea

Shainee Saha, Research Scholar, Department of Statistics, Gauhati University, India

Zillur Rahman Shabuz, Senior Research Associate, School of Mathematical Sciences, Lancaster University, United Kingdom

Santosh Kumar Sharma, Postdoctoral Researcher, School of Medicine, University of Limerick, Limerick, Ireland

Vivek Verma, Assistant Professor of Statistics, Department of Statistics, Assam University Silchar, Assam, India

Ramesh K. Vishwakarma, Senior Research Associate in Biostatistics, Norwich Medical School, University of East Anglia, Norwich, United Kingdom

## CHAPTER 1

Introduction to Biostatistics

Vivek Verma

Background

Biostatistics plays a critical role in health research, providing essential tools for the analysis and interpretation of data related to health, disease, and medical interventions. This introductory section of the book on biostatistics aims to provide a systematic exploration of the key pedagogical features that will guide readers through the fundamental concepts, importance, and practical applications of biostatistical methods in health research.

Definition of Biostatistics

Biostatistics is a specialized branch of statistics that applies statistical techniques to the collection, analysis, and interpretation of data related to biological, medical, and health-related fields. It is an interdisciplinary science that bridges the gap between biology, medicine, and statistical theory. By utilizing mathematical models and statistical tools, biostatistics helps researchers make sense of complex biological phenomena and health outcomes.

Importance of Biostatistics

Biostatistics is vital for several reasons in health research:

- **Evidence-Based Decision-Making:** In health research, biostatistics enables researchers and policymakers to make data-driven decisions, ensuring that conclusions drawn from health data are reliable and valid.
- **Designing Robust Studies:** It guides the design of health studies, such as clinical trials, observational studies, and epidemiological research, ensuring that the methodologies used are appropriate to the research objectives.

DOI: 10.4324/9781032701004-1

- **Analyzing Health Data:** Biostatistics helps in analyzing complex datasets, identifying patterns, and drawing meaningful conclusions about public health trends, risk factors, treatment efficacy, and disease prevention.
- **Policy Formulation:** Governments and health organizations rely on biostatistical methods to establish guidelines, regulations, and policies that promote health and prevent disease.

Applications of Biostatistics in Health Research

Biostatistics has vast applications in various aspects of health research, including but not limited to the following:

- **Epidemiology:** Biostatistics is crucial in the study of disease patterns, causes, and risk factors within populations. It supports epidemiological research in assessing the prevalence, incidence, and distribution of diseases.
- **Clinical Trials:** Biostatistical methods are essential for designing clinical trials, determining sample sizes, analyzing treatment effects, and interpreting trial results to determine the efficacy and safety of medical interventions.
- **Genetic and Molecular Studies:** In genomics, biostatistics aids in analyzing data from genetic studies, helping to identify genes associated with diseases and understanding genetic predispositions to certain conditions.
- **Public Health:** Biostatistics supports public health interventions by analyzing health surveys, evaluating health programs, and identifying health disparities among different populations.
- **Environmental Health:** Biostatistical techniques are used to examine the effects of environmental exposures (e.g., pollutants) on human health, helping to guide regulations and public health policies.

Pedagogical Approach Followed for Learning Biostatistics

The book will use an accessible pedagogical framework that includes the following features:

- **Clear Definitions and Terminology:** Every key term and concept will be defined concisely to ensure that readers build a strong foundation.
- **Step-by-Step Problem-Solving:** Real-life examples and practical exercises will guide readers through the process of applying statistical methods to health research data.
- **Graphical Representation:** Diagrams, charts, and tables will be used extensively to enhance understanding and provide visual clarity on statistical concepts and results.
- **Interactive Learning Tools:** The book will include practice problems, quizzes, and case studies that allow learners to apply statistical techniques in diverse health research scenarios.
- **Focus on Real-World Applications:** Emphasis will be placed on how biostatistical methods are directly applied in contemporary health research, such as in analyzing clinical trial data, understanding disease outbreaks, and public health studies.

Key Statistical Methods and Applications in Health Research

This section of the book outlines the essential statistical methods that are frequently used in health research. These techniques are foundational to analyzing data from clinical trials, epidemiological studies, and other health-related research areas. Each chapter is designed with a clear pedagogical approach to help readers build a comprehensive understanding of these important topics.

- **Probability and Distributions:** The book will start with the basic concepts of probability, including events, sample spaces, and probability laws. Clear, step-by-step examples will demonstrate how probabilities are calculated in the context of health research (e.g., probability of a disease occurrence or treatment success). The book will introduce the most commonly used probability distributions in health research, and each of them will be explained through real-world health examples.

- **Hypothesis Testing:** The book will break down the hypothesis testing procedure, from formulating the null and alternative hypotheses to choosing appropriate parametric and non-parametric tests. The concepts of significance levels, power of the test, and p-values will be explained in-depth, with a focus on their importance in medical decision-making. Real-life medical study examples will illustrate hypothesis testing.

- **Regression Analysis:** This chapter will cover simple and multiple linear regression analysis, teaching readers to model relationships between a continuous outcome and predictor variables. The book will introduce logistic regression for analyzing binary outcomes (e.g., presence or absence of a disease) and provide step-by-step guidance on model interpretation.

- **Survival Analysis:** This section will explain the unique nature of survival data and introduce key concepts such as censoring and hazard functions. The book will guide readers through constructing Kaplan-Meier survival curves and Cox model in interpreting survival probabilities over time.

- **Meta-Analysis and Systematic Reviews:** Introduction to meta-analysis and systematic reviews will explain their role in synthesizing evidence across multiple studies to draw more reliable conclusions. Techniques like fixed effects and random effects models for combining effect sizes will be explained with a focus on their applications in health research. Readers will be guided through the steps of conducting a meta-analysis, including data extraction, heterogeneity assessment, and interpretation of results. Real examples from medical literature will demonstrate how meta-analytic findings influence health policy.

- **Clinical Trials Design and Analysis:** The key aspects of clinical trial design, such as randomization, blinding, and control groups. It will explain how to determine sample size and statistical power before conducting a trial. The focus will be on analyzing the outcomes of clinical trials using methods such as t-tests, ANOVA, and survival analysis. Detailed case studies from clinical trials will illustrate the statistical methods and their application in assessing treatment effects.

- **Diagnostic Tests: Statistical Methods Specifically for Clinical Decisions:** This chapter will teach the reader about key statistical measures used to evaluate diagnostic tests, including sensitivity, specificity, positive predictive value, and negative predictive value. Readers will learn how to use receiver operating characteristic

(ROC) curves to assess and compare diagnostic test performance. Practical examples will show how these methods are used to evaluate diagnostic tools (e.g., blood tests) for diseases.

■ *Bayesian Methods and Machine Learning*: This chapter will introduce the concept of Bayesian inference, emphasizing how it differs from traditional frequentist statistics. Key concepts, such as prior distributions, posterior distributions, and Bayes' theorem, will be explained clearly. Practical applications of Bayesian methods in clinical trials and public health will be discussed, showing how Bayesian models allow for incorporating prior knowledge and uncertainty in health research. The book will also introduce basic machine learning techniques, explaining their growing role in biostatistics for predicting health outcomes, identifying risk factors, and analyzing large datasets.

Conclusion

The book provides a thorough, step-by-step exploration of advanced statistical methods used in biostatistics, with a focus on practical applications in health research. Each topic will include clear explanations, real-world examples, and exercises to ensure that readers not only grasp the theoretical aspects of these methods but also gain practical experience in applying them to improve public health decision-making. By the end of the book, readers will be well-equipped to understand, analyze, and interpret complex health data, with the skills needed to contribute meaningfully to health research and policy formulation.

PART I

Basic Statistics, Probability and Statistical Hypothetical Testing

Descriptive Statistics in Health Research

Methods for Summarizing Health-Related Data

Shafiqur Rahman

Learning Outcomes

Readers will gain foundational knowledge of descriptive statistics as essential tools for summarizing and presenting health-related data. They will learn to calculate and interpret measures of central tendency (mean, median, mode) and dispersion (range, variance, standard deviation, interquartile range). Emphasis will be placed on identifying data patterns, understanding distribution characteristics such as skewness and kurtosis, and selecting appropriate graphical displays like histograms, box plots, and scatterplots. By mastering these skills, learners will be equipped to translate raw data into meaningful summaries that support public health research, clinical decision-making, and effective communication of study findings.

Introduction

Health statistics is a part of statistics that deals with collection, presentation, analysis, and interpretation of data related to public health and healthcare (Heumann et al., 2022). It is used to understand risk factors for communities, track and monitor health events such as diseases, see the impact of government's policy changes, and assess the quality and safety of healthcare (Rosner, 2015).

The words data and statistics are closely related with each other. The main ingredient of the subject statistics is data. If there is no data, there is no statistics. The functions of statistics are as follows: It presents facts in a definite form, it simplifies mass of figures, it facilitates comparison, it helps in formulating and testing hypothesis, it helps in prediction, and it helps in policymaking. Health statistics is a branch of statistics (Agarwal, 2023) that deals with data relating to human biology, health, and medicine.

Data: Data are the observed values of a variable. Data can be either qualitative or quantitative.

Variable: Variable is a characteristic which varies from individual to individual or element to element.

Elements: The elements are the entries or issues on which data are collected.

Observations: The set of measurements collected for a particular element or individual is called observation.

Let us consider the following dataset on coronavirus cases for four countries to understand the aforementioned four terms:

Table 2.1 Coronavirus cases for four countries

Country	Continent	Total cases	Total deaths	Cases/1M	Deaths/1M
USA	North America	244,877	6,070	740	18
Italy	Europe	115,242	4,668	1,906	230
Spain	Europe	112,065	10,348	2,397	221
Germany	Europe	84,794	1,107	1,012	13

Source: https://www.worldometers.info/coronavirus/

For the earlier dataset, each country is an element. The dataset has four elements, five variables (Continent, Total cases, Total deaths, Cases per million, Deaths per million), and $4 \times 5 = 20$ observations.

Classification of Data

Qualitative Data: When the data being studied is non-numeric and used to identify an attribute of each element. In the earlier dataset in Table 2.1, the variable continent name is non-numeric. The name of continent is qualitative variable.

Quantitative Data: When the data studied is reported numerically, the data is called quantitative data. It indicates either how much or how many. In the previous table, the values 244,877, 6,070, 740, and so on are numerical values, and these are quantitative data, and the variables Total cases, Total deaths, Cases/one million, and Deaths/one million are quantitative variables. Quantitative data are either discrete or continuous.

Cross-Sectional and Time Series Data

Cross-Sectional Data: When the data is collected at the same point in time, then they are called cross-sectional data. The body temperatures of four patients (Table 2.2) taken by a nurse at around 8:00 A.M. from a hospital room on the 15th of November 2025 are cross-sectional data because they are collected at the same point in time.

Time Series Data: When the data are collected over several periods of time, then they are called time series data. The following is a time series data.

Data Collection/Sources

Data can be collected from two sources: (a) primary source and (b) secondary source

Table 2.2 Body temperature of a patient at different times of the day

Time	Body temperature (in degree centigrade) of a patient
5:00 A.M.	38.1°
6:00 A.M.	37.5°
7:00 A.M.	38.2°
8:00 A.M.	38.9°
9:00 A.M.	39.4°
10:00 A.M.	38.3°
11:00 A.M.	37.9°

Primary date: These are original/raw data. It can be collected by the following techniques

(i) Direct personal interview
(ii) Indirect sources
(iii) Local agency
(iv) Questionnaire method

Direct Personal Interview: In this case, the researcher or the investigator collects data directly from the respondents. For example, if you want to know the health condition of cancer patients, you can contact them directly and collect your desired information.

Indirect Sources: In this case, data are collected from the third party. Sometimes the respondents do not want to give information about him; in this case, a third party can give information about him. For example, if you want to know some information about AIDS patients, you can collect it from the hospital, not from the patients, as the general tendency of patients with AIDS is to hide the information that they are suffering from the disease.

Local Agency: In this case, different local agencies are set up at different places. First, they collect data and then they send it to the central/head office. News media uses this system of collecting information.

Questionnaire Method: This is a very popular method. A formal list of questions is called a questionnaire. In this case, the investigator makes a questionnaire and sends it to the respondent to collect data.

Secondary Sources: In this case, data can be collected from the following published data:

(i) Government sources
(ii) Nongovernmental sources
(iii) Bureau of Statistics
(iv) Published journals/books
(v) Central bank, etc.

Tabular and Graphical Presentation of Data

After the raw data has been collected, the next step is to present them in some suitable form, either in a statistical table or in a graphical form.

Summarizing Qualitative Data

Frequency Distribution: A frequency distribution is a tabular summary of a set of data showing the frequency (or number) of items in each of several non-overlapping classes. The number of times a particular value is repeated is called frequency.

Objective: The main objective of frequency distribution is to provide real picture about the data that cannot be quickly obtained by looking only at the original data.

Example 2.2.1: suppose we ask 40 outdoor patients of a public hospital about their main health issues for visiting the hospital and receive the following responses:

Fever	Headache	Chest pain	Fever
Diarrhea	Fever	Fever	Diarrhea
Chest pain	Fever	Diarrhea	Headache
Diarrhea	Headache	Fever	Fever
Headache	Fever	Diarrhea	Diarrhea
Diarrhea	Chest pain	Diarrhea	Headache
Fever	Diarrhea	Fever	Headache
Diarrhea	Chest pain	Headache	Fever
Fever	Headache	Fever	Fever
Headache	Fever	Diarrhea	Diarrhea

It is difficult to understand the health issues pattern from this dataset. We need to organize the data to get a clear picture of the trend of the health issues' responses. The first step is to determine the frequency with which each health issue has been chosen. In this example, "fever" was selected by 15 patients. In statistical terms, we say that the category "fever" has a frequency of 15. We can determine the frequency of choice for each of the other health issues and list them in a frequency distribution, as shown in Table 2.3. Here, we have introduced our first two statistical symbols: f, meaning frequency, and N, meaning the total number of responses.

Display of Data

Relative Frequency Distribution: A relative frequency distribution of a class is the proportion of the total number of data items belonging to the class.

For a dataset with no observations, the relative frequency for each class is given by the formula (see Table 2.4).

$$\text{Relative Frequency of a Class} = \frac{Frequency\ of\ the\ class}{n}$$

Table 2.3 Frequency distribution of health issues of 40 patients

Health issues	f
Headache	9
Diarrhea	12
Chest pain	4
Fever	15
	$N = 40$

Table 2.4 Relative frequency distribution of health issues of 40 patients

Health issues	Relatively frequency
Headache	0.225
Diarrhea	0.3
Chest pain	0.1
Fever	0.375
Total	**1**

Table 2.5 Percent frequency distribution of pet choices of 40 children

Health issues	Percent frequency
Headache	22.5
Diarrhea	30
Chest pain	10
Fever	37.5
Total	**100**

Bar Graph

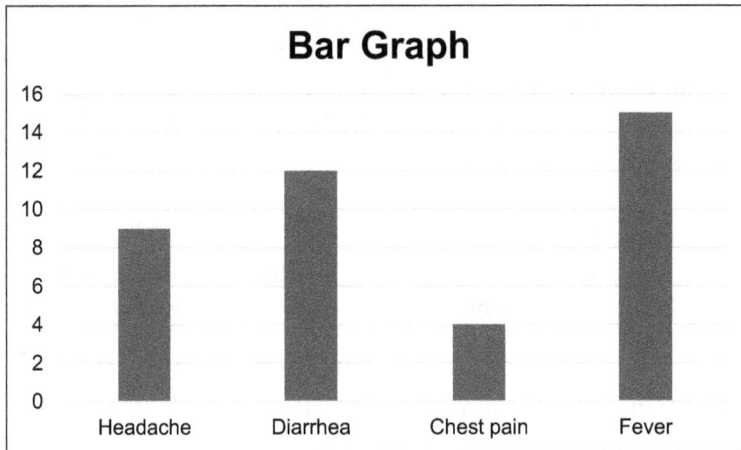

Figure 2.1 Bar chart.

Percent Frequency Distribution: A percent frequency distribution is a tabular summary of a dataset showing the percent frequency for each class. That is, the percent frequency of a class is the relative frequency multiplied by 100 (see Table 2.5).

Percent Frequency of a Class = Relative Frequency of the Class × 100

Bar Graphs: A bar graph is a graphical device for representing data that has been summarized in a frequency, relative frequency, or percent frequency distribution. On the horizontal axis of the graph, we specify the labels/class. On the other hand, we put frequency, relative frequency, or percent frequency on the vertical axis of the graph. The bars are separated to emphasize the fact that each class is a separate category. Each category is assigned a rectangular bar whose height is proportional to the observed value for that category (see Figure 2.1).

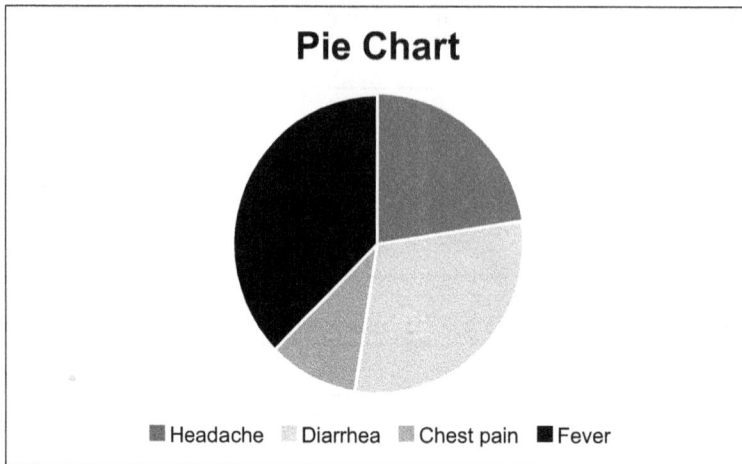

Figure 2.2 Pie chart.

Pie Chart: A pie chart is also a graphical device for presenting relative frequency distribution of data. It is commonly useful for qualitative data. It is based on the subdivision of a circle into different sectors. To draw a pie chart, first make a circle with an appropriate radius, then use the relative frequency to subdivide the circle into sectors/parts that correspond to the relative frequency for each class (see Figure 2.2).

Summarizing Quantitative Data

The definitions given earlier for qualitative data will remain the same for quantitative data as well. But here, we need to be very careful about the definition of classes. In such a case, we need to take thre important steps:

1. Determine the number of non-overlapping classes.
2. Determine the width of the classes.
3. Determine the class limits.

Number of Classes: Classes are formed by specifying the ranges of data values that will be used to group the elements in the dataset. In general, the recommended number of classes is between five and twenty. Datasets with a larger number of elements usually require a larger number of classes.

For example, we consider the following quantitative dataset representing the total cholesterol level of 26 patients:

281	193	296	268	195	215	160
212	216	236	271	215	207	222
151	277	260	180	164	206	204
226	322	217	301	284		

Since the dataset given earlier is relatively small, $(n = 26)$, we can choose only five classes to develop frequency distribution.

Width of the Classes: This is the second step for constructing a frequency distribution. In general, the width of the class should be same for each class. The formula for approximate class width is given next.

$$\text{Approximate Class Width} = \frac{largest\ data\ value - smallest\ data\ value}{Number\ of\ classes}$$

The approximate class width (ACW) can be rounded to a more convenient value.

For the earlier dataset, the ACW is $\frac{322-151}{5} = 34.2$. In such a fractional case, we may consider 34 or 35 as the class width.

Class Limits: Class limits should be chosen in such a way that each data value belongs to one and only one class. The lower-class limit identifies the smallest possible value, and the upper-class limit identifies the largest possible value assigned to the class.

Our previous dataset is rounded to the nearest integer, so we can define the class limits as 150–184, 185–219, 220–254, 255–289, and 290–324. The smallest data value, 151, is included in class 150–184, whereas the largest data value, 322, is included in the 290–324 class. The difference between the lower-class limits of adjacent classes provides the class width. Using the first two lower class limits of 185 and 150, we see that the class width is $185 - 150 = 35$.

After determining the number of classes, class width, and class limits, a frequency, relative frequency, and percent frequency distribution can be obtained by using the earlier (see Table 2.6) dataset as follows.

Histogram: Histogram is one of the most common graphical representations of quantitative data. If the classes in a frequency table all have the same width, then the table can be represented graphically by a simple modification of bar chart, and it is called histogram. It is constructed by placing the variable of interest on the horizontal axis and the frequency, relative frequency, or percent frequency on the vertical axis. The frequency, relative frequency, or percent frequency of each class is shown by drawing a rectangular bar whose base is the class interval on the horizontal axis and whose height is the corresponding frequency, relative frequency, or percent frequency.

Table 2.6 Frequency distribution of quantitative data

Cholesterol level	Frequency	Relative frequency	Percent frequency
150–184	4	4/26 = 0.15	0.15 × 100 = 15
185–219	10	10/26 = 0.38	0.38 × 100 = 38
220–254	3	3/26 = 0.12	0.12 × 100 = 12
255–289	6	6/26 = 0.23	0.23 × 100 = 23
290–324	3	3/26 = 0.12	0.12 × 100 = 12
Total	26	1.00	100

Measures of Location/Central Tendency

Mean is the average value of a variable. It is obtained by adding all the data values and dividing by the total number of values/items.

Population Mean

Suppose there are N data items/values in a population. Then the population mean μ is computed as follows.

$$\mu = \frac{\sum_{i=1}^{N} x_i}{N}$$

Sample Mean

Suppose there are n data items in a sample dataset and the value of each item is denoted as x_i, where i ranges from 1 to n. Then the sample mean is defined as follows.

$$\bar{x} = \frac{\sum_{i=1}^{n} x_i}{n}$$

Median is the value in the middle when the data items are arranged in ascending order (from low to high). If there is odd number of items, the median is the value of the middle item, and if the data list has an even number of values, then the average of the two middle values will be the median, after arranging the data values in ascending order.

Mode is the data value with the highest/largest frequency. There may be more than one mode for a dataset: that is bimodal or multimodal.

Example 2.3.1: Consider systolic blood pressure of 11 patients.
158, 165, 130, 159, 150, 140, 142, 125, 130, 120, and 128.
Mean. $\bar{x} = (158 + 165 + 130 + ... + 128)/11 = 140.64$
Median. The data items in ascending orders are 120, 125, 128, 130, 130, 140, 142, 150, 158, 159, 165.
The middle item is 140, which is the median.
Mode. 130, as it has the highest frequency.

Example 2.3.2: Suppose diastolic blood pressure of 12 people, arranged in ascending order, are as follows:

1	2	3	4	5	6	7	8	9	10	11	12
68	88	89	96	96	102	104	105	105	110	112	120

Mean. $\bar{x} = (68 + 88 + 89 + ... + 120)/11 = 99.58$
The average of the middle two items is (102 + 104)/2 = 103, which is the median.
The numbers 96 and 105 occur the maximum number of times – that is twice. Hence, the given data is bimodal, and it has modes as 96 and 105.

Percentiles: A percentile provides information about how the data items are spread over the interval from the smallest value to the largest value. The pth percentile is the data value such that p percent of the data items take this value or less and at least $(100 - p)$ percent of the items take this value or more.

How to Calculate the pth Percentile
1. Arrange the data in ascending order (from smallest value to largest value).
2. Compute the index i,

$$i = (\frac{p}{100})n$$

where p is the percentile of interest and n is the number of items.
3. (a) If i is not an integer, round it up. The next integer value greater than i denotes the position of the pth percentile.
(b) If i is an integer, the pth percentile is the average of the data values in positions i and $i + 1$.

Example 2.3.3. Find 85th percentile.
Step 1: Consider diastolic blood pressure of 12 people, arranged in ascending order, are as follows:

1	2	3	4	5	6	7	8	9	10	11	12
68	88	89	96	96	102	104	105	105	110	112	120

Step 2.

$$i = (p/100) \times n = (85/100) \times 12 = 10.2$$

Step 3. Here, i is not an integer; round it up. The position of the 85th percentile is the next integer greater than 10.2, the 11th position. We see that the 85th percentile corresponds to 11th data position, i.e., 112.

Quartiles
It divides data into four parts, with each part containing approximately one-fourth or 25% of the items.

The 25th percentile is also called the *first quartile* and may be denoted by Q_1.

The 50th percentile is also called the *second quartile* and may be denoted by Q_2. It is also the *median*.

The 75th percentile is called the *third quartile*, denoted by Q_3.

The computations of Q_1, Q_2, and Q_3 require the use of the rule of finding the 25th, 50th, and 75th percentiles. The calculations are as follows:

For Q_1,

$$i = (p/100) \times n = (25/100) \times 12 = 3$$

As i is an integer, step 3(b) indicates that Q_1 is the average of third and fourth data values, i.e., $Q_1 = (89 + 96)/2 = 92.5$.
For Q_2,

$$i = (50/100) \times 12 = 6$$

Here, also i is an integer, Q_2 is the average of sixth and seventh data values, i.e., $Q_2 = (102 + 104)/2 = 103$.
For Q_3,

$$i = (p/100) \times n = (75/100) \times 12 = 9$$

Again, since i is an integer, Q_3 is the average of ninth and tenth data values, i.e., $Q_3 = (105 + 110)/2 = 107.5$.

Measures of Variability
Measures of variability talk about the spread of the data. It means the extent to which the values/observations vary from one another and from some average value.

Numerical Measures of Variability
Simplest measure of variability/dispersion is as follows:

$$Range = \text{largest value} - \text{smallest value}$$

Example 2.4.1: Consider diastolic blood pressure of 12 people, arranged in ascending order, are as follows:

1	2	3	4	5	6	7	8	9	10	11	12
68	88	89	96	96	102	104	105	105	110	112	120

Range $= 120 - 68 = 52$.

Drawback: It depends on just two extreme values of the data.

Interquartile Range (IQR)
It is the difference $Q_3 - Q_1$.
For this data, $Q_3 = 107.5$ and $Q_1 = 92.5$. Thus IQR $= 107.5 - 92.5 = 15$.

Variance
It utilizes all data values. It is the average of squared deviations of the data values about the mean.

Population Variance

Suppose the population size is N, then the population variance, denoted as σ^2, is defined as follows:

$$\sigma^2 = \frac{\sum_{i=1}^{N}(x_i - \mu)^2}{N}$$

Another formula for *population variance* is as follows:

$$\sigma^2 = \frac{\sum_{i=1}^{N}x_i^2 - N\mu^2}{N}$$

Sample Variance

Suppose there are n items in the sample, then the sample variance, denoted as s^2 is defined as follows:

$$s^2 = \frac{\sum_{i=1}^{n}(x_i - \bar{x})^2}{n-1}$$

Where x_i $(i = 1, 2, \ldots, n)$ are the values in the sample.

Another formula for the *sample variance* is as follows:

$$s^2 = \frac{\sum_{i=1}^{n}x_i^2 - n\bar{x}^2}{n-1}$$

Example 2.4.2: Consider diastolic blood pressure of 12 people, arranged in ascending order, are as follows:

1	2	3	4	5	6	7	8	9	10	11	12
68	88	89	96	96	102	104	105	105	110	112	120

Here, sample mean $\bar{x} = 1195/12 = 99.58$

$(x_i - \bar{x}) = -31.58, -11.58, -10.58, -3.58, -3.58, 2.42, 4.42, 5.42, 5.42, 10.42, 12.42, 20.42$

$(x_i - \bar{x})^2 = 997.30, 134.10, 111.94, 12.82, 12.82, 5.86, 19.54, 29.38, 29.38, 108.58, 154.26, 416.98$

$\Sigma(x_i - \bar{x})^2 = 2032.92,$

$s^2 = 2{,}032.92/11 = 184.81$

Standard Deviation (SD)

It is the positive square root of the variance. Therefore, SD is measured in the same units as the original data.

Population standard deviation: $\sigma = \sqrt{\sigma^2}$
Sample standard deviation: $s = \sqrt{s^2}$

For Example 2.4.2, sample standard deviation, s = $\sqrt{(184.81)}$ = 13.59.

Coefficient of Variation (CV)

It is the relative measure of standard deviation, as compared to the mean. It is obtained by dividing the standard deviation by the mean and multiplying by 100. Thus:

Population CV: $\dfrac{\sigma}{\mu} \times 100$

Sample CV: $\dfrac{s}{\bar{x}} \times 100$

For Example 2.4.2, the CV is (13.59/99.58) × 100 = 13.65. It tells that the standard deviation of the sample is 13.65% of the value of the sample mean.

For two sets of data with the same means, we can look at the standard deviations to see which data is more dispersed. For data with different means, a better measure of dispersion is the coefficient of variation.

Measures of Relative Location and Detecting Outliers

For each data value x_i, there is a standardized score called *z-score*. It is found by dividing the deviation about the mean by the standard deviation. Thus:

$$z_i = \frac{x_i - \bar{x}}{s}$$

where z_i is the z-score for data value x_i, $\bar{x}$ is the sample mean, and s is the sample standard deviation. The z-score is called standardized value.

Detecting Outliers: Extreme values that are unusually large or small are called *outliers*. A data value with a *z-score* of more than 3 or less than –3 is considered as an outlier.

For Example 2.4.2, the z-scores are –2.32, –0.85, –0.78, –0.26, –0.26, 0.18, 0.33, 0.40, 0.40, 0.77, 0.91, and 1.50. It shows that outliers are not present in this dataset.

Measures of Association Between Two Variables

Covariance

A measure of the linear relationship between two variables, X and Y. The data items are shown as (x_1, y_1), (x_2, y_2), and so forth.

Sample Covariance

For a sample of n elements with the corresponding pairs of data values (x_1, y_1), (x_2, y_2), and so on in the sample. Then the sample covariance is defined as follows.

$$S_{xy} = \frac{\Sigma(x_i - \bar{x})(y_i - \bar{y})}{(n-1)}$$

where $\bar{x}$ is the mean of X and $\bar{y}$ is the mean of Y.

Population Covariance

$$\sigma_{xy} = \frac{\sum_{i=1}^{N}(x_i - \mu_x)(y_i - \mu_y)}{N} = \frac{\sum_{i=1}^{N}x_i y_i - n\mu_x\mu_y}{N}$$

where μ_x and μ_y are the population means of variables X and Y, respectively.

Interpretation of Covariance

A positive value of s_{xy} is indicative of a positive liner association between X and Y – that is, as the value of X increases, the value of Y also increases. A negative value indicates a negative linear association between X and Y – that is, as the value of X increases the value of Y decreases. The value zero indicates no linear association between X and Y.

Drawback: Covariance depends on the unit of measurements for X and Y. To avoid that, we have the *Pearson correlation coefficient*:

Correlation Coefficient

This measure standardizes covariance between –1 and 1.

Pearson Product Moment Correlation Coefficient

Pearson product moment *correlation coefficient* (for sample) is $r_{xy} = \dfrac{S_{xy}}{S_x S_y}$

where s_x and s_y are the sample standard deviations of X and Y, respectively.

Population correlation coefficient: $\rho_{xy} = \dfrac{\sigma_{xy}}{\sigma_x \sigma_y}$

Interpretation of Correlation Coefficient

Correlation coefficient lies between –1 and +1. When the coefficient is close to 0, the linear relationship between the two variables is weak or nonexistent. When the coefficient is close to 1 or –1, the linear relationship is strong. When a sample correlation coefficient is +1, it indicates a perfect positive *linear* relationship between the variables. When it is –1, it shows that the variables have a perfect negative *linear* relationship.

Example 2.6.1: The systolic and diastolic blood pressures of ten patients are as follows:

	1	2	3	4	5	6	7	8	9	10	Total
Sys_bp (x)	158	165	159	150	150	180	230	142	180	199	1,713
Dia_bp (y)	88	110	99	105	102	110	120	96	105	115	1,050
$x - \bar{x}$	-13.30	-6.30	-12.30	-21.30	-21.30	8.70	58.70	-29.30	8.70	27.70	0
$y - \bar{y}$	-17	5	-6	0	-3	5	15	-9	0	10	0
$(x - \bar{x})(y - \bar{y})$	226.10	-31.50	73.80	0.00	63.90	43.50	880.50	263.70	0.00	277.00	1,797
$(x - \bar{x})^2$	176.89	39.69	151.29	453.69	453.69	75.69	3,445.69	858.49	75.69	767.29	6,498.1
$(y - \bar{y})^2$	289	25	36	0	9	25	225	81	0	100	790

$\bar{x} = 1713/10 = 17.13$, $\bar{y} = 1050/10 = 105$

(a) Compute covariance and comment.

Covariance, $S_{xy} = 1{,}797/9 = 199.67$

Comment: There exists a positive linear relationship between systolic and diastolic blood pressures.

(b) Compute Pearson product-moment correlation coefficient (r_{xy}) and comment.

$S_x = \sqrt{(6{,}498.1/9)} = \sqrt{(722.01)} = 26.87$, $S_y = \sqrt{(790/9)} = \sqrt{(87.78)} = 9.37$

Correlation coefficient, $r_{xy} = \frac{S_{xy}}{S_x S_y} == 199.67 / (26.87 \times 9.37) = 0.79$

There exists a strong positive linear relationship between systolic and diastolic blood pressures.

Regression: The relationship between y and x can be formulated as a linear regression model given by $y_i = \beta_0 + \beta_1 x_i + u_i$, $i = 1, 2, \ldots, n$.

The basic assumptions of this model are as follows:

(i) u_i is a random variable with mean 0 and variance σ^2 (unknown), that is,

$E(u_i) = 0$ and $V(u_i) = \sigma^2 \ \forall \ i$.

(ii) u_i and u_j are uncorrelated $\forall$ i and j, so that $\text{Cov}(u_i, u_j) = 0$.
(iii) u_i is a normally distributed random variable.
(iv) x is a fixed variable.

Coefficient of determination R^2 measures the proportion of variation in the dependent variable explained by the model or independent variable.

The estimators of β_1 and β_0 are as follows:

$$b_1 = \frac{\sum x_i y_i - \frac{(\sum x_i \sum y_i)}{n}}{\sum x_i^2 - \frac{(\sum x_i)^2}{n}} = \frac{\sum(x_i - \bar{x})(y_i - \bar{y})}{\sum(x_i - \bar{x})^2} \text{ and } b_0 = \bar{y} - b_1\bar{x}.$$

$$R^2 = \frac{\sum(\hat{y}_i - \bar{y})^2}{\sum(y_i - \bar{y})^2}$$

where x_i = value of the independent variable for the ith observation

y_i = value of the dependent variable for the *i*th observation

$\bar{x}$ = mean value of $x_1, x_2, ..., x_n$

$\bar{y}$ = mean value of $y_1, y_2, ..., y_n$

n = total number of pairs of observations.

Example 2.6.2: The systolic and diastolic blood pressures of ten patients are as follows:

	1	2	3	4	5	6	7	8	9	10	Total
Sys_bp (x)	158	165	159	150	150	180	230	142	180	199	1,713
Dia_bp (y)	88	110	99	105	102	110	120	96	105	115	1,050
$x - \bar{x}$	-13.30	-6.30	-12.30	-21.30	-21.30	8.70	58.70	-29.30	8.70	27.70	0
$y - \bar{y}$	-17	5	-6	0	-3	5	15	-9	0	10	0
$(x - \bar{x})(y - \bar{y})$	226.10	-31.50	73.80	0.00	63.90	43.50	880.50	263.70	0.00	277.00	1797
$(x - \bar{x})^2$	176.89	39.69	151.29	453.69	453.69	75.69	3,445.69	858.49	75.69	767.29	6,498.1
$(y - \bar{y})^2$	289	25	36	0	9	25	225	81	0	100	790

a. Develop a scatter diagram for this data and comment on the relationship between the two variables (see Figure 2.3).

Comment: There appears to be a positive linear relationship between the two variables.

b. Develop the estimated regression equation for these data.

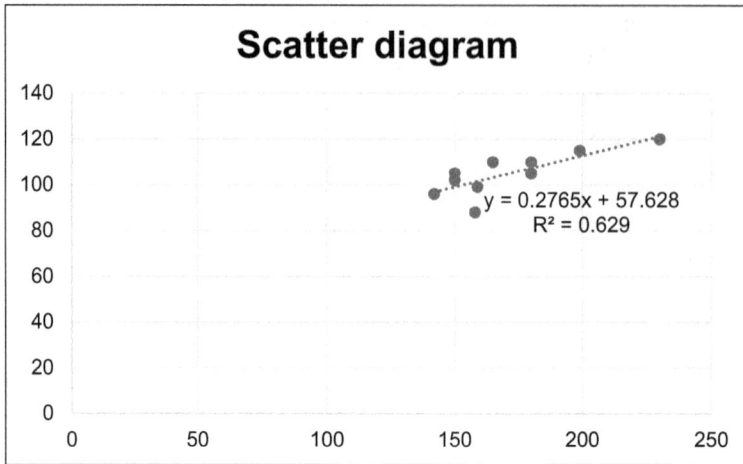

Figure 2.3 Scatter diagram.

The estimated regression equation is as follows:

$$\hat{y} = b_0 + b_1 x$$

where $b_1 = \dfrac{\sum x_i y_i - \frac{(\sum x_i \sum y_i)}{n}}{\sum x_i^2 - \frac{(\sum x_i)^2}{n}} = 1797 / 6498.1 = 0.2765$

and $b_0 = \bar{y} - b_1 \bar{x} = 105 - 0.2765 \times 171.3 = 57.63$

The estimated regression equation for the given data is as follows:

$$\hat{y} = 0.75 + 0.51x \ 57.63 + 0.28x$$

and $R^2 = \dfrac{\sum (\hat{y}_i - \bar{y})^2}{\sum (y_i - \bar{y})^2} = b_1 S_{xy}/S_{yy} = 0.2765 \times 1{,}797/790 = 0.6285$

Comment: 62.85% variation of diastolic blood pressure is explained by systolic blood pressure.

Data Source: The medical data used in this chapter was collected on some patients and is a subset of data collected from a health study on the prevalence of obesity, diabetes, and other cardiovascular risk factors in African-Americans living in Virginia.

The data contained in this part of the book relates to aspects of cardiovascular disease.
  These data are courtesy of Dr. John Schorling, Department of Medicine, University of Virginia School of Medicine.

Discussion Questions

- Why are descriptive statistics critical in the early stages of health research analysis?
- How do measures like mean and standard deviation help in understanding the nature of health data?
- In what ways can skewness and kurtosis affect data interpretation in clinical studies?
- What are the benefits of using data visualization tools like histograms and box plots when summarizing health outcomes?
- Lastly, how do descriptive statistics contribute to identifying trends, outliers, or inconsistencies that might influence further inferential analysis or research conclusions?

References

Agarwal, B.L. (2023). Basic Statistics, 8th edition, New Age International Publishers.
Heumann, C., Schomaker, M. and Shalabh. (2022). Introduction to Statistics and Data Analysis, 2nd edition, Springer Cham, Springer Nature.
Rosner, B. (2015). Fundamentals of Biostatistics, 8th edition, Cengage Learning.

## CHAPTER 3

Exploratory Data Analysis in Health Research – Describing Measures and Methods for Summarizing Health-Related Data

Nazim Husain

Learning Outcomes

By the end of this chapter, learners will be able to understand and apply key descriptive statistical methods for organizing, summarizing, and interpreting health research data. They will gain proficiency in measures of central tendency, dispersion, and distributional characteristics, as well as data visualization techniques. Learners will also be able to identify common pitfalls in data interpretation and utilize statistical software effectively. Through real-world case studies, they will develop the skills to transform raw health data into meaningful insights, supporting evidence-based decisions in clinical, epidemiological, and public health contexts.

Introduction to Descriptive Statistics

Descriptive statistics are essential techniques for summarizing and interpreting data, allowing researchers to present complex information in a structured and meaningful way. These methods provide clear and concise summaries of datasets, whether through numerical measures, such as mean, median, and mode, or visual representations, like histograms and pie charts (Vetter 2017). In health research, descriptive statistics serve a fundamental role by offering critical insights into study data, facilitating preliminary analysis, guiding hypothesis formulation, and enhancing the clarity of data presentation and comparison. Their application is crucial in understanding research findings, supporting evidence-based decision-making, and ultimately advancing medical knowledge and clinical practice (Grieve 2013; Vetter 2017).

Importance in Health Research

Initial Data Analysis: Descriptive statistics form the foundation of data analysis, offering a clear and concise summary of information collected from clinical trials, epidemiological investigations, and surveys. These methods help researchers grasp the fundamental characteristics of the dataset, guiding the selection of appropriate statistical tests for further inferential analysis (Vetter 2017; Grieve 2013).

Data Presentation: By structuring and summarizing data in a meaningful way, descriptive statistics facilitate better understanding of data distribution and characteristics. They serve as a crucial stepping stone for inferential statistics, which enable researchers to draw probability-based conclusions about populations and hypotheses (Rendón-Macías, Villasís-Keever, and Miranda-Novales 2016; Vetter 2017).

Hypothesis Generation: Identifying patterns and trends within data is essential for hypothesis formulation, and descriptive statistics provide a robust framework for this process. Particularly in descriptive epidemiology, these methods help in mapping disease distribution, identifying high-risk populations, and generating insights that inform further research (Mao and Huo 2023).

Data Comparison: Summarizing and categorizing data allows researchers to compare different datasets efficiently, helping to identify similarities, differences, and potential associations. In medical research, this is crucial for evaluating treatment outcomes, comparing patient responses, and assessing key clinical variables (Spina 2007).

Visual Representation: Graphical representations, such as histograms, box plots, and scatterplots, provide an intuitive way to communicate complex data. These visual tools enhance comprehension, making statistical findings more accessible not only to researchers but also to policymakers, healthcare professionals, and the general public, including those without a strong statistical background (Labreuche 2020).

Types of Data Commonly Encountered in Health Research

The application of descriptive statistics varies according to the type of data being analyzed. A comprehensive understanding of the different types of data and their corresponding subtypes is essential in health research, as this knowledge significantly impacts the selection of appropriate statistical methodologies and graphical representations utilized for analytical purposes (Labreuche 2010).

Quantitative Data

Quantitative data consist of numerical values that represent measurable quantities. It can be further divided into the following:

- **Continuous Data:** This type of data encompasses numerical data that can assume any value within a defined range. Examples include physiological measurements, such as blood pressure, cholesterol levels, and body weight.
- **Discrete Data:** This category refers to numerical data that can only assume specific values, frequently in the form of counts. Notable examples include the frequency of hospital visits, the total number of patients enrolled in a study, or the enumeration of particular symptoms.

Qualitative Data

Qualitative data can be divided into the following:

- **Nominal Data:** This type of data consists of categorical data that lacks a defined order. Representative examples include gender, blood type, and the presence or absence of a particular disease.
- **Ordinal Data:** This classification includes categorical data that possesses a meaningful order, albeit without a consistent interval between categories. Exemplary instances include pain scales (e.g., mild, moderate, severe) and classifications of cancer stages (Labreuche 2010).

Significance in Real-World Applications

Descriptive statistics play a fundamental role in various fields of health research, shaping the way data is interpreted and applied in real-world settings.

In clinical trials and epidemiological studies, descriptive statistics are used to describe the characteristics of patients, such as age, gender, and health status. This helps in understanding the sample population and ensuring the validity of the study. For example, a study on burns research highlighted the use of descriptive statistics to present data on patient demographics and outcomes, which is critical for understanding the scope and impact of the research (Al-Benna et al. 2010).

In public health and policymaking, descriptive statistics are essential for describing the distribution of diseases, identifying high-risk populations, and evaluating the effectiveness of interventions used in health research. For example, in a study, descriptive statistics were used to assess the quality of life in patients with hypertension, providing insights into the effectiveness of treatments and interventions (Gómez Gómez et al. 2011).

In medical research, descriptive statistics are used to summarize experimental data, which is crucial for hypothesis testing and determining the efficacy of treatments (Spina 2007; Grieve 2013). For example, in studies on dermatological diseases in the elderly, descriptive statistics helped in identifying the prevalence and types of conditions, aiding in better healthcare planning and resource allocation (Yorulmaz and Yalçin 2016).

Types of Descriptive Statistics

Descriptive statistics encompass various measures that summarize and describe the main features of a dataset. These measures can be broadly categorized into three types: measures of central tendency, measures of dispersion, and measures of the shape of the data distribution. Each plays a unique role in providing a comprehensive understanding of the dataset.

Measures of Central Tendency

Measures of central tendency are statistical tools used to describe the center or typical value of a dataset. The most commonly used measures are the mean, median, and mode, each of which has unique properties and applications.

Mean

The *mean* is a measure of central tendency that represents the average value of a set of numbers. It is calculated by summing all the values in a dataset and then dividing by the number of values (Martinez and Bartholomew 2017). There are various types of means, including the arithmetic mean, geometric mean, and harmonic mean, each serving distinct purposes and being suited to specific contexts (Drzymała 2021).

Arithmetic Mean

The arithmetic mean, commonly referred to as the average, is a fundamental statistical measure used extensively in health research to summarize data. It is simple to calculate, easy to interpret, and incorporates all data points, making it a comprehensive measure of central tendency. Additionally, its strong mathematical properties make it useful for further statistical analysis (Martinez and Bartholomew 2017).

However, the arithmetic mean has certain limitations. It is highly sensitive to outliers, which can distort the representation of the dataset, and may not always be the best indicator of central tendency in skewed distributions. Furthermore, it assumes that data is measured on an interval or ratio scale, which may not always be applicable.

For the arithmetic mean to be meaningful, specific assumptions must be met. The data should be measured on an *interval or ratio scale*, exhibit a *symmetric distribution*, and be free from *significant outliers* that could skew results. While these conditions are ideal, real-world health data often deviates from them, necessitating careful interpretation and, at times, alternative measures of central tendency (Speelman and McGann 2013).

CALCULATION OF ARITHMETIC MEAN

The formula for calculating the arithmetic mean is as follows:

$$\bar{x} = \frac{x_1 + x_2 + x_3 \ldots \ldots x_n}{n} = \frac{\sum_{i=1}^{n} x_i}{n}$$

Where,
$\bar{x}$ (x bar) = Arithmetic mean
x_i = Individual observations
n = *Number of observations*
Σ = *Greek letter sigma that denotes the sum of all values*

Geometric Mean

The geometric mean is a measure of central tendency calculated by taking the nth root of the product of n numbers. Unlike the arithmetic mean, it is particularly useful for datasets containing positive values, making it widely applicable in fields such as finance, economics, and environmental science.

For the geometric mean to be meaningful, certain assumptions must be met. It is only defined for positive values, is most applicable when data follows a lognormal distribution, and generally assumes that values are independent of each other.

This measure has several advantages. It is ideal for proportional growth calculations, making it useful for measuring average rates of return or environmental pollutant levels over time. Additionally, it is less affected by outliers, making it more robust than the arithmetic mean in certain datasets. For lognormal distributions, the geometric mean closely aligns with the median, providing an effective measure of central tendency.

However, the geometric mean has its limitations. It is more complex to compute, especially for large datasets, and can be unstable for small sample sizes or highly skewed data. Additionally, it cannot be used for datasets containing zero or negative values, restricting its applicability in some contexts. Despite these limitations, when used appropriately, the geometric mean offers a more accurate representation of central tendency in datasets involving growth rates or multiplicative relationships (Vogel 2022).

CALCULATION OF GEOMETRIC MEAN

The geometric mean (GM) of a set of n positive numbers $(x_1, x_2, x_3 \ldots \ldots x_n)$ is calculated as follows:

$$\left(\prod_{i=1}^{n} x_i \right)^{\frac{1}{n}} = \sqrt[n]{x_1 \times x_2 \times x_3 \ldots \ldots x_n}$$

Where:
Π = Geometric mean
n = Number of values
x_i = Values to average

$$GM = exp\left[\sum_{i=1}^{n} In(x_i) \right]$$

Harmonic Mean

The harmonic mean (HM) is a type of average, typically used for sets of numbers where the numbers are defined in relation to some unit, such as rates or ratios. It is calculated as the reciprocal of the arithmetic mean of the reciprocals of the given set of observations (Feng and Wang 2024). For the harmonic mean to be valid, the dataset must consist of positive real numbers, and it is most appropriate when values are expressed as rates or ratios without zero or negative values.

One of its key advantages is that it provides a more accurate measure for rates and ratios compared to the arithmetic mean. Additionally, it is less affected by large outliers, making it useful in cases where extremely high values could distort other measures of central tendency.

Despite these benefits, the harmonic mean has limitations. It is highly sensitive to very small values, which can disproportionately influence the result, making it less reliable in datasets with extreme low values. Furthermore, it cannot be applied to datasets containing zero or negative values, as these would render the calculation meaningless.

While not suitable for all types of data, the harmonic mean is an essential tool in scenarios where rates and ratios need to be averaged in a mathematically meaningful way (Rao, Shi, and Wu 2014; Lann and Falk 2006).

CALCULATION OF HARMONIC MEAN

The harmonic mean (HM) of a set of n numbers $(x_1, x_2, x_3 \ldots \ldots x_n)$ is calculated using the formula:

$$HM = \frac{n}{\sum_{i=1}^{n} \frac{1}{x_i}} = \frac{n}{\frac{1}{x_1} + \frac{1}{x_1} + \frac{1}{x_1} + \ldots + \frac{1}{x_n}}$$

Where:

n is the number of observations.

x_i represents the individual observations.

Mode

The *mode* is a measure of central tendency that represents the most frequently occurring value in a dataset. It is particularly useful for nominal data and is not influenced by the tail of the distribution (Kamanchi et al. 2019).

For the mode to be effective, certain conditions should be met. It is most applicable for nominal data, though it can be used for other types as well. Since it is not affected by extreme values, it is particularly useful when data distributions are skewed. Additionally, traditional mode estimation assumes that all data points are available, which is necessary for accurate identification of the most common value.

The mode has several advantages. It is simple to understand and calculate, especially when dealing with categorical data. Unlike the mean, it remains unaffected by outliers, making it a robust measure of central tendency. It also finds applications in various fields, including clustering and regression analysis, where identifying the most common category or value is essential.

However, the mode also has limitations. It may not always be unique, as datasets can be bimodal or multimodal, leading to multiple values representing central tendency. In some cases, particularly in small or highly skewed datasets, the mode may not provide a meaningful summary of the data. Additionally, computing the mode for large datasets, especially in continuous data, can be computationally intensive, requiring sorting and frequency analysis (Samawi et al. 2018; Chacón 2020).

Calculation of Mode

1. **For Discrete Data:**
   - **Frequency Distribution:** Identify the value(s) that appear most frequently in the dataset.
   - **Example:** In the dataset [1, 2, 2, 3, 4], the mode is 2.
2. **For Continuous Data:**
   - **Histogram Method:** Construct a histogram and identify the interval with the highest frequency.

- **Kernel Density Estimation**: Use non-parametric methods like kernel density estimation to find the peak of the density function.
- **Optimization Techniques**: If the analytical form of the density function is known, apply optimization techniques to find the argument of the maximum value of the density function (Kamanchi et al. 2019; Samawi et al. 2018).

Median

The *median* is a measure of central tendency that represents the middle value in a dataset when the values are arranged in ascending or descending order. If the dataset has an odd number of observations, the median is the middle value. If the dataset has an even number of observations, the median is the average of the two middle values (Madrid et al. 2022). Unlike the mean, which considers all data points, the median provides a positional measure that is particularly useful in non-normally distributed data.

Certain conditions ensure the meaningful use of the median. The data must be at least ordinal, meaning it can be ranked or ordered. Since it does not rely on any assumptions about the underlying distribution, it is considered a non-parametric measure. While the median is robust to outliers, it is most informative when the dataset exhibits a symmetric distribution (Jankowski and Flannelly 2015).

One of the key advantages of the median is its robustness. It remains unaffected by extreme values or skewed data, making it a more reliable measure of central tendency in such cases. Additionally, it is simple to understand and compute, especially in small datasets. Its applicability extends to ordinal data and non-normally distributed datasets, making it a preferred choice in many real-world scenarios (Buckley 2006).

However, the median has some limitations. Since it does not consider all data points, it may not provide as much information as the mean. For large datasets, calculating the median can be computationally demanding, especially when sorting is required. Furthermore, in datasets with an even number of observations, the median is not unique, as it is derived from the average of two middle values rather than a single definitive figure (Khorana et al. 2023).

Calculation of Median

1. **Order the data:** Arrange the data points in ascending or descending order.
2. **Identify the middle value:**
   - **Odd number of observations:** The median is the middle value.

$$Median = \left(\frac{n+1}{2}\right)^{th} observation\, of\, the\, series$$

   - **Even number of observations:** The median is the average of the two middle values.

$$Median = \frac{\left(\frac{n}{2}\right)^{th} observation + \left(\frac{n}{2}+1\right)^{th} observation}{2}$$

Measures of Dispersion

Measures of dispersion are statistical tools used to describe the variability or spread of a dataset, providing insights into how data points are distributed around a central value. These measures are essential for understanding the distribution and reliability of data. Commonly used measures of dispersion include the *range, interquartile range (IQR), variance, mean absolute deviation (MAD), median absolute deviation (MAD),* and *standard deviation (SD).* Additionally, advanced measures, such as the *coefficient of variation (CV), entropy-based dispersion (ED),* and *fisher information-based dispersion,* provide deeper assessments of variability in specific contexts.

Range

The range is the simplest measure of dispersion, calculated as the difference between the maximum and minimum values in a dataset. It defines the smallest interval that encompasses all data points and provides a quick snapshot of statistical variability. While straightforward, the range is highly sensitive to extreme values and does not account for the distribution of data between the two extremes.

For the range to be meaningful, certain assumptions are often considered. In some cases, statistical methods assume that the data follows a normal distribution, particularly in engineering and measurement contexts. Alternatively, in cases where data is assumed to be uniformly distributed, the accuracy of the range as a dispersion measure may be affected. Additionally, the range is often interpreted under the assumption that data points are independently drawn from the population, ensuring that the measure reflects true variability (Schwarz 2011).

Despite its simplicity, the range has several advantages. It is easy to calculate, requiring only the maximum and minimum values, making it particularly useful for quick estimations in preliminary data analysis. Under specific conditions, such as normally distributed data, the range can also serve as an unbiased estimator of population standard deviation when adjusted appropriately.

However, the range has notable limitations. It is highly sensitive to outliers, meaning a single extreme value can significantly distort its representation of dispersion. Additionally, it can lead to biased variance estimates, particularly when data does not follow a normal distribution. Its applicability is further limited by its reliance on distribution-specific coefficients, making it unsuitable as a universal measure of spread (Schwarz 2006; Piliposyan 2018).

Calculation of Range

The range is calculated as the difference between the maximum and minimum values in the dataset:

$$Range = Maximum\,value - Minimum\,value$$

Interquartile Range (IQR)

The interquartile range (IQR) is a measure of statistical dispersion, which is the spread of the middle 50% of the data. It is calculated as the difference between the third quartile (Q_3) and the first quartile (Q_1). For the IQR to be meaningful, the data should be at least ordinal, though it is useful for skewed distributions and datasets with outliers, as it is not influenced by extreme values that might otherwise distort measures like the mean or standard deviation.

One of the primary advantages of the IQR is its robustness. Since it excludes extreme values, it provides a stable measure of dispersion even in datasets with significant outliers. It is also simple to calculate and interpret, making it widely applicable in various fields. Additionally, it is particularly useful when comparing variability across different datasets, especially when the data is not normally distributed.

Despite its strengths, the IQR has some limitations. Since it only considers the middle 50% of the data, it ignores information in the tails, which could be significant in some analyses. In normally distributed data, the standard deviation may provide a more informative measure of variability since it accounts for all data points. Furthermore, the IQR may be less reliable in very small datasets, as quartile-based calculations require a sufficient number of observations for meaningful interpretation (Greco, Luta, and Wilcox 2024).

Calculation of IQR
To calculate the IQR:

1. **Order the data**: Arrange the data in ascending order.
2. **Find Q_1**: The first quartile (Q_1) is the median of the lower half of the data.
3. **Find Q_3**: The third quartile (Q_3) is the median of the upper half of the data.
4. **Subtract Q_1 from Q_3**(Greco, Luta, and Wilcox 2024).

$$IQR = Q_3 - Q_1$$

$$Q_3 = \left(\frac{3(n+1)}{4} \right) th \; value \, of \, the \, observation$$

$$Q_1 = \left(\frac{n+1}{4} \right) th \; value \, of \, the \, observation$$

Variance
Variance is a statistical measure that quantifies the degree of dispersion or spread in a set of data points. It is defined as the average of the squared differences between each data point and the mean of the dataset. Variance helps in understanding how much the data points deviate from the mean, providing insights into the variability within the data (Joarder 2014).

Certain assumptions are often made when using variance in statistical analysis. Many classical models assume homoscedasticity, meaning variance remains constant across all observations. Additionally, in many cases, normality is assumed, as variance-based methods often rely on the assumption that data follows a normal distribution. Another key assumption is independence, where each data point is considered separate from others in the dataset (Watthanacheewakul 2010; Oddi et al. 2020).

Variance has several advantages. It provides a quantitative measure of dispersion, essential for decision-making in various fields. In finance, variance is used to assess investment risk and volatility, while in quality control, it helps monitor and maintain consistency in manufacturing processes. Additionally, variance is a key component of statistical methods like ANOVA, which compares means across different groups to determine significant differences (Cheng, Feng, and Ahmadzade 2020; Braun 2012).

However, variance also has limitations. The calculation can be complex, particularly for large datasets or when dealing with uncertain variables. It is highly sensitive to outliers, meaning a few extreme values can disproportionately impact the results. Additionally, the squared nature of variance makes interpretation less intuitive, as it does not retain the same units as the original data. In practical applications, standard deviation is often preferred, as it represents variability in the same units as the dataset. Furthermore, assumptions such as homoscedasticity may not always hold, leading to potential inaccuracies in statistical models (Yi et al. 2016; Schumm, Bosch, and Doolittle 2009).

Calculation of Variance

The basic formula for calculating *population variance* (σ^2) is as follows:

$$\sigma^2 = \frac{1}{N} \sum_{i=1}^{N} (x_i - \mu)^2$$

where:
- N is the total number of data points,
- x_i represents each data point, and
- μ is the mean of the dataset (population mean).

For *sample variance* (s^2), the formula is slightly adjusted to account for sample size:

$$s^2 = \frac{1}{n-1} \sum_{i=1}^{n} (x_i - \bar{x})^2$$

where:
- n is the sample size, and
- $\bar{x}$ is the sample mean.

Mean Absolute Deviation

Mean absolute deviation (MAD) is a measure of dispersion that calculates the average absolute deviations of data points from the mean. Unlike variance, which squares deviations, MAD considers the absolute differences, making it a simple way to assess variability within a dataset. It provides a clear measure of how much data points typically differ from the average value (Yager and Alajlan 2014).

For MAD to be meaningful, the data must be numerical, whether continuous or discrete. The mean serves as the central reference point, and all deviations are measured in absolute terms, ensuring that negative and positive differences do not cancel each other out (Yager and Alajlan 2014).

One of the biggest advantages of MAD is its simplicity, making it easy to understand and compute, even for those new to statistical analysis. Additionally, it is more robust to outliers compared to variance and standard deviation, as extreme values have a lesser impact on the overall measure. This makes it particularly useful in datasets where outliers may distort results (Gorard 2005).

However, MAD has some limitations. It is less informative than variance and standard deviation when analyzing the shape of a distribution. Additionally, because it relies on absolute values, it is non-differentiable, making it less useful in some mathematical and statistical modeling applications. Furthermore, it is not as widely used or accepted as standard deviation in traditional statistical methods, which can limit its applicability in certain fields (Gorard 2005; Yager and Alajlan 2014).

Calculation of Mean Absolute Deviation
1. **Compute the mean:** Calculate the mean (average) of the dataset.
2. **Calculate deviations:** Subtract the mean from each data point to find the deviations.
3. **Absolute deviations:** Take the absolute value of each deviation.
4. **Average absolute deviations:** Sum the absolute deviations and divide by the number of data points.

$$Mean\ Absolute\ Deviation = \frac{1}{n}\sum_{i=1}^{n}|x_i - \mu|^2$$

where
- x_i represents each data point,
- μ is the mean of the dataset, and
- n is the total number of data points (Yager and Alajlan 2014; Gorard 2005).

Median Absolute Deviation

Median absolute deviation is a robust measure of statistical dispersion. It is defined as the median of the absolute deviations from the median of the dataset. This measure assumes that the dataset may contain outliers or be non-normally distributed, making it particularly useful in scenarios where extreme values could distort traditional dispersion measures. Although it is highly robust, it is most effective when the data is symmetrically distributed around the median, ensuring a balanced representation of variability (Liu, Liu, and Hu 2024).

One of the key strengths of this measure is its resilience to outliers and skewed data, which makes it particularly valuable in health research and other scientific disciplines where normal distribution cannot always be assumed. Additionally, it is simple to compute and interpret, making it accessible for various statistical applications. Beyond basic variability assessment, it is widely used in outlier detection and robust statistical procedures, further enhancing its practical utility (Liu, Liu, and Hu 2024; Elamir 2012).

However, this measure has certain limitations. Traditional implementations do not provide confidence intervals, which can make statistical inference more challenging. In small sample sizes, it can be biased, though correction factors can help address this issue. Additionally, while modifications exist for multivariate data, the standard median absolute deviation is primarily a univariate measure, meaning it may not fully capture the complexity of datasets with multiple variables (Hayes 2014; Arachchige and Prendergast 2024).

Calculation of Median Absolute Deviation
1. **Find the median:** Determine the median of the dataset.
2. **Calculate deviations:** Compute the absolute deviations of each data point from the median.
3. **Median of deviations:** Find the median of these absolute deviations.

Standard Deviation

Standard deviation (SD) is a statistical measure that quantifies the amount of variation or dispersion in a set of data values. It indicates how much individual data points deviate from the mean of the dataset (Lee, In, and Lee 2015). In a normal distribution, approximately 68% of values lie within one SD of the mean, 95% within two SDs, and 99.7% within three SDs, making it a key tool for understanding data spread (Jankowski and Flannelly 2015).

For SD to be meaningful, several assumptions are considered. It is often assumed that data follows a normal distribution, meaning most values cluster around the mean. Additionally, SD calculations typically assume that data points are independent of each other and that the variability remains consistent across the dataset, a condition known as homogeneity of variance (Darling 2022).

One of the greatest strengths of SD is its ability to quantify variability in a clear and interpretable manner, making it essential in statistical analysis. It allows researchers to compare the spread of different datasets, which is particularly useful in meta-analyses and systematic reviews. Moreover, SD is a critical component of statistical inference, playing a crucial role in hypothesis testing and confidence interval estimation (Darling 2022; Lee, In, and Lee 2015).

Despite its importance, SD has several limitations. It is highly sensitive to outliers, meaning that extreme values can significantly distort the measure of variability. Additionally, the assumption of normality may not always hold, potentially leading to inaccurate interpretations in skewed datasets. The calculation and interpretation of SD can be complex, particularly for individuals without a strong statistical background. Furthermore, misinterpretation is common, especially in distinguishing between standard deviation and the standard error of the mean (SEM), which serve different statistical purposes (Darling 2022; Lee, In, and Lee 2015).

Calculation of Standard Deviation

The basic formula for calculating *population standard deviation* (σ) is as follows:

$$\sigma = \sqrt{\frac{\sum(x_i - \mu)^2}{N}}$$

where:
- N is the total number of data points,
- x_i represents each data point, and
- μ is the mean of the dataset (population mean).

For *sample standard deviation* (s), the formula is slightly adjusted to account for sample size:

$$s = \sqrt{\frac{\sum(x_i - \bar{x})^2}{n-1}}$$

where:
- n is the sample size, and
- $\bar{x}$ is the sample mean.

Advanced Measures of Dispersion

Coefficient of Variation (CV)

The coefficient of variation (CV) is a standardized measure of dispersion of a probability distribution or frequency distribution. It is defined as the ratio of the standard deviation to the mean. CV is extensively used in applied statistics, including quality control and sampling, to measure stability or uncertainty. It indicates the relative dispersion of data in relation to the population mean. It is useful for comparing the degree of variation from one data series to another, even if the means are drastically different (Soliman et al. 2012).

Entropy-Based Dispersion

Entropy-based dispersion measures the uncertainty or randomness in a probability distribution. It is derived from the concept of Shannon entropy, which quantifies the unpredictability of information content. This measure is particularly useful in contexts where understanding the degree of randomness or disorder is crucial, such as in neuronal firing patterns or complex systems analysis. Entropy-based dispersion provides a different perspective on variability compared to traditional measures like standard deviation, capturing aspects of randomness that standard deviation might miss (Kostal, Lansky, and Pokora 2013).

Fisher Information-Based Dispersion

Fisher information-based dispersion measures the amount of information that an observable random variable carries about an unknown parameter upon which the probability depends. It is related to the precision of parameter estimates. This measure is used in statistical estimation and information theory to assess the quality of estimators and the amount of information present in the data about the parameter of interest. Fisher information-based dispersion is particularly useful in contexts where the accuracy of parameter estimation is critical. It is often used alongside entropy-based measures to provide a comprehensive view of information content and uncertainty (Kostal, Lansky, and Pokora 2013).

Additional Descriptive Statistics

Skewness

Skewness is a statistical measure that describes the asymmetry of a distribution around its mean. It indicates whether the data points are skewed to the left (negative skewness) or to the right (positive skewness). It is crucial in various fields, as it helps in understanding the distribution shape and potential outliers (Klein and Doll 2021).

Classical measurement methods include Pearson skewness, quartile skewness, and octile skewness, which are based on higher moments of the random variable about its mean. However, these measures are sensitive to extreme outliers and may be inefficient for small or medium-sized samples (Adil, Wahid, and Mantell 2021).

Skewness measures for ordered categorical variables are less developed but are essential for these fields. New classes of skewness functionals have been proposed to address this gap. Despite its importance, skewness is often underreported in psychological studies. Standardized indexes for skewness can help in better interpreting data. Accurate skewness measurement is vital for predicting phenomena like wind pressure on buildings and extreme precipitation events, which can significantly impact structural integrity and environmental modeling (Nejadseyfi, Geijselaers, and van den Boogaard 2019; Klein and Doll 2021).

Kurtosis

Kurtosis is a statistical measure that describes the distribution of data points in a dataset, particularly focusing on the tails and the peak of the distribution. *Kurtosis* is defined as the ratio of statistical moments and is used to describe the "peakedness" or tail extremity of a distribution. It is calculated using the fourth central moment of the data. For a normal distribution, the kurtosis value is 3, and the excess kurtosis ($\kappa - 3$) is zero (Baren 2005).

Kurtosis is more realistic and accurate for describing real-world data distributions compared to Gaussian distributions. It helps in understanding the distribution of data in various scenarios, such as vibration analysis. Additionally, kurtosis is used in normality tests to determine if a dataset deviates from a normal distribution. It is particularly useful in identifying non-normality in small samples (Westfall 2014; Van Baren 2005).

Misconceptions: A common misconception is that kurtosis measures the "peakedness" of a distribution. However, it actually provides information about the tails of the distribution, indicating the presence of outliers or the propensity to produce outliers. High kurtosis indicates heavy tails and a higher likelihood of outliers, while low kurtosis suggests light tails (Westfall 2014).

Methods for Summarizing Quantitative Data

Frequency Distributions

A frequency distribution is a summary of how often different values occur within a dataset. It is often represented in a table or graphically. It helps in understanding the distribution and patterns within the data, making it easier to identify trends, outliers, and the overall shape of the data distribution (Falk et al. 2020).

Relative Frequencies

Relative frequency is the proportion of the total number of data points that fall within a particular category or interval. It is calculated by dividing the frequency of a specific category by the total number of data points. Relative frequencies are useful for comparing different datasets or categories within the same dataset, as they provide a normalized measure of frequency (Sbert et al. 2021).

Cumulative Frequencies

Cumulative frequency is the sum of the frequencies for all categories up to a certain point. It shows the accumulation of frequencies as you move through the data. Cumulative frequency distributions are often used in statistical analysis to understand the distribution of data over a range and to identify trends and patterns (Sbert et al. 2021).

Presentation of Data

Data can be organized into tables where each row represents a different value or range of values, and columns show the frequency of these values. This tabular form is essential for summarizing large datasets in a comprehensible manner (Table 3.1) (Thrusfield and Christley 2017).

- **Interval:** The range of values.
- **Frequency:** The count of data points within each interval.
- **Relative Frequency:** Frequency divided by the total number of data points.
- **Cumulative Frequency:** Running total of frequencies up to the current interval.

Graphical Presentation of Data

These graphical representations are essential tools in data analysis, each with its own strengths and weaknesses. Understanding when and how to use them effectively can greatly enhance the clarity and impact of your data visualizations.

Table 3.1 Frequency distribution table

Interval	Frequency	Relative frequency	Cumulative frequency
0–10	5	0.10	5
10–20	15	0.30	20
20–30	20	0.40	40
30–40	10	0.20	50

Histograms

Histograms are used to visualize the distribution of a continuous variable by dividing the data into bins and counting the number of observations in each bin (Figure 3.1). Histograms provide a clear visual representation of the data distribution and are widely used due to their simplicity. The choice of bin size can significantly affect the interpretation of the data, potentially leading to misleading conclusions (Chekanov 2016).

Box Plots

Box plots, also known as box-and-whisker plots, summarize the distribution of a dataset by displaying its median, quartiles, and potential outliers (Figure 3.2). These plots are effective for comparing distributions between multiple groups and identifying outliers. Misinterpretation can occur if not used carefully, and they may not always provide a complete picture of the data distribution (Reese 2005).

Stem-and-Leaf Plots

Stem-and-leaf plots organize large amounts of numeric data to form visual distributions, making them useful for detailed data analysis (Table 3.2). These plots retain the original data values while providing a visual summary, which can be useful for small to moderate-sized datasets. They can become cumbersome and less informative with very large datasets (Brath and Banissi 2018).

Interpretation
- Stems (left side): Represent the tens digit (e.g., "12" means 120–129 mmHg).
- Leaves (right side): Represent the ones digit (e.g., "4" next to "12" means 124 mmHg).

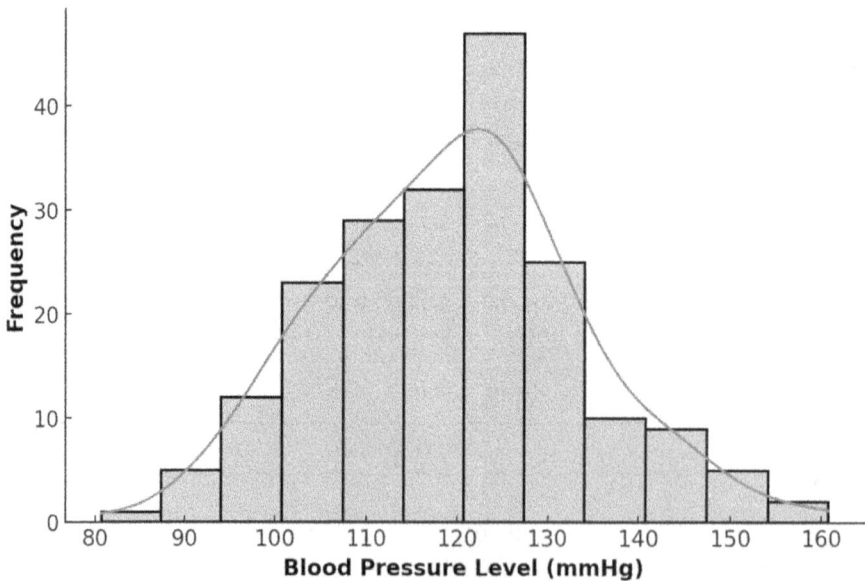

Figure 3.1 Histogram representing the distribution of blood pressure levels in a sample population.

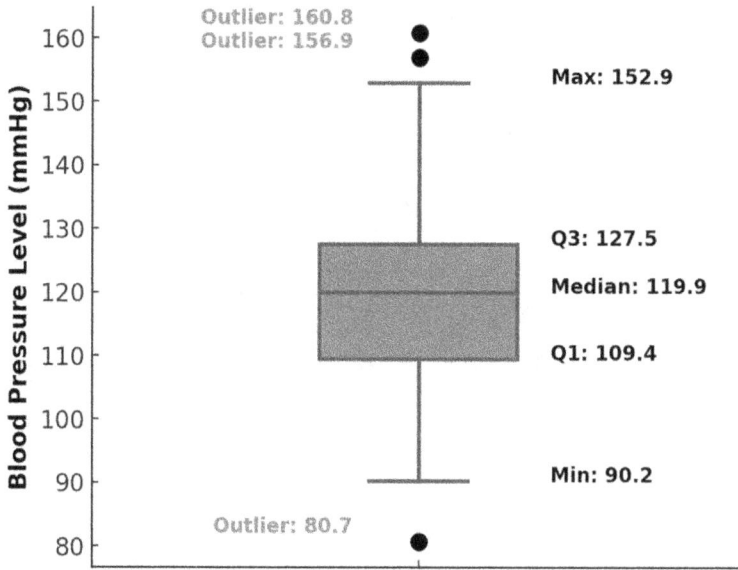

Figure 3.2 Box plot representing the distribution of blood pressure levels in a sample population.

Table 3.2 Stem-and-leaf plot for the blood pressure levels dataset.

Stem	Leaves
8	1
9	011144677889999
0	0011222223334445556667777788889999
11	000112222333333444555556666677777788899
12	00001111112233334444444455555555666677 7788999
13	001112222222222234445555677
14	001222333348888
15	3 7
16	

Example Interpretation:

- The row "12 | 0 0 0 0 1 1 1 1 1 1 1 1" means multiple patients have blood pressure values in the range of 120–121 mmHg.
- The row "15 | 3 7" means patients have readings of 153 mmHg and 157 mmHg.
- The most common values are around 120–129 mmHg.

Scatterplots

Scatterplots are used to visualize the relationship between two continuous variables, often to identify correlations or patterns (Figure 3.3). These plots are straightforward and effective for showing the relationship between variables, making them a staple in exploratory data analysis. Scatterplots can become cluttered with large datasets, making it difficult to discern patterns without additional techniques like smoothing or subsetting (Unwin 2015).

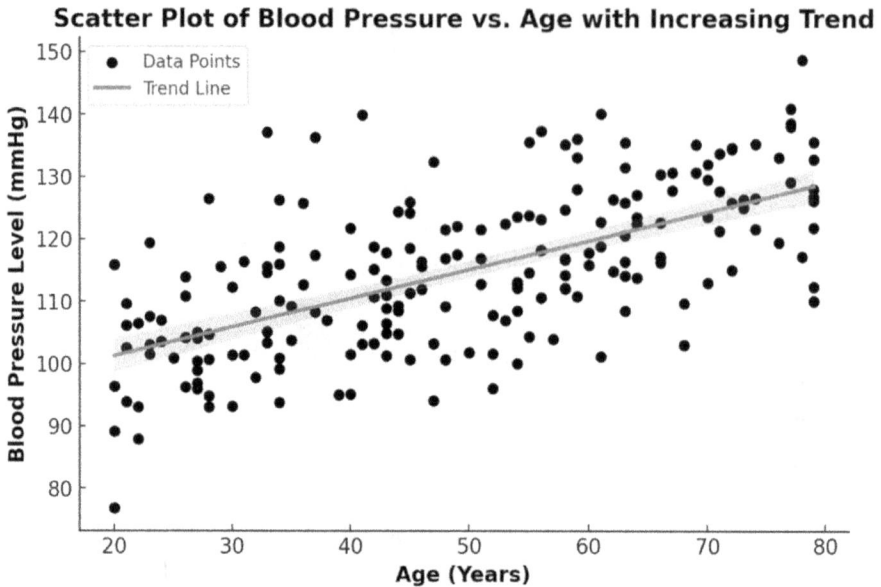

Figure 3.3 Scatterplot with a trend line, illustrating the relationship between blood pressure and age.

Descriptive Tables

Descriptive statistics are essential for summarizing and presenting research data in a clear and concise manner. These statistics can be presented in various forms, including tables, which are particularly useful for displaying numerical data. Descriptive tables play a crucial role in summarizing data and are essential for exploratory data analysis (Ali, Lulseged, and Medhin 2018).

Summary Statistics Tables

Summary statistics tables are used to describe characteristics within a study population and compare characteristics of two or more groups. They provide a quick and easy way to summarize different types of data within one table, allowing for the comparison of characteristics across groups. The tables can include both continuous variables (summarized by mean, standard deviation, etc.) and categorical variables (summarized by percentages and frequencies).

They are used to summarize and cross-tabulate data, offering a range of summary statistics and facilitating the exploration, summarization, and presentation of data from different angles (Scott and Rogers 2015).

Cross-Tabulations (Contingency Tables)

Cross-tabulations, also known as contingency tables, are a fundamental tool in statistical analysis used to summarize the relationship between two or more categorical variables. They are widely used due to their simplicity and effectiveness in displaying the distribution and association of variables (Lu et al. 2008). For example, cross-tabulating smoking status (smoker, non-smoker) with the incidence of lung cancer.

Stratified Summaries

Stratified summaries in descriptive statistics involve breaking down data into subgroups or strata, such as age, gender, or disease severity, to provide more detailed insights. This approach is particularly useful when analyzing heterogeneous datasets, as it allows for the examination of patterns and trends within specific subgroups. Example: Summarizing medication adherence rates by demographic categories.

Methods for Summarizing Qualitative Data

Frequency and Proportion Tables

These tables are used to display the frequency distribution of variables. They can show both absolute and relative frequencies, facilitating the analysis of relationships between categorical variables

Absolute Frequencies

Absolute frequency refers to the count of occurrences of each category in a dataset. It is used to show the raw number of times each category appears, providing a straightforward count without any adjustments or comparisons. If a survey records the number of people who prefer different types of fruits, the absolute frequency would be the actual number of people who prefer apples, oranges, bananas, etc. (Gries 2014).

Relative Frequencies (Percentages)

Relative frequency is the proportion of the total number of occurrences that each category represents, often expressed as a percentage. This helps in understanding the distribution of categories in relation to the whole dataset, making it easier to compare different categories. It is calculated by dividing the absolute frequency of a category by the total number of observations and then multiplying by 100 to get a percentage (Knapp 2015).

Example: If 20 out of 100 participants in a study prefer vegetarian diet, the relative frequency would be $\frac{20}{100} \times 100 = 20\%$. The table will be constructed as Table 3.2:

Table 3.3 Relative frequencies

Participants diet preference	Frequency
Vegetarian diet	20%
Mixed diet	80%

Graphical Representations
Bar Charts
Bar charts are commonly used for comparison purposes, allowing viewers to compare different categories or groups. These charts are particularly effective in representing negative values and identifying extreme values such as minimums and maximums (Figure 3.4).

Bar charts provide a clear visual comparison between different categories. They facilitate the rapid and accurate identification of extreme values. Bar charts are frequently used to display univariate data, making them one of the most common graphical representations in health research (Sandnes et al. 2020).

Pie Charts
Pie charts are used to illustrate part-whole relationships, showing how different parts contribute to a whole. These charts are visually appealing and easy to understand for showing proportions. Studies have shown that pie charts can be more accurate than bar charts for certain tasks, such as identifying parts of a whole (Figure 3.5). However, pie charts require more cognitive effort to interpret compared to bar charts and other visualizations like treemaps. Pie charts are used to represent the proportion of different categories within a whole (Sandnes et al. 2020).

Pareto Charts
Pareto charts are a specialized type of bar chart combined with a line graph (Figure 3.6). They are used to identify the most significant factors in a dataset by highlighting the

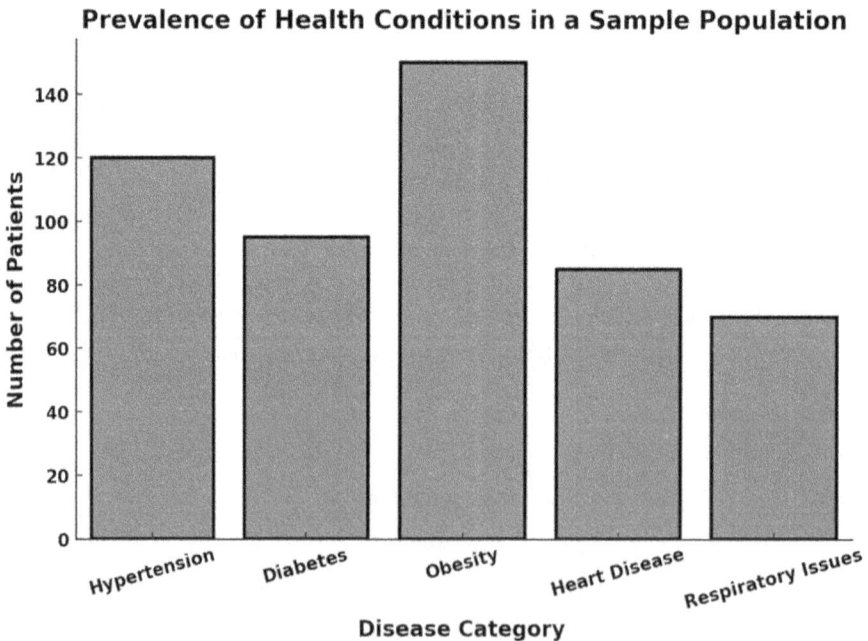

Figure 3.4 Bar chart illustrating the prevalence of health conditions in a sample population.

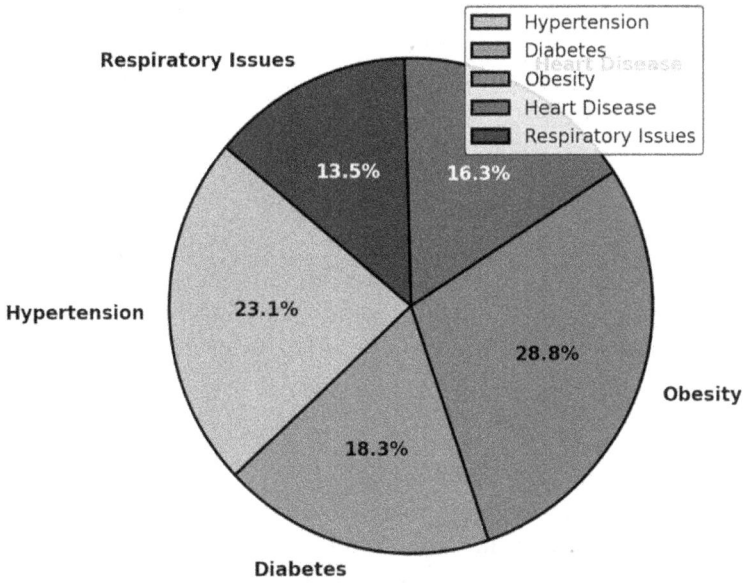

Figure 3.5 Pie chart illustrating the prevalence of health conditions in a sample population.

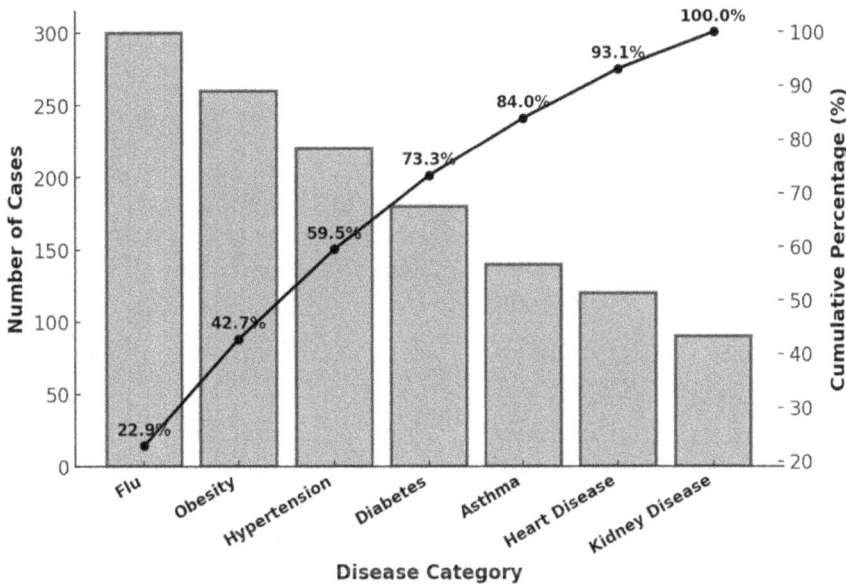

Figure 3.6 Pareto chart representing the prevalence of various diseases in a sample population.

cumulative impact of the factors. They help in prioritizing issues or causes by showing which factors have the most significant cumulative effect. Useful in quality control and business decision-making to focus on the most critical issues. Pareto charts combine bar and line graphs to highlight the most significant factors in a dataset (Labreuche 2020).

Data Presentation Principles in Health Research
Effective data presentation in health research is crucial for clear communication, influencing policy, and driving insights. Here are some key principles and considerations based on the provided abstracts:

Importance of Effective Data Presentation
Effective data presentation helps in creating insights and influencing change. It is essential for communicating complex health data clearly and effectively. Data should be presented in a way that is tailored to the needs of the target audience, whether they are policymakers, clinicians, or the general public (Flowers and Johnson 2016).

Key Principles
- **Simplicity and Precision**: Simple formats of tables and graphs with precise information are recommended. Avoid misleading formats, and clearly convey any uncertainties in the findings.
- **Appropriate Chart Selection**: Selecting the right type of chart or graph is crucial. The chosen method should best fit the data and the message intended to be communicated.
- **Avoiding Misinterpretation**: Care should be taken to avoid overcalling causality and confusing statistical significance with clinical significance (Flowers and Johnson 2016; Sabharwal 2023).

Benefits of Interactive Data Visualization
Interactive visualizations can help in understanding complex relationships and trends within the data. They are particularly useful for exploring multiple related facets simultaneously. These methods can engage users more effectively and provide powerful tools for knowledge discovery and hypothesis testing (Chishtie et al. 2022).

Ethical Considerations
Ensure that personal health information is protected and not unintentionally disclosed in presentations. This includes being cautious with data embedded in files. Present data ethically, especially when using statistics for advocacy. Use absolute risks or benefits in clinical situations to avoid misinterpretation (Dahl and Vedsted 2008).

Case Studies in Descriptive Statistics for Health Data
Case Study 1: Summarizing Patient Demographic Data in a Clinical Trial
A clinical trial was conducted to evaluate the effectiveness of a new antihypertensive medication. As part of the study, *20 participants* were enrolled, and their demographic data, including *age, gender, and body mass index (BMI)*, were collected.

Sample Data: The collected data from 20 patients is summarized in Table 3.3:

Table 3.4 Sample data for case study – 1

Patient ID	Age (Years)	Gender	BMI (kg/m²)
1	28	Female	22.1
2	47	Male	30.5
3	35	Female	25.6
4	60	Male	27.3
5	42	Female	24.9
6	50	Male	32.8
7	31	Female	23.4
8	55	Male	29.2
9	40	Female	28.7
10	36	Male	26.8
11	63	Female	31.4
12	29	Male	21.9
13	45	Female	27.8
14	70	Male	33.6
15	48	Female	30.1
16	39	Male	25.7
17	57	Female	28.4
18	34	Male	24.2
19	53	Female	29.6
20	64	Female	34.5
Total	926		558.5

Descriptive Statistics
Age Distribution

- Mean Age ($\bar{x}$) = **46.3 years**

$$\bar{x} = \frac{\Sigma x}{n} = \frac{926}{20} = 46.3$$

- Median Age = **46 years**
  - Ordered ages: 28, 29, 31, 34, 35, 36, 39, 40, 42, 45, 47, 48, 50, 53, 55, 57, 60, 63, 64, 70
  - Median = *Average of 10th and 11th values:*

$$Median = \frac{45+47}{2} = \frac{92}{2} = 46$$

- Range = **42 years**
  - *Maximum value* (70) *– Minimum value* $(28) = 42$

- IQR = **21.25**
  - Ordered Ages: 28, 29, 31, 34, 35, 36, 39, 40, 42, 45, 47, 48, 50, 53, 55, 57, 60, 63, 64, 70

- $Q3 = \left(\frac{3(n+1)}{4}\right)$ th value of the observation
- $= \left(\frac{3 \times 21}{4}\right)$ th value $= (15.75)$ th value $= 15th + 0.75[16th - 15th]$
- $= 55 + 0.75[57 - 55] = 56.5$
- $Q3 = \left(\frac{n+1}{4}\right)$ th value of the observation
- $= \left(\frac{21}{4}\right)$ th value $= (5.25)$ th value $= 5th + 0.25[6th - 5th]$
- $= 35 + 0.25[36 - 35] = 35.25$
- $IQR = Q_3 - Q_1 = 56.5 - 35.25$

- **Standard Deviation (SD) = 12.5 years**

  - $\Sigma(x_i - \bar{x})^2 = (28 - 46)^2 + (47 - 46)^2 + (35 - 46)^2 + (60 - 46)^2 + (42 - 46)^2 +$
  $(50 - 46)^2 + (31 - 46)^2 + (55 - 46)^2 + (40 - 46)^2 + (36 - 46)^2 + (63 - 46)^2 +$
  $(29 - 46)^2 + (45 - 46)^2 + (70 - 46)^2 + (48 - 46)^2 + (39 - 46)^2 + (57 - 46)^2 +$
  $(34 - 46)^2 + (53 - 46)^2 + (64 - 46)^2 = \mathbf{2962}$
  - The absolute value of the mean (46) is used for simpler calculations.

$$SD = \sqrt{\frac{\Sigma(x_i - \bar{x})^2}{n-1}} = \sqrt{\frac{2962}{20-1}} = \sqrt{\frac{2962}{20-1}} = 12.5$$

- **Graphical Representation of Age Distribution:**

The age distribution is visually depicted in Figure 3.7.

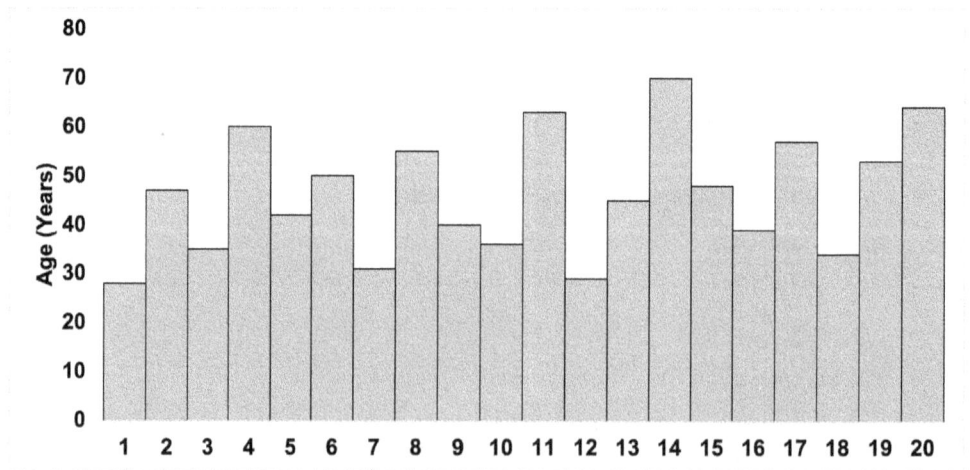

Figure 3.7 Histogram for age distribution.

Gender Distribution
- Frequency of Male and Female Patients
    - Male Patients = 8 (40%)
    - Female Patients = 12 (60%)
- Graphical Representation of Gender Distribution

The gender distribution is visually depicted in Figure 3.8.

BMI Distribution
- Summary statistics:
    - Mean BMI = 27.9 kg/m²
    - Median BMI = 28.1 kg/m²
    - Range = 34.5 – 21.9 = 12.6 kg/m²
    - IQR $= Q3 - Q1 = 30.4 - 25.1 = 5.3$
    - Standard Deviation (SD) = 3.7 kg/m²
    - Minimum BMI = 21.9 kg/m²
    - Maximum BMI = 34.5 kg/m²
- Visual Representation

The BMI distribution is visually depicted in Figure 3.9.

Interpretation and Key Findings
1. Age Analysis
    - The mean age (46.3 years) suggests that most participants are middle aged.
    - The mean (46.3 years) and median (46 years) are close, indicating a fairly symmetrical distribution.
    - The standard deviation (12.5 years) suggests moderate variability in participant ages.
    - The minimum and maximum age (28–70 years) confirms that the study includes both young and elderly participants.

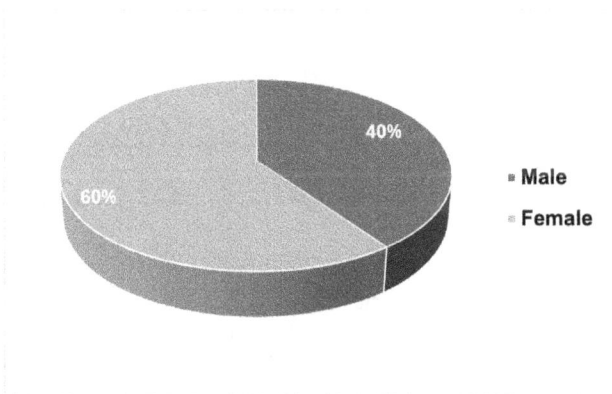

Figure 3.8 Pie chart for gender distribution.

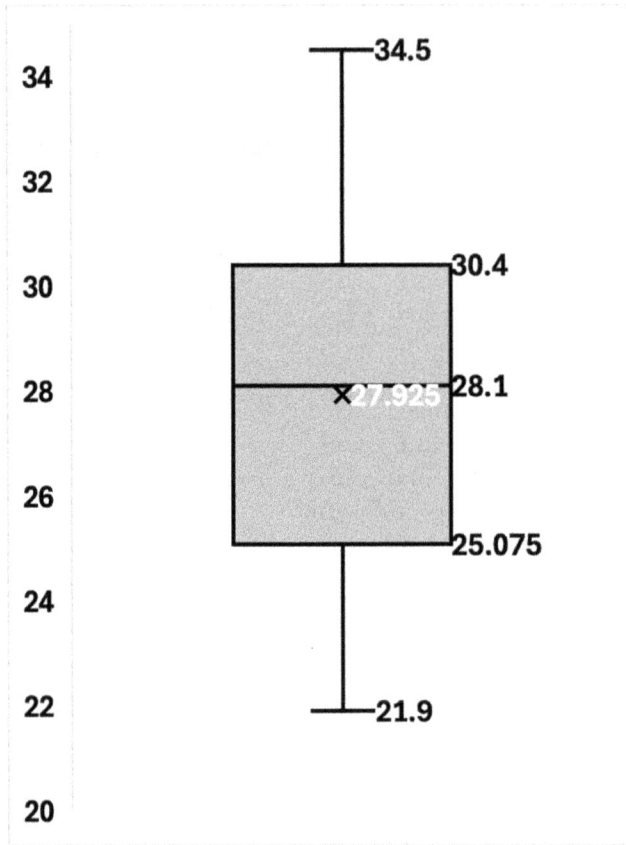

Figure 3.9 Box plot visualizing BMI variability.

2. **Gender Representation**
   - The study has more female participants (60%) than male participants (40%).
   - The gender balance is not perfectly equal, which may have implications for generalizability.
3. **BMI Analysis**
   - The mean BMI (27.9 kg/m²) suggests that most participants are overweight or obese.
   - The standard deviation (3.7 kg/m²) suggest that around 68% patients are within the range of 24.2–31.6.
   - Box plot visualization helps in identifying outliers and distribution trends.

Case Study 2: Analyzing Skewness and Kurtosis in Fasting Blood Sugar Levels
A study was conducted to evaluate the distribution of fasting blood sugar (FBS) levels among 20 patients. The objective was to determine whether the FBS values follow a normal distribution and to assess the skewness and kurtosis of the dataset.

Sample Data: The following 20 FBS readings (mg/dL) were recorded from the study participants:

FBS (mg/dL): 112.3, 98.7, 105.6, 121.2, 109.4, 133.7, 81.3, 94.2, 119.6, 101.4, 107.9, 111.2, 115.8, 108.5, 102.1, 126.3, 113.6, 89.5, 97.2, 110.1

Descriptive Analysis (Sample Estimates)

- Mean FBS Level: 107.98 mg/dL
- Median FBS Level: 108.95 mg/dL
- Standard Deviation (Sample): 12.49 mg/dL
- Min-Max: 81.3–133.7 mg/dL
- Range: 52.4

Skewness Analysis

Using the Fisher-Pearson Standardized Third Moment Coefficient Formula (Doane and Seward 2011):

$$G_1 = \frac{n}{(n-1)(n-2)} \sum_{i=1}^{n} \left(\frac{x_i - \bar{x}}{s} \right)^3$$

$$G_1 = \frac{20}{(20-1)(20-2)} \sum_{i=1}^{20} \left(\frac{x_i - 107.98}{12.49} \right)^3 = -0.079$$

Interpretation:

- If Sample Skewness > 0, the distribution is right-skewed (longer right tail).
- If Sample Skewness < 0, the distribution is left-skewed (longer left tail).
- If Sample Skewness ≈ 0, the data is symmetric.

Since Sample Skewness = –0.079, the distribution is slightly negatively (left) skewed, indicating a minor shift towards lower values but still close to symmetry.

Kurtosis Analysis

Using the Fisher's Excess Kurtosis with Small Sample Bias Correction (DeCarlo 1997):

$$G_2 = \left[\frac{n(n+1)}{(n-1)(n-2)(n-3)} \right] \sum_{i=1}^{n} \left(\frac{x_i - \bar{x}}{s} \right)^4 - \left[\frac{3(n-1)^2}{(n-2)(n-3)} \right]$$

$$G_2 = \left[\frac{20(20+1)}{(20-1)(20-2)(20-3)} \right] \sum_{i=1}^{n} \left(\frac{x_i - 107.98}{12.49} \right)^4 - \left[\frac{3(20-1)^2}{(20-2)(20-3)} \right]$$

$$G_2 = 0.282$$

Interpretation:

- If Sample Kurtosis > 0, the distribution is leptokurtic (heavier tails, more extreme values).
- If Sample Kurtosis < 0, the distribution is platykurtic (lighter tails, fewer extreme values).
- If Sample Kurtosis ≈ 0, the distribution has a normal-like shape.

Since Sample Kurtosis = 0.282, the distribution has moderate tails, slightly heavier than a normal distribution, meaning extreme values are less frequent than in a normal distribution.

Histogram and Interpretation
Figure 3.10 illustrates the distribution of FBS levels:

Practical Implications
Since skewness is low, standard statistical techniques, like mean and standard deviation, can be reliably used without transformations.

Case Study 3: Analyzing Blood Pressure Readings in a Cohort Study
A cohort study examines the impact of a *lifestyle intervention program* on *systolic blood pressure (SBP)* over time. The study tracks *ten patients* at three time points:

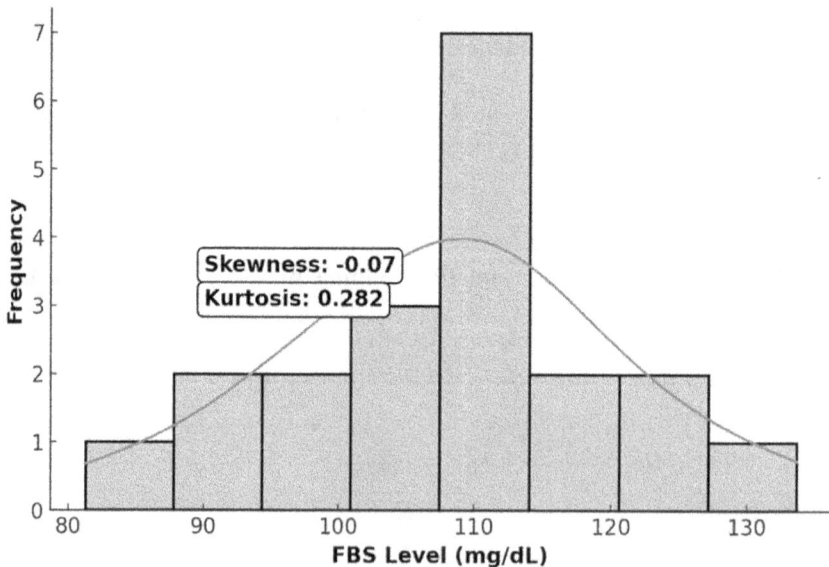

Figure 3.10 The histogram illustrating the distribution of FBS levels.

Table 3.5 SBP readings of the ten patients at different time points

Patient	Baseline SBP (mmHg)	Three-month SBP (mmHg)	Six-month SBP (mmHg)
P1	145	135	128
P2	160	150	142
P3	155	145	138
P4	148	140	133
P5	135	128	122
P6	165	155	147
P7	152	143	136
P8	140	130	123
P9	138	128	120
P10	158	148	139

Table 3.6 Summary statistics of the sample data

Statistic	Baseline SBP	Three-month SBP	Six-month SBP
Mean (mmHg)	149.60	140.20	132.80
Standard Deviation (mmHg)	10.08	9.64	9.20
Median (mmHg)	150.00	141.50	134.50
Range (mmHg)	30 (135–165)	27 (128–155)	27 (120–147)

baseline (before intervention), three months post-intervention, and six months post-intervention.

The goal is to assess whether the intervention effectively reduces blood pressure over time.

Sample Data: Table 3.4 next presents the *SBP readings* of the ten patients at the three time points.

Descriptive Statistics of SBP
The following summary provides central tendency and variability measures for SBP at each time point (Table 3.5).

Key Insights From Descriptive Statistics
- The mean SBP decreases from 149.6 mmHg at baseline to 132.8 mmHg at six months, indicating an overall improvement.
- Variability (standard deviation) also decreases over time, suggesting more consistent blood pressure control among participants.
- The range of SBP remains stable, but individual reductions vary.

Graphical Representation of Blood Pressure Trends
1. **SBP Trends Over Time (Bar Diagram)**
   The following *bar diagram* visualizes mean (SD) *SBP changes* over time (Figure 3.11).

2. **SBP Distribution at Different Time Points**

   The following *box plot* compares the *spread of SBP values* at Baseline, 3 Months, and 6 Months (Figure 3.12).

   ■ *Median SBP decreases* over time.

   ■ The *spread (IQR) narrows*, suggesting better blood pressure control.

   ■ No extreme *outliers*, indicating a consistent trend.

Case Study 4: Tracking Treatment Satisfaction Scores in a Patient Survey

A hospital conducts a *patient satisfaction survey* to evaluate the effectiveness of a *new outpatient appointment scheduling system*. The survey collects *feedback from ten patients*, assessing their satisfaction levels on a *five-point scale*.

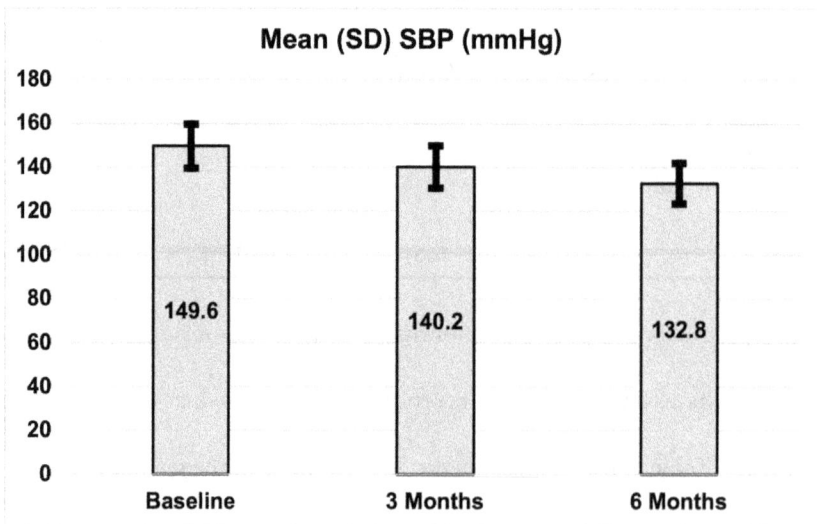

Figure 3.11 SBP trends over time.

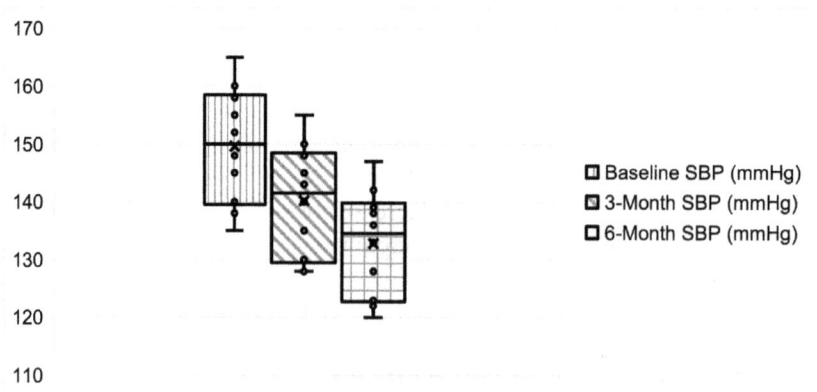

Figure 3.12 Box plot comparing the spread of SBP values at different time points.

Sample Data:
The following table presents the *satisfaction levels* recorded from ten patients (Table 3.6).

Descriptive Statistics of Patient Satisfaction
The following table summarizes the *frequency and proportion* of each satisfaction level (Table 3.7).

Key Insights From the Data
- 60% of patients (Very Satisfied + Satisfied) reported positive experiences.
- 20% (Neutral) had neither a positive nor negative opinion.
- 20% (Dissatisfied + Very Dissatisfied) were unhappy, indicating potential areas for improvement.

Graphical Representation of Patient Satisfaction
1. Satisfaction Level Distribution (Pie Chart)
   The following *pie chart* (see Figure 3.13) displays the frequency distribution of satisfaction scores.

- The highest number of patients (three each) were Very Satisfied and Satisfied.
- The Neutral group had two patients, indicating mixed feedback.
- One patient each was Dissatisfied and Very Dissatisfied, highlighting concerns.

Table 3.7 Satisfaction levels recorded from ten patients

Patient	Satisfaction level
P1	Very Satisfied
P2	Satisfied
P3	Neutral
P4	Satisfied
P5	Dissatisfied
P6	Very Satisfied
P7	Satisfied
P8	Neutral
P9	Very Satisfied
P10	Very Dissatisfied

Table 3.8 Frequency and proportion of each satisfaction level

Satisfaction level	Frequency	Percentage
Very Satisfied	3	$3/10 \times 100 = 30\%$
Satisfied	3	30.0%
Neutral	2	20.0%
Dissatisfied	1	10.0%
Very Dissatisfied	1	10.0%

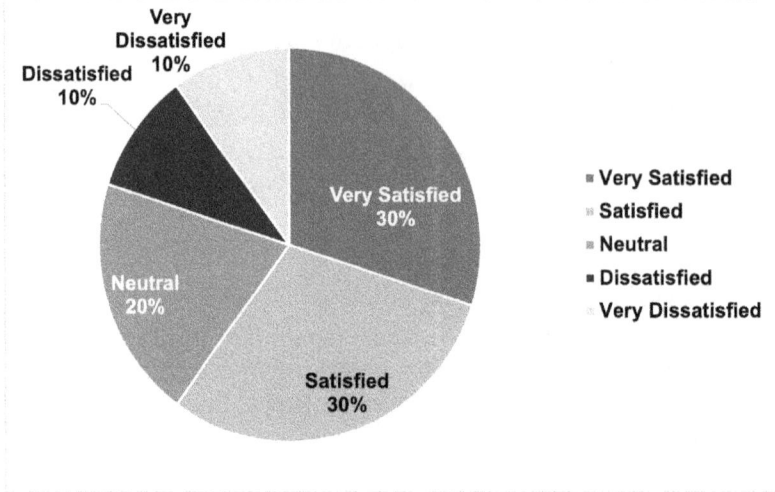

Figure 3.13 Pie chart displaying the frequency distribution of satisfaction scores.

Case Study 5: Evaluating Weight Loss in a Diet Intervention Program
A 12-week diet program enrolls ten participants. Researchers record baseline weight and weight at week 12 to evaluate the intervention's effectiveness.

Sample Data and Calculations
The following table (Table 3.8) presents the sample data along with the percentage change observed after the intervention in ten patients.

Table 3.9 Percentage weight change after a 12-week diet program

Participant	Baseline weight (kg)	Week 12 weight (kg)	Change (kg)	% Change
P1	80	75	−5	$(-5/80)\times100 = -6.25\%$
P2	92	88	−4	$(-4/92)\times100 \approx -4.35\%$
P3	70	68	−2	$(-2/70)\times100 \approx -2.86\%$
P4	85	82	−3	$(-3/85)\times100 \approx -3.53\%$
P5	100	95	−5	$(-5/100)\times100 = -5\%$
P6	77	73	−4	$(-4/77)\times100 \approx -5.19\%$
P7	90	84	−6	$(-6/90)\times100 \approx -6.67\%$
P8	82	79	−3	$(-3/82)\times100 \approx -3.66\%$
P9	76	74	−2	$(-2/76)\times100 \approx -2.63\%$
P10	88	84	−4	$(-4/88)\times100 \approx -4.55\%$
Total	840	802	−38	$(-38/840)\times100 \approx -4.52\%$

- Mean baseline weight: $= 84.0\,kg$
- Mean weight at week 12: $= 80.2\,kg$
- Mean % change: $\approx -4.52\%$

Visual Summaries

1. **Histogram of % Weight Change**

The percentage of weight change after the intervention is illustrated in Figure 3.14.

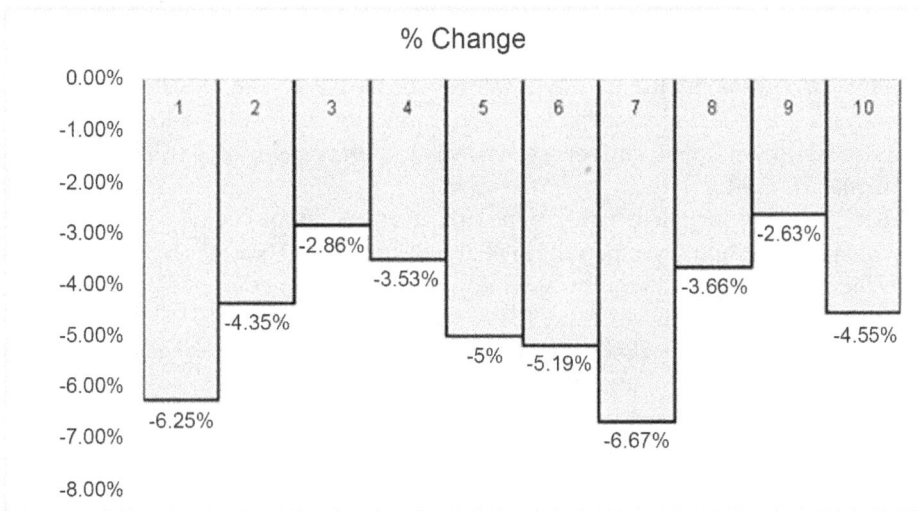

Figure 3.14 % Weight change in the participants.

Interpretation

- All participants experienced weight loss, with an average reduction of about 4.5%.
- Individual results varied (–2.63% to –6.67%), indicating different responses to the diet.
- The consistent downward trend supports the program's overall effectiveness.

Statistical Software for Descriptive Statistics

Statistical software applications provide a set of statistical toolboxes for analyzing data and presenting it through plots and graphs. Commonly used statistical software packages include SAS, SPSS, R, and STATA, each with its own advantages and disadvantages. These software packages offer capabilities such as handling large databases, graphing, compatibility with different operating systems, customization, and customer support. Descriptive statistics in these software packages include measures such as minimum, maximum, range, percentile, mean, median, mode, standard deviation, variance, skewness, and kurtosis (Shen et al. 2023).

Popular Statistical Software for Descriptive Statistics

1. **R:** *Strengths* included extensive packages for descriptive statistics and visualization. Open-source and widely used in academia and research. Strong data analysis and visualization capabilities. *Weaknesses* included steeper learning curve due to programming requirements (Li et al. 2021; Shen et al. 2023).
2. **SPSS (Statistical Package for the Social Sciences):** *Strengths* included user-friendly with point-and-click interface. Suitable for beginners and widely used in educational settings. Good for generating transparent graphs and visualizations. *Weaknesses* included costly compared to open-source alternatives (Loffing 2022; Shen et al. 2023).
3. **Excel:** *Strengths* included widely accessible and familiar to many users. Useful for basic descriptive statistics and data visualization. *Weaknesses* limited in handling large datasets and advanced statistical analyses (Quintela-del-Río and Francisco-Fernández 2017; Shen et al. 2023).
4. **Stata:** *Strengths* included powerful for both basic and advanced statistical analyses. User-friendly with both programming and point-and-click options. *Weaknesses* included can be expensive and may require additional training (Shen et al. 2023).
5. **SAS:** *Strengths* included highly powerful and capable of handling large datasets. Widely used in industry, especially in pharmaceuticals and biotechnology. *Weaknesses* included high cost and requires significant training (Shen et al. 2023).
6. **Open-Source Alternatives (e.g., PSPP, JASP, SOFA):** *Strengths* included free and open-source, making them cost-effective. Increasingly user-friendly with good documentation and community support. *Weaknesses* lack some advanced features found in commercial software (Wu, Zhao, and Niu 2021).

Common Pitfalls and Challenges in Descriptive Statistics in Health Research

Misinterpretation of descriptive statistics: One of the most significant challenges is the misinterpretation of descriptive statistics. Many medical practitioners and researchers lack formal statistical training, which can result in misunderstanding statistical vs. practical significance or confusing correlation with causation (Parks and Yeh 2021). Additionally, there is a widespread overreliance on p-values, often leading to conclusions based solely on statistical significance without considering confidence intervals or effect sizes. This narrow focus can obscure the real-world relevance of research findings (Pryjmachuk and Richards 2007).

Overgeneralization from summary measures: Another common issue is the overgeneralization from summary measures. Researchers sometimes fail to explore raw data thoroughly before analysis, leading to overgeneralized conclusions that do not capture important patterns or variations. Furthermore, the misuse of averages such as applying the mean in skewed distributions where the median would be more appropriate can create misleading interpretations (Parks and Yeh 2021).

Errors in graphical representations: Errors in graphical representations also contribute to miscommunication of findings. Bias in data presentation occurs when researchers use misleading scales, inappropriate graph types, or selectively present data, intentionally or unintentionally distorting the message. Additionally, lack of clarity and accuracy in visualizations can lead to confusion, making it difficult for readers to extract meaningful insights from the data (Parks and Yeh 2021).

Recommendations to Avoid These Pitfalls

To mitigate these challenges, several best practices should be followed. Early involvement of statisticians in study design ensures that appropriate statistical methods are applied from the outset. Providing comprehensive statistical training for medical practitioners and researchers can significantly reduce misinterpretations and enhance analytical rigor. Before conducting full-scale analysis, thorough data exploration, including cleaning, screening, and exploratory analysis, helps uncover hidden patterns and prevents erroneous conclusions. Finally, careful graphical design, with well-chosen scales, graph types, and unbiased data presentation, enhances the clarity and accuracy of statistical communication (Strasak et al. 2007; Pryjmachuk and Richards 2007; Parks and Yeh 2021).

Conclusion

Descriptive statistics constitute a foundational element within the health research, providing indispensable tools for the organization, summarization, and interpretation of data. These statistics facilitate the identification of trends, the assessment of variability, and the formulation of hypotheses that direct subsequent analytical endeavours. Beyond numerical representation, measures of central tendency and dispersion play a vital role in clinical decision-making, public health monitoring, and epidemiological research. When applied correctly, descriptive statistics enhance research clarity and ensure accurate communication of medical data. However, misinterpretations such as relying solely on summary measures, using means in skewed datasets, or misrepresenting trends can lead to flawed conclusions. Thus, proficiency in statistical concepts is essential for navigating these challenges.

Recent advancements in statistical software, like SPSS, SAS, R, and Python, have improved data analysis efficiency, but technology alone cannot replace a solid understanding of statistical principles. The effective utilization of these tools necessitates sound reasoning and methodological rigor. Ultimately, descriptive statistics function as the cornerstone of evidence-based medicine, influencing patient care, clinical protocols, and healthcare policies. As the complexity of medical research continues to escalate, the mastery of these principles remains a scientific obligation, ensuring that data-driven decisions are precise, transparent, and clinically pertinent.

Discussion Questions

- How can descriptive statistics be effectively utilized to enhance the interpretation and communication of health research findings, particularly in clinical and public health settings?
- Discuss the role of data visualization and summary measures in conveying complex information to diverse stakeholders, including policymakers, healthcare providers, and patients.
- Additionally, reflect on the potential consequences of misinterpreting descriptive statistics and how the use of statistical software can both aid and complicate this process. Use examples from real-world case studies or your own experience to support your discussion.

References

Adil, I.H., A. Wahid, and E.H. Mantell. 2021. "Split Sample Skewness." Communications in Statistics – Theory and Methods 50 (22): 5171–88. https://doi.org/10.1080/03610926.2020.1804588.

Al-Benna, S., Y. Al-Ajam, B. Way, and L. Steinstraesser. 2010. "Descriptive and Inferential Statistical Methods Used in Burns Research." Burns 36 (3): 343–6. https://doi.org/10.1016/j.burns.2009.04.030.

Ali, M.S., S. Lulseged, and G. Medhin. 2018. "EMJ Series on Methods and Statistics: Presenting and Summarizing Data – Part I." Ethiopian Medical Journal 56 (4): 375–88.

Arachchige, C.N.P.G., and L.A. Prendergast. 2024. "Confidence Intervals for Median Absolute Deviations." Communications in Statistics: Simulation and Computation. https://doi.org/10.1080/03610918.2024.2376198.

Brath, R., and E. Banissi. 2018. "Stem and Leaf Plots Extended for Text Visualizations." In Proceedings – 2017 14th International Conference on Computer Graphics, Imaging and Visualization, CGiV 2017, 99–104. https://doi.org/10.1109/CGiV.2017.32.

Braun, W.J. 2012. "Naive Analysis of Variance." Journal of Statistics Education 20 (2). https://doi.org/10.1080/10691898.2012.11889638.

Buckley, J.J. 2006. "Fuzzy Estimator for the Median." Studies in Fuzziness and Soft Computing. Vol. 196. https://doi.org/10.1007/11598152_28.

Chacón, J.E. 2020. "The Modal Age of Statistics." International Statistical Review 88 (1): 122–41. https://doi.org/10.1111/insr.12340.

Chekanov, S.V. 2016. "Histograms." Advanced Information and Knowledge Processing. https://doi.org/10.1007/978-3-319-28531-3_7.

Cheng, G., Y. Feng, and H. Ahmadzade. 2020. "On the Dispersion Measures of Complex Uncertain Random Variables." IEEE Access 8: 135700–705. https://doi.org/10.1109/ACCESS.2020.3011255.

Chishtie, J., I.A. Bielska, A. Barrera, J.-S. Marchand, M. Imran, S.F. Ali Tirmizi, L.A. Turcotte, et al. 2022. "Interactive Visualization Applications in Population Health and Health Services Research: Systematic Scoping Review." Journal of Medical Internet Research 24 (2). https://doi.org/10.2196/27534.

Dahl, M.R., and P. Vedsted. 2008. "Personal Data and Confidentiality on the Internet | Personhenførbare Og Fortrolige Data Og Resultater På Internettet." Ugeskrift for Laeger 170 (49): 4027–9.

Darling, H.S. 2022. "Do You Have a Standard Way of Interpreting the Standard Deviation? A Narrative Review." Cancer Research, Statistics, and Treatment 5 (4): 728–33. https://doi.org/10.4103/crst.crst_284_22.

DeCarlo, Lawrence T. 1997. "On the Meaning and Use of Kurtosis." Psychological Methods 2 (3): 292–307. https://doi.org/10.1037/1082-989X.2.3.292.

Doane, D.P., and L.E. Seward. 2011. "Measuring Skewness: A Forgotten Statistic?" Journal of Statistics Education 19 (2). https://doi.org/10.1080/10691898.2011.11889611.

Drzymała, J. 2021. "Universal Equations for Pythagorean and Sauter-Type Formulas of Mean Value Calculation and Classification of the Extended Pythagorean Means." Mining Science 24:227–35. https://doi.org/10.5277/msc172416.

Elamir, E.A.H. 2012. "Mean Absolute Deviation about Median as a Tool of Explanatory Data Analysis." In Lecture Notes in Engineering and Computer Science 2197: 324–29.

Falk, M., P. Ljung, C. Lundström, A. Ynnerman, and I. Hotz. 2020, September. "Feature Exploration Using Local Frequency Distributions in Computed Tomography Data." In Eurographics Workshop on Visual Computing for Biomedicine: 13–24. https://doi.org/10.2312/vcbm.20201166.

Feng, C., and H. Wang. 2024. "Harmonic Mean and Geometric Mean of a Non Negative Random Variable." Communications in Statistics – Theory and Methods. https://doi.org/10.1080/03610926.2024.2349713.

Flowers, J., and K. Johnson. 2016. "Data Presentation." Public Health Intelligence: Issues of Measure and Method. https://doi.org/10.1007/978-3-319-28326-5_11.

Gómez Gómez, M.D.R., C. García Reza, V. Gómez Martínez, and P.B. Mondragón Sánchez. 2011. "Life Quality in Patients Suffering from High Systemic Blood Pressure | Calidad de Vida En Pacientes Que Viven Con Hipertensión Arterial Sistémica." Revista Mexicana de Enfermeria Cardiologica 19 (1): 7–12.

Gorard, S. 2005. "Revisiting a 90-Year-Old Debate: The Advantages of the Mean Deviation." British Journal of Educational Studies 53 (4): 417–30. https://doi.org/10.1111/j.1467-8527.2005.00304.x.

Greco, L., G. Luta, and R. Wilcox. 2024. "On Testing the Equality between Interquartile Ranges." Computational Statistics 39 (5): 2873–98. https://doi.org/10.1007/s00180-023-01415-8.

Gries, Stefan Th. 2014, November. "Frequency Tables.", 365–89. https://doi.org/10.1075/HCP.43.14GRI/HTML.

Grieve, A.P. 2013. "Medical Statistics." The Textbook of Pharmaceutical Medicine. https://doi.org/10.1002/9781118532331.ch9.

Hayes, K. 2014. "Finite-Sample Bias-Correction Factors for the Median Absolute Deviation." Communications in Statistics: Simulation and Computation 43 (10): 2205–12. https://doi.org/10.1080/03610918.2012.748913.

Jankowski, K.R.B., and K.J. Flannelly. 2015. "Measures of Central Tendency in Chaplaincy, Health Care, and Related Research." Journal of Health Care Chaplaincy 21 (1): 39–49. https://doi.org/10.1080/08854726.2014.989799.

Joarder, A.H. 2014. "An Algorithm for Sample Variance." International Journal of Mathematical Education in Science and Technology 45 (1): 145–9. https://doi.org/10.1080/0020739X.2013.790517.

Kamanchi, C., R.B. Diddigi, K.J. Prabuchandran, and S. Bhatnagar. 2019. "An Online Sample-Based Method for Mode Estimation Using ODE Analysis of Stochastic Approximation Algorithms." IEEE Control Systems Letters 3 (3): 697–702. https://doi.org/10.1109/LCSYS.2019.2916467.

Khorana, A., A. Pareek, M. Ollivier, S.J. Madjarova, K.N. Kunze, B.U. Nwachukwu, J. Karlsson, E.M. Marigi, and R.J. Williams. 2023. "Choosing the Appropriate Measure of Central Tendency: Mean, Median, or Mode?" Knee Surgery, Sports Traumatology, Arthroscopy 31 (1): 12–15. https://doi.org/10.1007/s00167-022-07204-y.

Klein, I., and M. Doll. 2021. "Tests on Asymmetry for Ordered Categorical Variables." Journal of Applied Statistics 48 (7): 1180–98. https://doi.org/10.1080/02664763.2020.1757045.

Knapp, Thomas R. 2015. "'Percentaging' Contingency Tables: It Really Does Matter How You Do It." Research in Nursing & Health 38 (4): 323–5. https://doi.org/10.1002/NUR.21666.

Kostal, L., P. Lansky, and O. Pokora. 2013. "Measures of Statistical Dispersion Based on Shannon and Fisher Information Concepts." Information Sciences 235: 214–23. https://doi.org/10.1016/j.ins.2013.02.023.

Labreuche, J. 2010. "Variables: Their Graphical Representations and Descriptive Statistics | Les Différents Types de Variables, Leurs Représentations Graphiques et Paramètres Descriptifs." Sang Thrombose Vaisseaux 22 (10): 536–43. https://doi.org/10.1684/stv.2010.0541.

Labreuche, J. 2020. "Variables: Their Graphical Representations and Descriptive Statistics | Les Différents Types de Variables, Leurs Représentations Graphiques et Paramètres Descriptifs." Sang Thrombose Vaisseaux 32 (2): 62–9. https://doi.org/10.1684/stv.2020.1111.

Lann, A., and R. Falk. 2006. "Tell Me the Method, I'll Give You the Mean." American Statistician 60 (4): 322–7. https://doi.org/10.1198/000313006X151460.

Lee, D.K., J. In, and S. Lee. 2015. "Standard Deviation and Standard Error of the Mean." Korean Journal of Anesthesiology 68 (3): 220–3. https://doi.org/10.4097/kjae.2015.68.3.220.

Li, D., X. Yu, S. Han, H. Zhu, Y. Yuan, J. Shen, J. Lin, X. Li, Y. Gan, and J. Liu. 2021. "Data Visualization of Multiple Linear Regression Analysis Practiced by R Studio Software | 多元线性回归分析数据可视化的R Studio 软件实践." Chinese Journal of Evidence-Based Medicine 21 (4): 482–90. https://doi.org/10.7507/1672-2531.202008172.

Liu, Q., X. Liu, and Z. Hu. 2024. "Bahadur Representations for the Bootstrap Median Absolute Deviation and the Application to Projection Depth Weighted Mean." Metrika. https://doi.org/10.1007/s00184-024-00958-0.

Loffing, F. 2022. "Raw Data Visualization for Common Factorial Designs Using SPSS: A Syntax Collection and Tutorial." Frontiers in Psychology 13. https://doi.org/10.3389/fpsyg.2022.808469.

Lu, H., X. He, J. Vaidya, and N. Adam. 2008. "Secure Construction of Contingency Tables from Distributed Data." Lecture Notes in Computer Science (Including Subseries Lecture Notes in Artificial Intelligence and Lecture Notes in Bioinformatics) 5094 LNCS. https://doi.org/10.1007/978-3-540-70567-3_11.

Madrid, A.E., S.M. Valenzuela-Ruiz, C. Batanero, and J.A. Garzón-Guerrero. 2022. "University Students' Understanding of Median | Comprensión de La Mediana Por Estudiantes Universitarios." Avances de Investigacion En Educacion Matematica (22): 1–21. https://doi.org/10.35763/aiem22.3902.

Mao, Z., and W. Huo. 2023. "Descriptive Study." Textbook of Clinical Epidemiology: For Medical Students. https://doi.org/10.1007/978-981-99-3622-9_3.

Martinez, M.N., and M.J. Bartholomew. 2017. "What Does It 'Mean'? A Review of Interpreting and Calculating Different Types of Means and Standard Deviations." Pharmaceutics 9 (2). https://doi.org/10.3390/pharmaceutics9020014.

Nejadseyfi, O., H.J.M. Geijselaers, and A.H. van den Boogaard. 2019. "Evaluation and Assessment of Non-Normal Output during Robust Optimization." Structural and Multidisciplinary Optimization 59 (6): 2063–76. https://doi.org/10.1007/s00158-018-2173-2.

Oddi, F.J., F.E. Miguez, G.G. Benedetti, and L.A. Garibaldi. 2020. "When Variability Varies: Heteroscedasticity and Variance Functions | Cuando La Variabilidad Varía: Heterocedasticidad y Funciones de Varianza." Ecologia Austral 30 (3): 438–53. https://doi.org/10.25260/10.25260/EA.20.30.3.0.1131.

Parks, J., and D.D. Yeh. 2021. "How to Lie with Statistics and Figures." Surgical Infections 22 (6): 611–19. https://doi.org/10.1089/sur.2021.065.

Piliposyan, T.V. 2018. "The Distribution of the Maximum, Minimum and Range of a Sample." Journal of Contemporary Mathematical Analysis 53 (3): 180–6. https://doi.org/10.3103/S1068362318030093.

Pryjmachuk, S., and D.A. Richards. 2007. "Look before You Leap and Don't Put All Your Eggs in One Basket: The Need for Caution and Prudence in Quantitative Data Analysis." Journal of Research in Nursing 12 (1): 43–54. https://doi.org/10.1177/1744987106070260.

Quintela-del-Río, A., and M. Francisco-Fernández. 2017. "Excel Templates: A Helpful Tool for Teaching Statistics." American Statistician 71 (4): 317–25. https://doi.org/10.1080/00031305.2016.1186115.

Rao, C.R., X. Shi, and Y. Wu. 2014. "Approximation of the Expected Value of the Harmonic Mean and Some Applications." Proceedings of the National Academy of Sciences of the United States of America 111 (44): 15681–6. https://doi.org/10.1073/pnas.1412216111.

Reese, R.A. 2005. "Boxplots." Significance 2 (3): 134–35. https://doi.org/10.1111/j.1740-9713.2005.00118.x.

Rendón-Macías, M.E., M.Á. Villasís-Keever, and M.G. Miranda-Novales. 2016. "Descriptive Statistics | Estadística Descriptiva." Revista Alergia Mexico 63 (4): 397–407. https://doi.org/10.29262/ram.v63i4.230.

Sabharwal, S. 2023. "Presenting Data." Translational Sports Medicine. https://doi.org/10.1016/B978-0-323-91259-4.00002-3.

Samawi, H., H. Rochani, J.J. Yin, D. Linder, and R. Vogel. 2018. "Notes on Kernel Density Based Mode Estimation Using More Efficient Sampling Designs." Computational Statistics 33 (2): 1071–90. https://doi.org/10.1007/s00180-017-0787-2.

Sandnes, F.E., A. Flønes, W.T. Kao, P. Harrington, and M. Issa. 2020. "Searching for Extreme Portions in Distributions: A Comparison of Pie and Bar Charts." Lecture Notes in Computer Science (Including Subseries Lecture Notes in Artificial Intelligence and Lecture Notes in Bioinformatics) 12341 LNCS: 342–51. https://doi.org/10.1007/978-3-030-60816-3_37.

Sbert, M., C. Ancuti, C.O. Ancuti, J. Poch, S. Chen, and M. Vila. 2021. "Histogram Ordering." IEEE Access 9: 28785–96. https://doi.org/10.1109/ACCESS.2021.3058577.

Schumm, W.R., K.R. Bosch, and A.W. Doolittle. 2009. "Explaining the Importance of Statistical Variance for Undergraduate Students." Psychology and Education 46 (3–4): 1–7.

Schwarz, C.R. 2006. "Statistics of Range of a Set of Normally Distributed Numbers." Journal of Surveying Engineering 132 (4): 155–9. https://doi.org/10.1061/(ASCE)0733-9453(2006)132:4(155).

Schwarz, C.R. 2011. "Statistics of Range of a Set of Normally Distributed Numbers." CORS and OPUS for Engineers: Tools for Surveying and Mapping Applications. https://doi.org/10.1061/9780784411643.ch06.

Scott, L.J., and C.A. Rogers. 2015. "Creating Summary Tables Using the Sumtable Command." Stata Journal 15 (3): 775–83. https://doi.org/10.1177/1536867x1501500310.

Shen, C., R. Klein, P. Holguin, and A.N. Kulaylat. 2023. "Statistical Software." Handbook for Designing and Conducting Clinical and Translational Surgery. https://doi.org/10.1016/B978-0-323-90300-4.00065-3.

Soliman, A.A., A.H. Abd Ellah, N.A. Abou-Elheggag, and A.A. Modhesh. 2012. "Estimation of the Coefficient of Variation for Non-Normal Model Using Progressive First-Failure-Censoring Data." Journal of Applied Statistics 39 (12): 2741–58. https://doi.org/10.1080/02664763.2012.725466.

Speelman, C.P., and M. McGann. 2013, July. "How Mean Is the Mean?" Frontiers in Psychology 4. https://doi.org/10.3389/fpsyg.2013.00451.

Spina, D. 2007. "Statistics in Pharmacology." British Journal of Pharmacology 152 (3): 291–93. https://doi.org/10.1038/sj.bjp.0707371.

Strasak, A.M., Q. Zaman, K.P. Pfeiffer, G. Göbel, and H. Ulmer. 2007. "Statistical Errors in Medical Research – A Review of Common Pitfalls." Swiss Medical Weekly 137 (3–4): 44–9.

Thrusfield, M., and R. Christley. 2017. "Presenting Numerical Data." Veterinary Epidemiology: Fourth Edition. https://doi.org/10.1002/9781118280249.ch12.

Unwin, A. 2015. "Graphical Methods, Analytic." International Encyclopedia of the Social & Behavioral Sciences: Second Edition. https://doi.org/10.1016/B978-0-08-097086-8.42131-8.

Van Baren, J., 2005. "Kurtosis-the missing dashboard knob." TEST Engineering and Management, 67(5), p.14.

Vetter, T.R. 2017. "Descriptive Statistics: Reporting the Answers to the 5 Basic Questions of Who, What, Why, When, Where, and a Sixth, so What?" Anesthesia and Analgesia 125 (5): 1797–802. https://doi.org/10.1213/ANE.0000000000002471.

Vogel, R.M. 2022. "The Geometric Mean?" Communications in Statistics – Theory and Methods 51 (1): 82–94. https://doi.org/10.1080/03610926.2020.1743313.

Watthanacheewakul, L. 2010. "Analysis of Variance with Weibull Data." In Proceedings of the International MultiConference of Engineers and Computer Scientists 2010, IMECS 2010, 2051–6.

Westfall, P.H. 2014. "Kurtosis as Peakedness, 1905–2014. R.I.P." American Statistician 68 (3): 191–5. https://doi.org/10.1080/00031305.2014.917055.

Wu, Z., Z. Zhao, and G. Niu. 2021. "Introduction to the Popular Open Source Statistical Software (OSSS)." Research Anthology on Usage and Development of Open Source Software. Vol. 1. https://doi.org/10.4018/978-1-7998-9158-1.ch040.

Yager, R.R., and N. Alajlan. 2014. "A Note on Mean Absolute Deviation." Information Sciences 279: 632–41. https://doi.org/10.1016/j.ins.2014.04.016.

Yi, X., Y. Miao, J. Zhou, and Y. Wang. 2016. "Some Novel Inequalities for Fuzzy Variables on the Variance and Its Rational Upper Bound." Journal of Inequalities and Applications (1): 1–18. https://doi.org/10.1186/s13660-016-0975-6.

Yorulmaz, A., and B. Yalçin. 2016. "Investigating the Frequency of Dermatological Diseases in the Oldest Old | İleri Yaşlilarda Dermatolojik Hastaliklarin Sikliğinin Araştirilmasi." Turk Geriatri Dergisi 19 (4): 211–16.

## CHAPTER 4

Introduction to Probability

Gholamreza Oskrochi

Learning Outcomes

By the end of this chapter, readers will understand key probability principles, including outcomes, events, and conditional probability. They will be able to identify and apply common probability distributions such as binomial, Poisson, and normal distributions in health research. The chapter will equip learners with the ability to model health data, estimate risks, and make predictions using probability concepts.

Definitions

Experiment

A process of taking measurements, often under controlled conditions. Examples include the following:

- Throwing a die or spinning a wheel.
- Conducting a medical trial.

Sample Space

The set of all possible outcomes resulting from an experiment. Examples:

- Rolling a die: S = {1, 2, 3, 4, 5, 6}.
- Outcomes of a medical trial: S = {success, failure, no difference, measured difference}.

Event

One or more outcomes or results of an experiment. Examples:

- Rolling a six on a die.
- Observing no change in blood pressure during a medical trial.

DOI: 10.4324/9781032701004-5

Event Relations

Two events, A and B, each contain respective outcomes. Their relationships can be expressed as follows:

- A ∩ B: All outcomes that are in event A, event B, or both.
- A ∩ B: All outcomes that are in both event A and event B.
- A' is the complement of event A, which is all elements in the sample space that is not in A, hence A ∪ A' = S.

Mutually Exclusive Events

Events A and B are mutually exclusive if they share no common outcomes. This means the occurrence of one event precludes the occurrence of the other at the same time. Symbolically:

A ∩ B = ∅. Hence, A ∩ A' = ∅

Example 1.1:

- Rolling a die: Event A – even numbers, A = {2, 4, 6}. Event B – rolling a three or five, B = {3, 5}. Then, A ∩ B = ∅.

Example 1.2:

- Event A: Patient admitted with broken bones.
- Event B: Patient admitted with a headache.
- Here, A ∩ B can occur, so A and B are not mutually exclusive.

Independent Events

Events A and B are independent if the occurrence of one does not affect the probability of the other.

Example 1.3: Independent Events

- Two (or more) flips of a coin.
- Weekly draws in lottery games.
- The chance of rain in London and the chance of an accident in Paris.

Example 1.4: Non-Independent Events

- Weather on two consecutive days.
- The airlines we choose for holidays.
- The weather report and the clothes we wear.

Random Variables

A random variable (RV) represents a measurable characteristic of something (event, object, process, person, etc.) that can take different values at different times or for different cases. Random variables are often denoted by capital letters, such as X or Y, and can be the following:

1. **Continuous Random Variables**
   Variables that take uncountable outcomes, such as the following:
   - Height, weight, distance, time.
2. **Discrete Random Variables**
   Variables that take countable outcomes, such as the following:
   - Number of children in a household.
   - Number of car accidents in a city in one day.
   - Number of patients visiting an emergency room in one hour.

Assigning Probabilities

Probability values can be determined using three main approaches:

1. **Theory (Classical Approach):**
   - Probability is calculated based on theoretical reasoning and simple mathematical principles.
   - Example: The chance of getting no heads when flipping a coin three times is $P(\{T \cap T \cap T\}) = 0.5 \times 0.5 \times 0.5 = 0.125$.
2. **Observation (Relative Frequency or Empirical Approach):**
   - Probability is determined by observing how often an event occurs in a large sample.
   - Example: The probability of testing positive for COVID-19 (event A) is the ratio of positive tests $[n(A)]$ to the total number of tests (n), as the number of tests becomes very large. Mathematically, $P(A) = lim_{n \to \infty} \frac{n(A)}{n}$
3. **Opinion (Subjective Approach):**
   - Probability represents a "degree of belief."
   - Example: "There is a 50% chance that I will join the meeting."

Key Principles:

- All probability values must lie between 0 and 1.
- The sum of probabilities of all possible outcomes in the sample space must equal to 1.

Axioms of Probability

Probability is a number that is assigned to each event of a random experiment, satisfying the following properties:

1. If S is the sample space and E is any event of the random experiment:
   - $P(S) = 1$
   - $0 \leq P(E) \leq 1$
2. Implications of the axioms:
   - $P(\varnothing) = 0$, where $\varnothing$ is the empty set.

- $P(E') = 1 - P(E)$, where E' is the complement of E.
- If E_1 is a subset of E_2 ($E_1 \subseteq E_2$), then $P(E_1) \leq P(E_2)$.

Addition Rules
Joint events are formed by combining individual events using set operations:

Probability of a Union: For any two events A and B:
$P(A \cup B) = P(A) + P(B) - P(A \cap B)$
If A and B are mutually exclusive ($A \cap B = \varnothing$): $P(A \cup B) = P(A) + P(B)$

Therefore, the probability of joint events can often be calculated using individual probabilities:

Conditional Probability Rule
The conditional probability of event B given event A, denoted $P(B \mid A)$, is as follows:

$P(B \mid A) = P(A \cap B)/P(A)$, for $P(A) > 0$.

Multiplication Rule
The formula for conditional probability can be rearranged to derive the multiplication rule:

$P(A \cap B) = P(B \mid A) \cdot P(A) = P(A \mid B) \cdot P(B)$

If A and B are independent events, then $P(B \mid A) = P(B)$, and thus: $P(A \cap B) = P(A) \cdot P(B)$

Conditional probability from a relative frequency perspective:

- $P(A) = $ (Number of outcomes in A)$/n$
- $P(A \cap B) = $ (Number of outcomes in A and B)$/n$
- $P(B \mid A) = $ (Number of outcomes in A and B)/(Number of outcomes in A)

Part 2: Probability Distributions
Discrete Probability Distribution
Suppose past experience shows that the number of patients arriving in the A&E ward of a particular hospital in an hour follows the following pattern (see Table 4.1):

Table 4.1 Number of patients arriving in the A&E ward

# Patients Arriving (x)	0	1	2	3	4	5+
Probability, $P(X = x)$	0.05	0.10	0.15	0.35	0.25	0.10

This is a discrete probability distribution, as there are countable possible outcomes.

Interpreting the Probabilities

■ 15% of the time, one or fewer patients arrive per hour.
■ Most of the time, three or four patients arrive per hour.

In practice, probabilities are often estimated from relative frequencies. For instance, consider the following data (see Table 4.2):

The number of patients waiting in the A&E ward was recorded every half hour over a week (24 hours × 2 × 7 = 336 observations). The data was summarized as follows:

Table 4.2 Number of patients waiting in the A&E ward, recorded every half hour over a week

Patients waiting	0	1	2	3	4	Total
Frequency	15	50	120	100	51	336

Probability Mass Function (PMF)

If X is the number of patients waiting, the probability of three patients waiting is as follows:

$$P(X = 3) = \frac{100}{336} = 0.298$$

For discrete distributions, this is known as probability mass function (PMF)

Cumulative Distribution Function (CDF)

The probability that at most two patients are waiting is as follows:

$$P(X \leq 2) = \frac{15 + 50 + 120}{336} = F_X(2) = 0.55.$$

This is known as *cumulative distribution function (CDF)* at point x = 2.

The probabilities for the entire distribution are calculated as follows (see Table 4.3):

Table 4.3 Probabilities for the entire distribution

Patients waiting	0	1	2	3	4	Total
Frequency	15	50	120	100	51	336
PMF: $P(X = x)$	0.0446	0.1488	0.357	0.298	0.1517	1
CDF: $P(X \leq x)$	0.0446	0.1934	0.5504	0.8484	1	

Measures of Center and Spread

A probability distribution represents a model of a particular population. To describe such populations, we compute the following:

- **Mean (or Expected Value):** A measure of the center.
- **Variance:** A measure of spread around the mean.
- **Standard Deviation:** The square root of the variance.

Mean or Expected Value

The management of the A&E ward wanted to estimate the average number of patients waiting at any given time. This is called the *expected value* or *mean* of the distribution, denoted as or μ (see Table 4.4):

$$E(X) = \sum_{\text{for all } i} x_i \times P(X = x_i)$$

Example 2.1: In the earlier experiment, what is the expected number of patients waiting?

$$E(X) = \sum xP(X = x) = 0*0.0446 + 1*0.1488 + 2*0.357$$
$$+ 3*0.298 + 4*0.1517 = 2.36$$

Thus, on average, more than two patients are waiting at any time. This information can assist in planning resource allocation in the A&E ward.

Variance and Standard Deviation

The *variance* of a discrete random variable is defined as follows (see Table 4.4):

$$Var(X) = E(X^2) - [E(X)]^2$$

Where:

$$E(X^2) = \sum_{\text{for all } i} x_i^2 \times P(X = x_i)$$

Example 2.2: What is the variance and standard deviation?

$$E(X^2) = \sum x^2 P(X = x) = 0*0.0446 + 1*0.1488 + 4*0.357$$
$$+ 9*0.298 + 16*0.1517 = 6.686$$

$$Var(X) = E(X^2) - [E(X)]^2 = 6.686 - 2.364^2 = 1.097$$

The **standard deviation** is the square root of the variance:

$$\text{Hence: } \sigma = \sqrt{Var(X)} = \sqrt{1.097} = 1.047$$

Table 4.4 Laws of expected value and variance

Laws of expected value (C is a constant)	Laws of variance (C is a constant) (if X and Y are independent)
■ $E(c) = c$	
■ $E(X + c) = E(X) + c$	■ $V(c) = 0$
■ $E(cX) = cE(X)$	■ $V(X + c) = V(X)$
■ $E(X + Y) = E(X) + E(Y)$	■ $V(cX) = c2V(X)$
■ $E(X - Y) = E(X) - E(Y)$	■ $V(X + Y) = V(X) + V(Y)$
	■ $V(X - Y) = V(X) + V(Y)$

Expected values, variances, and standard deviations provide valuable insights into the number of patients waiting in the A&E ward, aiding in effective decision-making and resource planning.

Specific Discrete Probability Distributions

Certain discrete probability distributions possess specific characteristics that make them well-suited for modeling particular types of random variables. Next, we introduce some fundamental distributions.

Bernoulli Distribution: Describes a single trial with two outcomes, often labeled as success (X = 1) and failure (X = 0).
Binomial Distribution: Models the number of successes in a fixed number (n) of independent Bernoulli trials.
Geometric Distribution: Represents the probability of the first success occurring on the xth trial.
Poisson Distribution: Captures the likelihood of a certain number of events happening in a fixed interval, assuming events occur independently and at a constant rate.

These distributions are foundational in probability theory and have wide applications in various fields, like clinical data analysis, risk assessment, and operations research. In what follows, we explain briefly these distributions.

Bernoulli Distribution

The Bernoulli distribution describes a single trial with two outcomes, commonly labelled as success (X = 1) and failure (X = 0). The probability mass function (PMF) of a Bernoulli random variable is given by the following:

$$P(X = x) = p^x (1-p)^{1-x} \qquad x = 0,1$$

where:
■ p is the probability of success, and
■ $(1-p)$ is the probability of failure.

Expected value and variance:

$$E(X) = p, \quad V(X) = p(1-p)$$

Binomial Distribution

The binomial distribution models the number of successes in a fixed number (n) of independent Bernoulli trials. The PMF of a binomial random variable is given by the following:

$$P(X = x) = \binom{n}{x} p^x (1-p)^{n-x} = \frac{n!}{(n-x)!x!} p^x (1-p)^{n-x} \quad x = 0, 1, 2, \ldots n$$

where:

$\binom{n}{x}$ is the binomial coefficient.

Expected value and variance:

$$E(X) = np \quad , \quad V(X) = np(1-p)$$

Example 2.2: Suppose 5% of a clinical test is unreliable (0.95 are reliable). For a sample of ten independent tests ($n = 10$), find the probability of exactly eight reliable tests ($x = 8$).

$$P(X = 8) = \binom{10}{8} 0.95^8 (0.05)^{10-8} = \frac{10!}{(10-8)!8!} 0.95^8 (0.05)^{10-8}$$

$$= \frac{10 \times 9 \times 8 \times \ldots \times 1}{(2 \times 1) \times (8 \times 7 \times 6 \times \ldots \times 1)} 0.95^8 (0.05)^{10-8} = 0.075$$

Geometric Distribution

The geometric distribution models the number of trials until the first success. The PMF of a geometric random variable is given by the following:

$$P(X = x) = p(1-p)^{x-1}$$

Expected value and variance: $E(X) = 1/p$, $V(X) = 1/p^2$

Example: Suppose 5% of clinical tests are unreliable ($p = 0.05$). Find the probability that the first unreliable test occurs on the seventh trial ($x = 7$).

$$P(X = 7) = 0.05(1 - 0.05)^{7-1} = 0.037$$

Poisson Distribution

The Poisson distribution is used to model the number of rare events occurring in a fixed interval or region, assuming events occur independently and at a constant rate. The PMF of a Poisson random variable is given by the following:

$$P(X = x) = \frac{e^{-\mu}\mu^x}{x!} \quad x = 0, 1, 2, \ldots.$$

where:

μ is the average rate of occurrence.

Expected value and variance:

$$E(X) = \mu, \ V(X) = \mu$$

Examples 2.3:

Suppose the average number of patients visiting an A&E ward is three per hour ($\mu = 3$).

a) Find the probability of exactly 5 patients arriving in the next hour.

$$P(X = 5) = \frac{e^{-3} 3^5}{5!} = 0.1$$

b) Find the probability of more than five patients arriving in the next hour.

$$P(X > 5) = \frac{e^{-3} 3^5}{5!} = 1 - P(X \leq 5) = 1 - \sum_{x=0}^{5} \frac{e^{-3} 3^x}{x!} = 1 - 0.916 = 0.0839$$

These discrete distributions are foundational in probability theory and have widespread applications in fields such as clinical data analysis, risk assessment, and operations research.

Continuous Probability Distributions

A *continuous random variable (RV)* takes values in an uncountable set, often used to measure physical characteristics, such as height, weight, time, or volume.

Characteristics of Continuous Random Variables

- A continuous RV can take fractional values (e.g., 5.67, 123.45), unlike discrete RVs, which can only take integer values.
- Examples:
  - **Discrete RV:** The number of babies delivered yesterday in a hospital is a discrete RV since it can only be an integer (e.g., 1, 2, 3).
  - **Continuous RV:** The heights and weights of babies are continuous RVs, as they can have infinite possible values (e.g., 3.150 kg, 51.62 cm).

Graphical Representation

For continuous RVs, the graph is a curve due to the infinite data points they can assume. Probabilities are determined by areas under the curve between two points, not at a single point.

Probability Distributions for Continuous RVs

The *probability density function (PDF)* $f(x)$ of a continuous RV X satisfies the following (see Figure 4.1):

- $f(x) \geq 0$ for all x
- The total area under $f(x)$ is 1: $P(-\infty \leq X \leq \infty) = \int_{-\infty}^{\infty} f(x)dx = 1$
- $P(a \leq X \leq b) = \int_{a}^{b} f(x)dx$

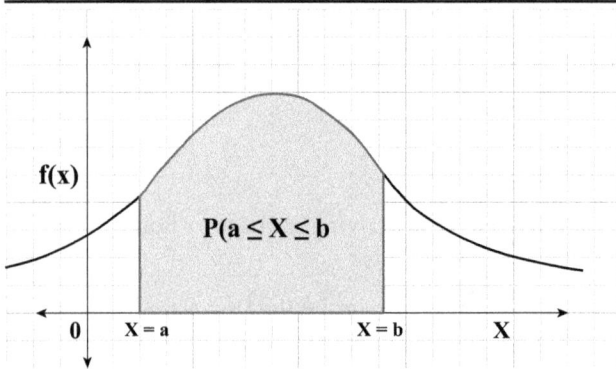

$$P(a < X < b) = \int_{a}^{b} f(x)dx$$

Where $f(x)$ is the *probability density function (PDF)* of RV X.

Figure 4.1 Probability density function (PDF) plot.

Example 2.4: Suppose $f(x) = \frac{3}{2}(1 - x^2)$ for $0 \leq x \leq 1$, find $P(0.1 \leq X \leq 0.5)$.

$$P(0.1 \leq X \leq 0.5) = \frac{3}{2} \int_{0.1}^{0.5} (1 - x^2) dx = \frac{3}{2} \left[x - \frac{x^3}{3} \right]_{x=0.1}^{x=0.5}$$

$$= \frac{3}{2} \left[\left(0.5 - \frac{(0.5)^3}{3} \right) - \left(0.1 - \frac{(0.1)^3}{3} \right) \right] = \frac{3}{2} \left[\left(0.5 - \frac{0.125}{3} \right) - \left(0.1 - \frac{0.001}{3} \right) \right]$$

$$= \frac{3}{2} \left(\frac{1.375}{3} - \frac{0.299}{3} \right) = \frac{3}{2} \times \frac{1.076}{3} = \frac{1.076}{2} = 0.538$$

Cumulative Distribution Function (CDF)
The *CDF* $F_X(x)$ represents the probability that X is less than or equal to a specific value:

$$F_X(x) = P(X \leq x) = \int_{-\infty}^{x} f(x)dx$$

For continuous RVs, the following probabilities are equivalent:

$$P(a \leq X \leq b) = P(a < X < b) = P(a < X \leq b) = P(a \leq X < b)$$

That means the probability of a single point is zero: $P(X=a)=0$ for any a.

Expected Value and Variance

For continuous RV X, the expected value and the variance are calculated by the following:

$$E(X) = \int_{-\infty}^{\infty} xf(x)dx \quad \text{and} \quad V(X) = E(X^2) - [E(X)]^2$$

Specific Continuous Probability Distributions

Some continuous distributions have well-defined forms that make them particularly useful for modeling specific types of random variables. For example:

■ **Uniform Distribution:** Assumes that all outcomes within a given interval are equally likely, often used when there is no prior information favouring one outcome over another within the range.

■ **Normal Distribution:** Characterized by its bell-shaped curve, this distribution models many natural phenomena, such as heights, test scores, or measurement errors.

■ **Exponential Distribution:** Describes the time between events in a Poisson process, often used in reliability analysis and queuing theory.

These continuous distributions are fundamental in probability theory, forming the basis for statistical modeling and inference in fields such as engineering, economics, and environmental science. Next, we briefly explain these distributions.

Uniform Distribution

A continuous RV X has a uniform distribution on [a, b] if:

$$f(x) = \tfrac{1}{b-a} \text{ and } F(x) = P(X \le x) = \tfrac{x-a}{b-a} \quad \text{for} \quad a \le X \le b$$

■ Expected value: $E(X) = \frac{b+a}{2}$

■ Variance: and $V(X) = \frac{(b-a)^2}{12}$

Example 2.5: Suppose a clinic schedules appointment for a patient between 9:00 to 9:30 A.M. to arrive, and the patient is equally likely to arrive at any time within this interval. The arrival time can be modelled using a uniform continuous distribution, with a $= 0$ and b $= 30$ minutes after 9:00 A.M.

Calculate the probability that the patient will arrive before 9:20. What is the expected and variance of arrival time?

$$P(X \le 20) = \frac{20-0}{30-0} = 0.667;$$

$$E(X) = \frac{30+0}{2} = 15; \quad Var(X) = \frac{(30-0)^2}{12} = 75$$

Normal Distribution

The most useful continuous probability model as many naturally occurring measurements (heights, weights, normal BP, etc.) are approximately normally distributed. Normal distribution has a smooth, symmetrical, bell-shaped curve (see Figure 4.2), generated by the density function given by the following:

$$f(x) = \frac{1}{\sqrt{2\pi}\sigma} e^{\frac{-(x-\mu)^2}{2\sigma^2}}$$

Each combination of mean and standard deviation generates a unique normal curve. Unfortunately, the PDF of normal distribution is not easily tractable. However, any normal distribution can be transformed into a specific normal distribution called the *standard normal distribution* (see Figure 4.3) with $\mu = 0$, and $\sigma = 1$. By using the following conversation, any normal distribution can be converted to standard normal (Z), where the cumulative probabilities for all values of Z are available in standard normal probability tables (see Table 4.5).

$$Z = \frac{x - \mu}{\sigma}$$

Example 2.6:

The weight of a medication pack is normally distributed with $\mu = 60$ gm and $\sigma = 1.5$ gm

- What is the probability that a random pack of this medication is less than 61.5 gm?
- What is the probability that a random pack weight is more than 62.34 gm?

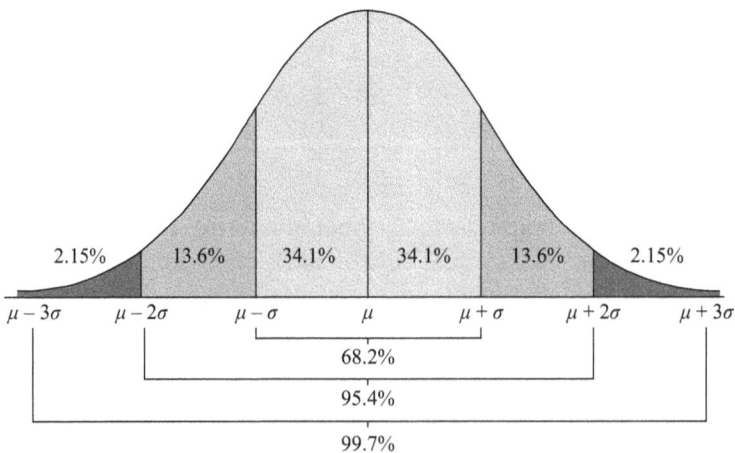

Figure 4.2 Probability density function (PDF) plot for normal distribution.

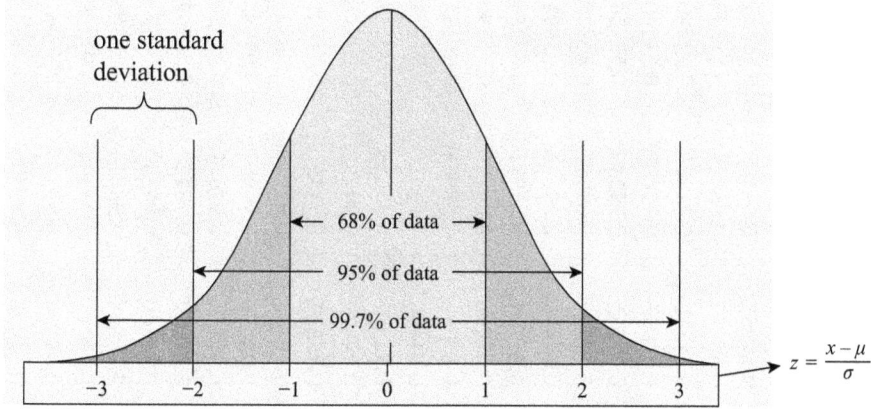

Figure 4.3 Probability density function (PDF) plot for standard normal distribution.

$$X \sim N(\mu = 60, \sigma^2 = (1.5)^2) \rightarrow$$

$$P(X < 61.5) = P\left(\frac{x - \mu}{\sigma} < \frac{61.5 - 60}{1.5}\right) = P(Z < 1) = 0.8413$$

$$(X > 62.34) = P\left(\frac{x - \mu}{\sigma} > \frac{62.34 - 60}{1.5}\right) = P(Z > 1.56) = 1 - P(Z < 1.56)$$

$$= 1 - 0.9404 = 0.0594$$

A sample of a Z table

z	.00	.01	.02	.03	.04	.05	.06	.07	.08	.09
.0	.5000	.5040	.5080	.5120	.5160	.5199	.5239	.5279	.5319	.5359
.1	.5398	.5438	.5478	.5517	.5557	.5596	.5636	.5675	.5714	.5753
.2	.5793	.5832	.5871	.5910	.5948	.5987	.6026	.6064	.6103	.6141
.3	.6179	.6217	.6255	.6293	.6331	.6368	.6406	.6443	.6480	.6517
.4	.6554	.6591	.6628	.6664	.6700	.6736	.6772	.6808	.6844	.6879
.5	.6915	.6950	.6985	.7019	.7054	.7088	.7123	.7157	.7190	.7224
.6	.7257	.7291	.7324	.7357	.7389	.7422	.7454	.7486	.7517	.7549
.7	.7580	.7611	.7642	.7673	.7704	.7734	.7764	.7794	.7823	.7852
.8	.7881	.7910	.7939	.7967	.7995	.8023	.8051	.8078	.8106	.8133
.9	.8159	.8186	.8212	.8238	.8264	.8289	.8315	.8340	.8365	.8389
1.0	.8413	.8438	.8461	.8485	.8508	.8531	.8554	.8577	.8599	.8621
1.1	.8643	.8665	.8686	.8708	.8729	.8749	.8770	.8790	.8810	.8830
1.2	.8849	.8869	.8888	.8907	.8925	.8944	.8962	.8980	.8997	.9015
1.3	.9032	.9049	.9066	.9082	.9099	.9115	.9131	.9147	.9162	.9177
1.4	.9192	.9207	.9222	.9236	.9251	.9265	.9279	.9292	.9306	.9319
1.5	.9332	.9345	.9357	.9370	.9382	.9394	.9406	9418	.9429	.9441

Table 4.5 Standard normal probability table (Z)

Z	0.00	0.01	0.02	0.03	0.04	0.05	0.06	0.07	0.08	0.09
0.0	0.50000	0.50399	0.50798	0.51197	0.51595	0.51994	0.52392	0.52790	0.53188	0.53586
0.1	0.53983	0.54380	0.54776	0.55172	0.55567	0.55962	0.56356	0.56749	0.57142	0.57535
0.2	0.57926	0.58317	0.58706	0.59095	0.59483	0.59871	0.60257	0.60642	0.61026	0.61409
0.3	0.61791	0.62172	0.62552	0.62930	0.63307	0.63683	0.64058	0.64431	0.64803	0.65173
0.4	0.65542	0.65910	0.66276	0.66640	0.67003	0.67364	0.67724	0.68082	0.68439	0.68793
0.5	0.69146	0.69497	0.69847	0.70194	0.70540	0.70884	0.71226	0.71566	0.71904	0.72240
0.6	0.72575	0.72907	0.73237	0.73565	0.73891	0.74215	0.74537	0.74857	0.75175	0.75490
0.7	0.75804	0.76115	0.76424	0.76730	0.77035	0.77337	0.77637	0.77935	0.78230	0.78524
0.8	0.78814	0.79103	0.79389	0.79673	0.79955	0.80234	0.80511	0.80785	0.81057	0.81327
0.9	0.81594	0.81859	0.82121	0.82381	0.82639	0.82894	0.83147	0.83398	0.83646	0.83891
1.0	0.84134	0.84375	0.84614	0.84849	0.85083	0.85314	0.85543	0.85769	0.85993	0.86214
1.1	0.86433	0.86650	0.86864	0.87076	0.87286	0.87493	0.87698	0.87900	0.88100	0.88298
1.2	0.88493	0.88686	0.88877	0.89065	0.89251	0.89435	0.89617	0.89796	0.89973	0.90147
1.3	0.90320	0.90490	0.90658	0.90824	0.90988	0.91149	0.91308	0.91466	0.91621	0.91774
1.4	0.91924	0.92073	0.92220	0.92364	0.92507	0.92647	0.92785	0.92922	0.93056	0.93189
1.5	0.93319	0.93448	0.93574	0.93699	0.93822	0.93943	0.94062	0.94179	0.94295	0.94408
1.6	0.94520	0.94630	0.94738	0.94845	0.94950	0.95053	0.95154	0.95254	0.95352	0.95449
1.7	0.95543	0.95637	0.95728	0.95818	0.95907	0.95994	0.96080	0.96164	0.96246	0.96327
1.8	0.96407	0.96485	0.96562	0.96638	0.96712	0.96784	0.96856	0.96926	0.96995	0.97062
1.9	0.97128	0.97193	0.97257	0.97320	0.97381	0.97441	0.97500	0.97558	0.97615	0.97670
2.0	0.97725	0.97778	0.97831	0.97882	0.97932	0.97982	0.98030	0.98077	0.98124	0.98169
2.1	0.98214	0.98257	0.98300	0.98341	0.98382	0.98422	0.98461	0.98500	0.98537	0.98574
2.2	0.98610	0.98645	0.98679	0.98713	0.98745	0.98778	0.98809	0.98840	0.98870	0.98899
2.3	0.98928	0.98956	0.98983	0.99010	0.99036	0.99061	0.99086	0.99111	0.99134	0.99158
2.4	0.99180	0.99202	0.99224	0.99245	0.99266	0.99286	0.99305	0.99324	0.99343	0.99361
2.5	0.99379	0.99396	0.99413	0.99430	0.99446	0.99461	0.99477	0.99492	0.99506	0.99520
2.6	0.99534	0.99547	0.99560	0.99573	0.99585	0.99598	0.99609	0.99621	0.99632	0.99643
2.7	0.99653	0.99664	0.99674	0.99683	0.99693	0.99702	0.99711	0.99720	0.99728	0.99736

	.00	.01	.02	.03	.04	.05	.06	.07	.08	.09
2.8	0.99744	0.99752	0.99760	0.99767	0.99774	0.99781	0.99788	0.99795	0.99801	0.99807
2.9	0.99813	0.99819	0.99825	0.99831	0.99836	0.99841	0.99846	0.99851	0.99856	0.99861
3.0	0.99865	0.99869	0.99874	0.99878	0.99882	0.99886	0.99889	0.99893	0.99896	0.99900
3.1	0.99903	0.99906	0.99910	0.99913	0.99916	0.99918	0.99921	0.99924	0.99926	0.99929
3.2	0.99931	0.99934	0.99936	0.99938	0.99940	0.99942	0.99944	0.99946	0.99948	0.99950
3.3	0.99952	0.99953	0.99955	0.99957	0.99958	0.99960	0.99961	0.99962	0.99964	0.99965
3.4	0.99966	0.99968	0.99969	0.99970	0.99971	0.99972	0.99973	0.99974	0.99975	0.99976
3.5	0.99977	0.99978	0.99978	0.99979	0.99980	0.99981	0.99981	0.99982	0.99983	0.99983
0.0	0.50000	0.49601	0.49202	0.48803	0.48405	0.48006	0.47608	0.47210	0.46812	0.46414
0.1	0.46017	0.45621	0.45224	0.44828	0.44433	0.44038	0.43644	0.43251	0.42858	0.42466
0.2	0.42074	0.41683	0.41294	0.40905	0.40517	0.40129	0.39743	0.39358	0.38974	0.38591
0.3	0.38209	0.37828	0.37448	0.37070	0.36693	0.36317	0.35942	0.35569	0.35197	0.34827
0.4	0.34458	0.34090	0.33724	0.33360	0.32997	0.32636	0.32276	0.31918	0.31561	0.31207
0.5	0.30854	0.30503	0.30153	0.29806	0.29460	0.29116	0.28774	0.28434	0.28096	0.27760
0.6	0.27425	0.27093	0.26763	0.26435	0.26109	0.25785	0.25463	0.25143	0.24825	0.24510
0.7	0.24196	0.23885	0.23576	0.23270	0.22965	0.22663	0.22363	0.22065	0.21770	0.21476
0.8	0.21186	0.20897	0.20611	0.20327	0.20045	0.19766	0.19489	0.19215	0.18943	0.18673
0.9	0.18406	0.18141	0.17879	0.17619	0.17361	0.17106	0.16853	0.16602	0.16354	0.16109
1.0	0.15866	0.15625	0.15386	0.15151	0.14917	0.14686	0.14457	0.14231	0.14007	0.13786
1.1	0.13567	0.13350	0.13136	0.12924	0.12714	0.12507	0.12302	0.12100	0.11900	0.11702
1.2	0.11507	0.11314	0.11123	0.10935	0.10749	0.10565	0.10384	0.10204	0.10027	0.09853
1.3	0.09680	0.09510	0.09342	0.09176	0.09012	0.08851	0.08692	0.08534	0.08379	0.08226
1.4	0.08076	0.07927	0.07780	0.07636	0.07493	0.07353	0.07215	0.07078	0.06944	0.06811
1.5	0.06681	0.06552	0.06426	0.06301	0.06178	0.06057	0.05938	0.05821	0.05705	0.05592
1.6	0.05480	0.05370	0.05262	0.05155	0.05050	0.04947	0.04846	0.04746	0.04648	0.04551
1.7	0.04457	0.04363	0.04272	0.04182	0.04093	0.04006	0.03920	0.03836	0.03754	0.03673
1.8	0.03593	0.03515	0.03438	0.03363	0.03288	0.03216	0.03144	0.03074	0.03005	0.02938
1.9	0.02872	0.02807	0.02743	0.02680	0.02619	0.02559	0.02500	0.02442	0.02385	0.02330

(Continued)

Table 14.1 (Continued)

z	0.00	0.01	0.02	0.03	0.04	0.05	0.06	0.07	0.08	0.09
2.0	0.02275	0.02222	0.02169	0.02118	0.02068	0.02018	0.01970	0.01923	0.01876	0.01831
2.1	0.01786	0.01743	0.01700	0.01659	0.01618	0.01578	0.01539	0.01500	0.01463	0.01426
2.2	0.01390	0.01355	0.01321	0.01287	0.01255	0.01222	0.01191	0.01160	0.01130	0.01101
2.3	0.01072	0.01044	0.01017	0.00990	0.00964	0.00939	0.00914	0.00889	0.00866	0.00842
2.4	0.00820	0.00798	0.00776	0.00755	0.00734	0.00714	0.00695	0.00676	0.00657	0.00639
2.5	0.00621	0.00604	0.00587	0.00570	0.00554	0.00539	0.00523	0.00509	0.00494	0.00480
2.6	0.00466	0.00453	0.00440	0.00427	0.00415	0.00403	0.00391	0.00379	0.00368	0.00357
2.7	0.00347	0.00336	0.00326	0.00317	0.00307	0.00298	0.00289	0.00280	0.00272	0.00264
2.8	0.00256	0.00248	0.00240	0.00233	0.00226	0.00219	0.00212	0.00205	0.00199	0.00193
2.9	0.00187	0.00181	0.00175	0.00170	0.00164	0.00159	0.00154	0.00149	0.00144	0.00140
3.0	0.00135	0.00131	0.00126	0.00122	0.00118	0.00114	0.00111	0.00107	0.00104	0.00100
3.1	0.00097	0.00094	0.00090	0.00087	0.00085	0.00082	0.00079	0.00076	0.00074	0.00071
3.2	0.00069	0.00066	0.00064	0.00062	0.00060	0.00058	0.00056	0.00054	0.00052	0.00050
3.3	0.00048	0.00047	0.00045	0.00043	0.00042	0.00040	0.00039	0.00038	0.00036	0.00035
3.4	0.00034	0.00033	0.00031	0.00030	0.00029	0.00028	0.00027	0.00026	0.00025	0.00024
3.5	0.00023	0.00022	0.00022	0.00021	0.00020	0.00019	0.00019	0.00018	0.00017	0.00017

Exponential Distribution

The *exponential probability distribution* is widely used to model the time until the occurrence of an event, such as the time required to complete a procedure. It is particularly useful in scenarios where events occur independently and at a constant average rate.

Applications of the Exponential Distribution
- *Time between patient arrivals* at a hospital or clinic.
- *Duration to complete a task*, such as filling out a questionnaire.
- *Waiting time management*, including service times in queues or customer support systems.

Probability Density Function (PDF)
The PDF of an exponential random variable X is defined as follows:

$$f(x) = \lambda e^{-\lambda x} \text{ and } F(x) = 1 - e^{-\lambda x}$$

$$E(X) = \mu = \frac{1}{\lambda} \text{ and } V(X) = \mu^2 = \frac{1}{\lambda^2}$$

Where:
- λ is the rate parameter (the reciprocal of the mean, $\lambda = 1/\mu$).

This distribution is often used in reliability analysis, queuing theory, and other areas requiring the modeling of time intervals.

The mathematical constant e (approximately 2.71828) is the base of natural logarithms and is fundamental in calculus and mathematical modeling.

Example Exponential Distribution
The time between arrivals of patients to an A&E follows an exponential probability distribution with a mean time between arrivals of 15 minutes. We would like to know the probability that the time between two successive arrivals will be the following:

a) 20 minutes or less.
b) 10 minutes or more.

$$X \sim Exp(\mu = 15) - \rightarrow \lambda = \frac{1}{\mu} = \frac{1}{15}$$

a) $P(X \leq 20) = F(20) = 1 - e^{-\frac{20}{15}} = 1 - 0.263 = 0.736$

b) $P(X \geq 10) = 1 - F(10) = 1 - \left[1 - e^{-\frac{10}{15}} \right] = e^{-\frac{10}{15}} = 0.513$

These distributions form the foundation of continuous probability modeling, widely applied in fields like medicine, engineering, and economics.

Discussion Questions

- How do different probability distributions (binomial, Poisson, normal) apply to health research scenarios?
- Why is understanding conditional probability important in clinical decision-making?
- In what ways can probability theory help manage uncertainty in health studies?

## CHAPTER 5

Statistical Hypothesis Testing for Health Sciences

Parametric and Non-Parametric

Dilip C. Nath and Dibyojyoti Bhattacharjee

Learning Outcomes

By the end of this chapter, readers will be able to do the following:

1. *Define* and *differentiate* between parametric and non-parametric statistical methods.
2. *Understand the assumptions* underlying parametric tests, such as normality, homogeneity of variances, and scale of measurement.
3. *Recognize when to use* non-parametric tests, particularly in cases where parametric assumptions are violated.
4. *Identify common parametric tests* (e.g., t-test, ANOVA) and *non-parametric counterparts* (e.g., Mann-Whitney U test, Kruskal-Wallis test).
5. *Interpret the results* of parametric and non-parametric tests correctly in the context of data analysis.
6. *Evaluate the advantages and limitations* of both approaches and make informed decisions on test selection based on data characteristics.

Introduction

In many situations, researchers have to take decision about various features of the population based on sample observations. The situation may be either estimating a value of some population characteristic called the parameter. The value of the parameter is estimated or is decided upon based on sample observations.

When the researcher is completely in the dark about the value of the parameter, then the problem is solved by applying the technique of estimation. However, if the problem is to check some existing beliefs of the researcher, about the parameter, based on the sample observations, then the technique applied is called 'hypothesis testing' or 'testing of hypothesis'. In this chapter, the two phrases shall be used alternatively, as they are synonymous.

DOI: 10.4324/9781032701004-6

Let us take an example to understand this. Suppose, a researcher wants to know the mean body mass index (BMI) of the patients showing up in the cardiology department of a hospital in a given calendar month. Then he can consider a sample of patients from those who show up and then, using their BMI, may estimate the mean BMI of the all the patients under consideration.

However, if he wants to check whether the mean BMI of the patients are not different from 19.5, then he can resort to 'hypothesis testing'. With Pearson (1900) being one of the earlier works, subsequent developments in statistical theory expanded on his ideas to establish a more rigorous framework. Here, the researcher is actually bestowed with the responsibility of checking a belief that the average BMI of the patients is 19.5.

The concept of hypothesis testing is better understood if we get acquainted with some related terminologies.

Definitions

Next, we provide the definition and explanation of some very basic terminologies related to test of significance. Without proper understanding of these concepts, it is difficult to take the point further.

Statistical Hypothesis

In many situations, the researchers are asked to make a decision about the parameters[1] of the population. In order to reach to such a decision, the researcher may take the help of some guesses. Such guesses are called statistical hypothesis or simply hypothesis.

Null Hypothesis

In tests of significance, we start with a certain hypothesis about the population characteristic. This hypothesis is called the null hypothesis. The null hypothesis is put to test and is ultimately either accepted or rejected. The null hypothesis is generally a hypothesis of no significant difference and is denoted by H_0. According to Prof. R. A. Fisher, "A null hypothesis is the hypothesis which is tested for possible rejection under the assumption that it is true."

Alternative Hypothesis

Any hypothesis that completely opposes what the null hypothesis states is called the alternative hypothesis. To every null hypothesis, there is at least one complementary hypothesis called the alternative hypothesis. For example, if the null hypothesis is that the population mean is not different from $H_0: \mu = 5$, the alternative hypothesis can be the following:

(i) $H_1: \mu \neq 5$ (ii) $H_1: \mu > 5$ (iii) $H_1: \mu < 5$

Actually (i) includes both (ii) and (iii).

The first alternative hypothesis is called a two-tailed alternative hypothesis, while (ii) and (iii) are called one-tailed alternative hypothesis. More precisely, H_1:

$\mu > 5$ is called the right-tailed hypothesis, while H_1: $\mu < 5$ is called the left-tailed hypothesis.

Test Statistic

Once the hypothesis to be tested is decided, the next step is to formulate a procedure to accept or reject the hypothesis. The straightforward procedure would be to examine each and every member of the population. But in most cases, the population is very large in size and so one has to depend on sample observations for such decisions. From the sample observations, a statistic is computed. The test statistic is then defined. It is a function of the statistic computed earlier. The test statistic is used to compare the results obtained from the sample with the expected results. If the difference is significant, the null hypothesis is rejected; else, it is accepted.

Errors in Hypothesis Testing (Type I and Type II Error)

In hypothesis testing, the decision about accepting or rejecting of a null hypothesis is taken based on sample observations. Thus, the decision taken may always not be correct. In testing a hypothesis, one and only one of the following situations may occur:

(i)   Accept H_0 when H_0 was actually true.
(ii) Reject H_0 when H_0 was actually true.
(iii) Accept H_0 when H_0 was actually false.
(iv) Reject H_0 when H_0 was actually false.

It may be noted that (i) and (iv) results in a correct decision while (ii) and (iii) results in an incorrect decision. The situations can be placed in tabular form as follows:

Table 5.1 Actual situation

Decision	Actual situation	
	H_0 is true	H_0 is false
Accept H_0	Correct Action	Error (Type II)
Reject H_0	Error (Type I)	Correct Action

The decision of rejecting H_0 when H_0 is actually true is called Type I error. The decision of accepting H_0 when H_0 is actually false is called Type II error. The consequence of Type I and Type II errors are different. In some cases, the Type I error may be more serious than the Type II error. The probability of Type I error is denoted by α, and the probability of Type II error is denoted by β. Thus:

$\alpha = P(\text{Type I error}) = P(\text{Rejecting } H_0 \text{ when } H_0 \text{ is true}) = P(\text{Rejecting } H_0 \mid H_0)$ and
$\beta = P(\text{Type II error}) = P(\text{Accepting } H_0 \text{ when } H_0 \text{ is false}) = P(\text{Accept } H_0 \mid H_1)$

The probability of Type I error is also called level of significance and is defined formally in the subsequent section.

Degrees of Freedom

A test statistic always depends on the sample vis-à-vis the size of the sample. Size of the sample here means the number of observations in the sample. The sample size takes a vital role in the test of significance. In most cases, it is found that the estimate approaches the true value of the parameter as the sample size increases. Thus, it is essential to take into consideration the sample size in tests of significance, especially in the case of a smaller-sized sample.[2] The sample size is considered in hypothesis testing through degrees of freedom or '*df*' as it is commonly called. The degree of freedom is defined as *the number of observations in a set minus the number of restrictions imposed on it.*

Level of Significance

The word 'significance' in hypothesis testing implies that we are going to accept the null hypothesis if the difference between the statistic and the corresponding parameter is not much significant. Thus, the level of significance in simple words is the amount of confidence the researcher wants to attach to the conclusions that s/he has drawn from the test. The level of significance is denoted by 'α' and is the probability of a Type I error. If $\alpha = 0.05$, then the level of significance expressed in percentage is 5%. The corresponding confidence is $100 \times (1 - \alpha)\%$, i.e., $100 \times (1 - 0.05)\% = 95\%$, which means that the researcher is 95% confident about the conclusion that s/he has taken on the performance of the test. Hence, the level of significance is defined by the maximum probability level below which we reject the null hypothesis.

Standard Error

The standard deviation of the sampling distribution of a statistic or any estimate of that standard deviation is known as the standard error. The standard error plays a vital role in sampling theory. The standard error acts as a vital tool for finding an interval in which the parameter is expected to fall with a certain degree of confidence. Such intervals are called confidence intervals.

However, the main purpose of standard error is in testing whether the difference between observed and expected values is due to chance and otherwise. The criteria usually adopted is that if the difference is less than three times of the standard error, then it may be due to chance, but if the difference exceeds that value, then the difference is considered to be significant and cannot be attributed to chance factors.

p-Value of a Test

The *p*-value is the probability that we would get the sample we have to give us something more extreme if the null hypothesis were true. So a smaller *p*-value of a test indicates that there is more evidence in the sample data against the null hypothesis, and the sample characteristics is in support of the opinion expressed in the alternative hypothesis. Thus, a small value of p leads to accepting the alternative hypothesis and rejecting the null hypothesis. In very simple words, it is the probability of accepting the null hypothesis given the sample under consideration. The researcher is to decide the level of significance for a test; generally, it is 5%, i.e., 0.05 if expressed in terms of probability. If the p-value of a test is less than 0.05, then we consider that the probability of accepting the null hypothesis given the sample is very low, and hence, we need to reject the null hypothesis and accept the alternative hypothesis. Depending on the purpose of the study, a researcher can take even 1% (0.01), 3% (0.03), and 10% (0.1) as the level of significance as well.

One-Tailed and Two-Tailed Tests

In testing a hypothesis, we are interested in testing the significance of the difference between the parameter and its corresponding statistic, which arises due to the fluctuations of random sampling.

Let μ be a population parameter and μ_0 be a fixed value. The null hypothesis to be tested is $H_0: \mu = \mu_0$ against an alternative hypothesis, $H_1: \mu \neq \mu_0$. Thus, assuming H_0 to be true, we would be looking for a large difference in both sides of the expected value, i.e., in both tails of the distribution. This test is therefore called the two-tailed test.

Sometimes we are interested to test large difference in one side only, i.e., in one tail of the distribution. These tests are known as 'one-tailed tests'. For testing the null hypothesis against a one-sided alternative hypothesis (right side), we have, $H_0: \mu = \mu_0$ against an alternative hypothesis, $H_1: \mu > \mu_0$. For a left-tailed test, we have the alternative hypothesis, $H_1: \mu < \mu_0$.

In case of a two-sided alternative hypothesis, the critical region lies on either side of the sampling distribution, and so the size of the critical region lies on both the tails.

In case the direction of difference is known, i.e., if the alternative hypothesis is of the form $H_1: \mu > \mu_0$ or $H_1: \mu < \mu_0$, then the critical region (region of rejection) lies in one

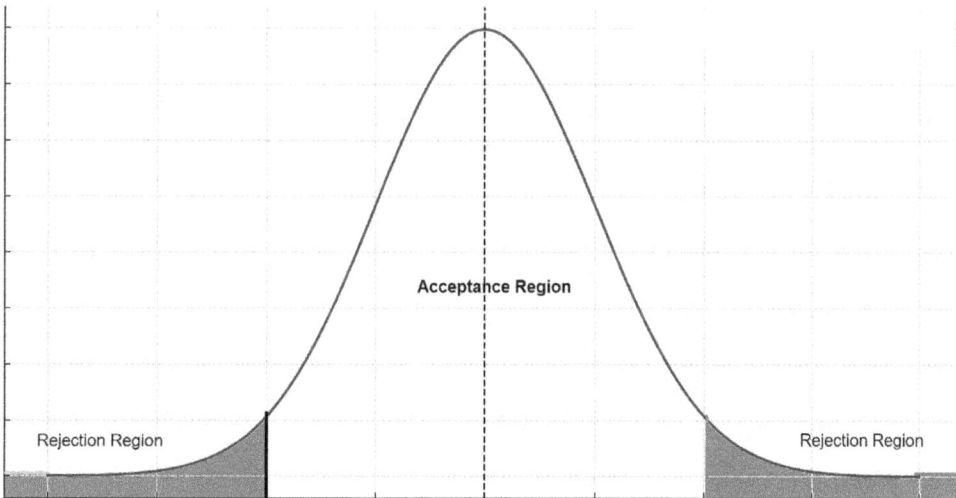

Figure 5.1 Acceptance and rejection region for a typical two-sided alternative hypothesis (left-tailed and right-tailed).

side of the sampling distribution (see Figure 5.1), and in such a case, we have the critical region in one of the tails, i.e., we have the see Figure 5.2:

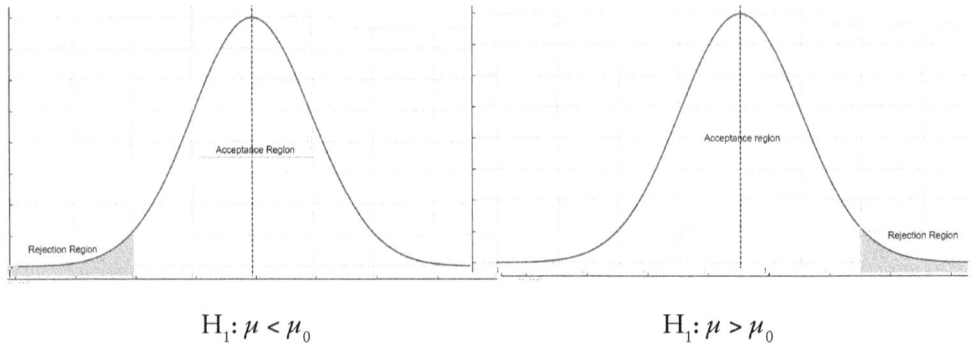

$$H_1: \mu < \mu_0 \qquad\qquad\qquad H_1: \mu > \mu_0$$

Figure 5.2 Acceptance and rejection region for a typical one-sided alternative hypothesis (left-tailed and right-tailed).

Steps in Hypothesis Testing

(i) To set up the 'null hypothesis' H_0 and the corresponding 'alternative hypothesis' H_1.

(ii) State the appropriate test statistic for the test. It is also important to derive the form of the test statistic under the null hypothesis. The test statistic generally used for the purpose of comparison for large samples are as follows:

$$Z = \frac{t - E(t)}{S.E(t)}$$

(iii) The value of $E(t)$ and S.E.(t) under the null hypothesis is determined if not known.

(iv) To select the level of significance, i.e., α for the test, if not specified. Most generally, 5% or 1% level of significance is used.

(v) After deciding about the level of significance, identify the critical region, i.e., that value of the test statistic beyond which the difference would be considered significant.

(vi) Compute the value of the test statistic based on the sampled data.

(vii) Compare the calculated value of the test statistic with the critical value. If the computed value falls in the critical region, then reject the null hypothesis; otherwise, accept it.

However, in case the computation is done with the help of any statistical package, the p-value of the test shall be generated. In case the p-value is low (less than the level of significance), then the null-hypothesis shall be rejected.

(viii) Draw the conclusion accordingly, avoiding the technical terms.

Parametric and Non-Parametric Tests

Methods of statistical inferences (Ferguson, 2014) can basically be divided into two categories 'parametric' and 'non-parametric' inferences. In parametric inferences, we generally assume the specific form of the distribution, and the problem comprises of estimating the parameters or/and testing certain hypothesis related to the parameters. Non-parametric procedures are concerned with the form of the population distribution and not with the values of the parameters of the distribution. Hence, these types of tests are called non-parametric tests because of Jacob Wolfowitz in 1942. In one of his works published in the *Annals of Mathematical Statistics* (now called *Annals of Statistics*), he explained that the parametric procedures signify those where one makes the assumption that distributions have known from, whereas non-parametric procedures are those that do not require such assumptions. During the 1940s, it was believed that non-parametric methods were understood as the 'Shortcuts for well-established parametric methods' to many, and in the 1950s, it was believed as 'Quick and inefficient methods that are wasteful of information'. However, in the 1960s, these tests grew over its criticisms and seemed to be hardly differentiable from parametric statistics at all. The next decade, that is, by the 1970s, this technique was recognized as a science of providing statistical inference procedures that depends on weaker assumptions of the underlying distributions.

Thus, non-parametric statistics is a subfield of statistics that provides statistical inference procedures which rely on weaker assumptions about the underlying distribution of the population than the parametric procedures. Since these types of procedures assume less about the underlying distribution, errors in correct assessment of the nature of the underlying distribution will usually have less effect on non-parametric procedures than on parametric procedures since the latter usually rely more heavily on the correct assessment of the nature of the underlying distribution. However, the more information we have about the underlying distribution, the better is the inference. So for a given situation, a non-parametric procedure will usually be the one with greater variance in case of point estimation, with less power in case of hypothesis testing, with wider intervals in case of confidence interval estimation, and with higher risk in decision theory when compared with a corresponding parametric procedure provided the assumptions are not violated.

Large Sample Parametric Tests

Z-test for Single Proportions

(i) Assumptions
    a) Independent Bernoulli trials are repeated a number of times.
    b) The number of repetitions is large, i.e., $n > 30$.

(ii) Hypothesis of the Test
    a) Null Hypothesis: $H_0: P = P_0$
    b) Alternative Hypothesis: $H_1: P \neq P_0$ or $H_1: P > P_0$ or $H_1: P < P_0$

(iii) Test Statistic

$$Z = \frac{p - P_0}{\sqrt{P_0 Q_0 / n}} \sim N(0,1), \text{ where } p = \frac{x}{n} \text{ (sample proportion)}$$

where x is the number of individuals possessing the particular attribute out of 'n' sampled observations.

(iv) *Reject H_0 if p*-value of the test statistics is less than 0.05 (if tested for 5% level of significance). For any other level of significance, decision is to be taken accordingly.

Illustration 4.1: In a sample of 200 people attacked by malaria, 180 of them survived. Will you reject the null hypothesis that the survival rate, if attacked by malaria, is 85% in favour of the hypothesis that it is not 85% at 5% level.

Solution: Null Hypothesis: H_0: $p = 0.85$

Alternative Hypothesis: H_1: $p \neq 0.85$

Here, the number of survivors is180 out of 200, so $x = 180$ and $n = 200$.

R Commands (Braun and Murdoch, 2007):

```
>ztest = prop.test(180, 200, p = 0.85, correct=FALSE)

# The above command computes the result of the test and save it in
'ztest'

>ztest # this command shall produce the output below

    One-sample proportions test

    data: 180 out of 200, null probability 0.85
    X-squared = 3.9216, df = 1, p-value = 0.04767
    alternative hypothesis: true p is not equal to 0.85
    95 percent confidence interval:
    0.8505942 0.9343296
    sample estimates:
    p
    0.9
```

Interpretation: Here, the result of the Z-test is approximated by a chi-square test in R. The calculated value of the X^2 statistic comes out to be 3.9216, and the corresponding *p*-value of the test is 0.04767. Since the *p*-value of the test is less than $0.05 = 1 - 0.95$ (1 – the confidence interval) of the test, we reject the null hypothesis and conclude that survival rate, if attacked by malaria, is not 85%.

NOTE: 1. The 'correct $=$ FALSE' option of the command is used to suppress the default behavior of R of adding a continuity correction.

Z-test for Equality of Two Proportions
   (i) Assumptions
      a) Both the samples are sufficiently large.
   (ii) Hypothesis of the Test
      a. Null Hypothesis: H_0: $P_1 = P_2$
      b. Alternative Hypothesis: H_1: $P_1 \neq P_2$ or H_1: $P_1 > P_2$ or H_1: $P_1 < P_2$
   (iii) Test Statistic

$$Z = \frac{p_1 - p_2}{\sqrt{PQ\left(\frac{1}{n_1} + \frac{1}{n_2}\right)}} \sim N(0,1), \text{ where } p_1 = \frac{x_1}{n_1} \text{ and } p_2 = \frac{x_2}{n_2}$$

If the value of P and Q are not known, then they are estimated by $\hat{P}$ and $\hat{Q}$, where: $\hat{P} = \frac{n_1 p_1 + n_2 p_2}{n_1 + n_2}$ and, $P_1 = \frac{x_1}{n_1}, P_2 = \frac{x_2}{n_2}$ with $\hat{Q} = 1 - \hat{P}$

(iv) *Reject H_0 if p*-value of the test statistics is less than 0.05 (if tested for 5% level of significance). For any other level of significance, decision is to be taken accordingly.

Illustration 5.1: In a large city, A, 20% of a random sample of 900 school children had defective eyesight. In the other large city, B, 15% of a random sample of 1,600 children had the same defect. Is this difference between the two proportions significant?

Solution: Hypothesis of the test is H_0: $P_1 = P_2$, and the alternative hypothesis is H_1: $P_1 \neq P_2$

Here, 20% of 900 is 180 and 15% of 1,600 is 240.

R Commands:
```
>ztest = prop.test(c(180,240), n = c(900, 1600), correct = FALSE)
# The above command computes the result of the test and save it in
'ztest'
>ztest# this command shall produce the output below
```

```
2-sample test for equality of proportions.
    data: c(180, 240) out of c(900, 1600)
    X-squared = 10.302, df = 1, p-value = 0.001329
    alternative hypothesis: two.sided
    95 percent confidence interval:
    0.01855096 0.08144904
    sample estimates:
    prop 1 prop 2
    0.20 0.15
```

Interpretation: Here, the result of the Z-test is approximated by a chi-square test in R. The calculated value of the X^2 statistic comes out to be 10.302, and the corresponding p-value of the test is 0.001329. Since the p-value of the test is less than $0.05 = 1 - 0.95$ (1 – the confidence interval) of the test, we reject the null hypothesis and conclude that the proportion of defective eyesight differs significantly at 5% level of significance.

NOTE: The 'correct = FALSE' option of the command is used to suppress the default behavior of R of adding a continuity correction.

Z-test for Single Mean
(i) **Assumptions**
   a. The samples are sufficiently large.
   b. Population variance is known.
(ii) **Hypothesis of the Test**
   a. Null Hypothesis: H_0: $\mu = \mu_0$
   b. Alternative Hypothesis: H_1: $\mu \neq \mu_0$ or H_1: $\mu > \mu_0$ or H_1: $\mu < \mu_0$

(iii) **Test Statistic**

$$Z = \frac{\bar{x}-\mu_0}{\sigma/\sqrt{n}} \sim N(0,1), \text{ where } \bar{x} = \frac{\sum x_i}{n}$$

(iv) *Reject H_0 if p-value of the test statistics is less than 0.05 (if tested for 5% level of significance). For any other level of significance, decision is to be taken accordingly.*

Illustration 6.1 Among 157 African-American men, the mean systolic blood pressure was 146 mmHg with a standard deviation of 27. We wish to know if on the basis of these data, we may conclude that the mean systolic blood pressure for a population of African-American men is greater than 140. Perform the test at 1% level of significance.[3]

Let us set up the null hypothesis.

Null Hypothesis: H_0: $\mu = 140$ (specified)

Alternative Hypothesis: H_1: $\mu > 140$

R-Code

```
>sample_mean= 146
>population_mean= 140
>sd= 27
> n = 157
> z = (sample_mean - population_mean) / (sd / sqrt(n))
>p_value = pnorm(z,mean = 0, sd = 1))
# for a two tailed test use p_value = 2*(pnorm(z,mean = 0,
sd = 1))
```

Results

z-value = 2.7844

p-value = 0.0027

Interpretation: Since the p-value for this test is less than 0.05, thus, we reject the null hypothesis and conclude that mean the systolic blood pressure for a population of African-American men is greater than 140 at 5% level of significance.

Z-test for Difference of Two Means

(Population variances are known and equal)

(i) **Assumptions**
  a. Both the samples are sufficiently large.
  b. Population variance is known and equal.

(ii) **Hypothesis of the Test**
  a. Null Hypothesis: H_0: $\mu_1 = \mu_2$
  b. Alternative Hypothesis: H_1: $\mu_1 \neq \mu_2$ or H_1: $\mu_1 > \mu_2$ or H_1: $\mu_1 < \mu_2$

(iii) **Test Statistic**

$$Z = \frac{\bar{x}_1 - \bar{x}_2}{\sigma\sqrt{\left(\frac{1}{n_1} + \frac{1}{n_2}\right)}} \sim N(0,1)$$

(iv) Reject H_0 if p-value of the test statistics is less than 0.05 (if tested for 5% level of significance). For any other level of significance, decision is to be taken accordingly.

When Population Variances Are Known and Unequal

In case the variances of the two populations are known and are unequal, the following change is made to the test statistic.

Test Statistic

$$Z = \frac{\bar{x}_1 - \bar{x}_2}{\sqrt{\left(\frac{\sigma_1^2}{n_1} + \frac{\sigma_2^2}{n_2}\right)}} \sim N(0,1)$$

Illustration 7.1: Imagine a researcher wants to determine whether or not a given drug has any effect on the scores of human subjects performing a task of ESP sensitivity. He randomly assigns his subjects to one of two groups. 900 subjects in group one (the experimental group) receive an oral administration of the drug prior to testing. In contrast, 1,000 subjects in group two (control group) receive a placebo. For the drug group, the mean score on the ESP test was 9.78 with a S.D. = 4.05, and for the no-drug group, the mean = 15.10 with a S.D. = 4.28. Perform hypothesis testing (at 5% level) to check if the mean ESP test scores for the two groups differ significantly.[4]

Solution:

Let us set up the null hypothesis.

Null Hypothesis:

H_0: Mean ESP test scores for the two groups do not differ significantly.

Alternative Hypothesis:

H_1: Mean ESP test scores for the two groups do differ significantly.

R-Code

```
>n1 = 900
>n2 = 1000
>mean1 = 9.78
>mean2 = 15.10
>sd1 = 4.05
>sd2 = 4.28

# Calculate the standard error of the difference of means
>se_diff= sqrt((((sd1)2 / n1) + ((sd2)2 / n2))
# Calculate the z-statistic

>z_stat= (mean1 - mean2) / se_diff
>p_value = 2*pnorm(z_stat, mean = 0, sd = 1)
# multiplied by 2 as the test is two tailed
```

Results

z-value = −27.82961

p-value = 1.90159e − 170 (1.90159 × 10^{-170})

Interpretation: The p-value of the test statistic is less than 0.05, so we reject the null hypothesis and conclude that the mean ESP test scores for the two groups differ significantly at 5% level of significance.

Small Sample Parametric Tests
Student's t-test (Test for Single Mean Specified)
The test is attributed to W S Gosset, who wrote using the pseudonym Student (1908).

(i) Assumptions
    a) The sample is drawn from a normal population.
    b) The observations are independent.
(ii) Hypothesis
    Null Hypothesis: H_0: $\mu = \mu_0$ (specified)
    Alternative Hypothesis: H_1: $\mu \neq \mu_0$ or H_1: $\mu > \mu_0$ or H_1: $\mu < \mu_0$
(iii) Test Statistic

$$t = \frac{\bar{x} - \mu_0}{S/\sqrt{n}} \sim t \text{ distribution with } (n-1) \text{ df}$$

where $\bar{x} = \frac{\sum x_i}{n}$ and $S^2 = \frac{1}{n-1}\sum(x_i - \bar{x})^2$

(iv) Reject H_0 if p-value of the test statistics is less than 0.05 (if tested for 5% level of significance). For any other level of significance, decision is to be taken accordingly.

Illustration 8.1: The life expectancy of people in the year 1971 in India is expected to be 50 years. A survey was conducted in randomly selected 11 states of India, and the data obtained are given next. Do the data confirm the expected view?
Life Expectancy (Years): 54.2, 50.4, 44.2, 49.7, 55.4, 57.0, 58.2, 56.6, 61.9, 57.5, 53.4.
Solution: The null hypothesis of the test is H_0: $\mu = 50$, and the alternative hypothesis is H_1: $\mu \neq 50$.

R Commands:

```
>x = c(54.2, 50.4, 44.2, 49.7, 55.4, 57.0, 58.2, 56.6, 61.9,
57.5, 53.4)
>ttest = t.test(x, alternative="two.sided", conf.level=0.95)
# stores the result of the test in 'ttest'
>ttest # this shall produce the result of the t test as follows
```

Result:

```
One Sample t-test
data: x - 50
t = 3.0097, df = 10, p-value = 0.01312
alternative hypothesis: true mean is not equal to 0
95 percent confidence interval:
  1.144976 7.673206
sample estimates:
mean of x
  4.409091
```

Interpretation: The calculated value of t comes out to be 3.0097, and the corresponding p-value of the test is 0.01312. Since, the p-value of the test is less than $0.05 = 1 - 0.95$ (1 – the confidence interval) of the test, we reject the null hypothesis and conclude that the data do not confirm the expected view.

NOTE: If the alternative hypothesis is two-tailed, i.e., of the form $H_1: \mu \neq \mu_0$, then use alternative = 'two sided', and if the alternative is of the form $H_1: \mu > \mu_0$ and $H_1: \mu < \mu_0$, use alternative = 'greater' or alternative = 'less' in the t-test command.

Illustration 8.2: The purpose of a study by Luglie was to investigate the oral status of a group of patients diagnosed with thalassemia major (TM). One of the outcome measures was the decayed, missing, filled teeth index (DMFT). In a sample of 18 patients, the mean DMFT index value was 10.3 with standard deviation of 7.3. Is this sufficient evidence to allow us to conclude that the mean DMFT index is greater than 9 in a population of similar subjects? (Perform the test at 10% level of significance.)[5]

Solution: The null hypothesis of the test is $H_0: \mu = 9$, and the alternative hypothesis is $H_1: \mu > 9$.

R Commands:

```
>sample_mean= 10.3
>population_mean= 9
>sd= 7.3
> n = 18
> t = (sample_mean - population_mean) / (sd / sqrt(n))
>t_test=round(t, digits = 4)
>df= n - 1
>p_value= 2 * (1 - pt(abs(t_test), df))
>p_value
```

Result:

t-test = 0.7555
p-value = 0.4603

Interpretation: The calculated value of t comes out to be 0.7555, and the corresponding p-value of the test is 0.4603. Since the p-value of the test is more than $0.10 = 1 - 0.90$ (1 – the confidence interval) of the test, we accept the null hypothesis and conclude that the mean DMFT index is not significantly different from 9 in a population of similar subjects.

Fisher's t-test (t-test for Two Population Means with Variance Unknown but Equal)

(i) **Assumptions**
   a. Both the populations are normally distributed.
   b. Population variances are unknown but equal.
   c. The samples are independent of each other.

(ii) **Hypothesis of the Test**
   Null Hypothesis: $H_0: \mu_1 = \mu_2$
   Alternative Hypothesis: $H_1: \mu_1 = \mu_2$ or $H_1: \mu_1 > \mu_2$ or $H_1: \mu_1 < \mu_2$

(iii) **Test Statistic**

$$t = \frac{\bar{x}_i - \bar{y}_i}{S\sqrt{\left(\frac{1}{n_1} + \frac{1}{n_2}\right)}} \sim t_{n_1 + n_2 - 2} \text{ df with } S^2 = \frac{1}{n_1 + n_2 - 1}\left[\sum_{i=1}^{n_1}(x_i - \bar{x})^2 + \sum_{i=1}^{n_2}(y_i - \bar{y})^2\right]$$

(iv) *Reject H_0* if *p*-value of the test statistics is less than 0.05 (if tested for 5% level of significance). For any other level of significance, decision is to be taken accordingly (Das and Bhattacharjee, 2008).

t-test for Two Population Means with Variance Unknown and Unequal (Welch Two-Sample t-Test)

The test was developed by B L Welch (1947).

(i) **Assumptions**
   a. Both the populations are normally distributed.
   b. Population variances are unknown, but it is known that they are unequal.
   c. The samples are independent of each other.

(ii) **Hypothesis of the Test**
   1. Null Hypothesis: H_0: $\mu_1 = \mu_2$
   2. Alternative Hypothesis: H_1: $\mu_1 \neq \mu_2$ or H_1: $\mu_1 > \mu_2$ or H_1: $\mu_1 < \mu_2$

(iii) **Test Statistic**

$$t = \frac{\bar{x}_i - \bar{y}_i}{\sqrt{\left(\frac{S_1^2}{n_1} + \frac{S_2^2}{n_2}\right)}} \sim t \text{ distribution with } v \text{ df}$$

with $S_1^2 = \frac{1}{n_1 - 1}\sum_{i=1}^{n_1}(x_i - \bar{x})^2$ and $S_2^2 = \frac{1}{n_2 - 1}\sum_{i=1}^{n_2}(y_i - \bar{y})^2$

(iv) *Reject H_0* if *p*-value of the test statistics is less than 0.05 (if tested for 5% level of significance). For any other level of significance, decision is to be taken accordingly.

NOTE: It may be seen that there are two options of the t-test for two samples. One is performed if the variances are unknown but equal, and the other is applied if the variances are unknown and unequal. Thus, it is better to perform a F-test to verify if the variances of the two populations from which the samples are drawn are equal or not and then perform the appropriate t-test, i.e., Fisher's or Welch.

Equality of Variance Test
F-test for Equality of Two Variances
(i) **Assumptions**
   a. The samples are independent.
   b. The samples come from normal population.

(ii) **Hypothesis of the Test**

Null Hypothesis:

H_0: There is no significant difference between the population variances, i.e., $\sigma_1^2 = \sigma_2^2$

Alternative Hypothesis:

H_1: The population variance differs significantly.

(iii) Test Statistic

$$F = \frac{S_X^2}{S_Y^2} \text{ if } S_X^2 > S_Y^2 \sim \text{F distribution with } (n_1 - 1, n_2 - 1) \text{ df}$$

$$= \frac{S_Y^2}{S_X^2} \text{ if } S_Y^2 > S_X^2 \sim \text{F distribution with } (n_2 - 1, n_1 - 1) \text{ df}$$

where, $S_X{}^2 = \frac{1}{n_1 - 1}\sum(x_i - \bar{x})^2$ and $S_Y{}^2 = \frac{1}{n_2 - 1}\sum(y_i - \bar{y})^2$

(iv) *Reject H_0* if *p*-value of the test statistics is less than 0.05 (if tested for 5% level of significance). For any other level of significance, decision is to be taken accordingly.

Illustration 11.1: To evaluate if drug Z reduces mean systolic blood pressure, a randomized clinical trial will be performed where 12 individuals receive drug Z and 8 receive a placebo. The null hypothesis to be tested is that there is no difference in the mean systolic blood pressure of the experimental and placebo groups. The alternative hypothesis is that there is a difference between the means of the two groups. The Type I error for your trial will be 5%. The systolic blood pressure of patients treated with drug Z and placebo are as follows:[6]

Drug Z: 100, 110, 112, 109, 108,111, 118, 105, 115, 119, 106, 109
Placebo: 129, 125,136, 129, 135, 134, 140, 128

Solution: The null hypothesis of the test is the following:

H_0: There is no significant difference in the mean systolic blood pressure of the experimental and placebo groups.

Alternative Hypothesis:

H_1: The difference in the mean systolic blood pressure of the experimental and placebo groups differ significantly.

Under the null hypothesis, we have to apply t-test for this problem. But first we need to ascertain whether we need to apply Fisher or Walch t-test. For this, we need to check whether variances of two groups are equal or not. For this, we perform a F-test for equality of variance. The null hypothesis of the F-test is as follows:

Null Hypothesis: H_0: $\sigma_1^2 = \sigma_2^2$
Alternative Hypothesis: H_1: $\sigma_1^2 \neq \sigma_2^2$

R-Code for F test
```
>x=c(100,110,112,109,108,111,118,105,115,119,106,109)
>y=c(129,125,136,129,135,134,140,128)
```

```
>Ftest=var.test(x,y,ratio=1,alternative="two.sided",conf.
level=0.95)
>Ftest
```

Results

```
F test to compare two variances

data: x and y
F = 1.1631, num df = 11, denomdf = 7, p-value = 0.8712
alternative hypothesis: true ratio of variances is not
equal to 1
95 percent confidence interval:
 0.2469601 4.3714875
sample estimates:
ratio of variances
          1.163051
```

Interpretation: The calculated value of F comes out to be 1.1631, and the corresponding p-value of the test is 0.8721. Since the p-value of the test is more than $0.05 = 1 - 0.95$ (1 – the confidence interval) of the test, we accept the null hypothesis and conclude that the variances of the two populations from which the samples are drawn do not differ significantly, i.e., they are equal.

NOTE:
(1) If the alternative hypothesis is one-tailed, i.e., of the form $H_1: \sigma_1^2 > \sigma_2^2$ or $H_1: \sigma_1^2 < \sigma_2^2$, then use alternative = 'greater' or alternative = 'less', respectively in the var.test command.
(2) In R, if the first and second samples are interchanged, even then, the p-value remains the same and so the conclusion does not change. However, the F-value will not be the same, but this does not influence the result.
(3) Since the F-test indicates that the variances of the two populations from which the samples are drawn do not differ significantly, one can use the Fisher's t-test for comparing the means of the two populations for the dataset provided earlier (Illustration 11.1).

R-Code for t test

```
>x=c(100,110,112,109,108,111,118,105,115,119,106,109)
>y=c(129,125,136,129,135,134,140,128)
# when done in unison with F test entering data is not required
>ttest= t.test(x, y, alternative = "two.sided", conf.
level=0.95, var.equal = TRUE)
>ttest
```

Results

```
Two Sample t-test

data: x and y
t = -9.0972, df = 18, p-value = 3.752e-08
alternative hypothesis: true difference in means is not equal to 0
95 percent confidence interval:
 -26.87556 -16.79111
sample estimates:
```

```
mean of x mean of y
110.1667 132.0000
```

Interpretation: The calculated value of t comes out to be −9.0972, and the corresponding p-value of the test is 3.752e − 08. Since the p-value of the test is less than $0.05 = 1 - 0.95$ (1 − the confidence interval) of the test, we reject the null hypothesis and conclude that there is a difference in the mean systolic blood pressure of the experimental and placebo groups.

NOTE:
(1) If the alternative hypothesis is one-tailed, i.e., of the form H1: $\mu_1 > \mu_2$ or H1: $\mu_1 < \mu_2$, then use alternative = 'greater' or alternative = 'less', respectively in the t.test command.
(2) In case the variances of the two populations from which the samples are drawn differ significantly, then we use var.equal = FALSE in the t.test command.

Illustration 11.2: Two patients reported to a doctor with some symptoms that indicated that they might be diabetic, which was later confirmed through some clinical tests. The doctor advised the patients to take to brisk walking early morning. Both the patients abided by the advice. But one of them took to brisk walking alone while the other walked with his pet dog. The dog stops occasionally and sometimes starts running, too, and so the patient has to keep pace with the dog while walking. The walking speed of the two individuals measured in terms of Kms/hour in some randomly picked-up days are as follows:

Patient 1: 2.7 4.8 3.6 5.3 5.1 4.3 2.9 4.1 5.1
Patient 2: 4.3 4.4 4.6 4.9 5.2 5.3 4.9

Test at 5% level of significance if the variation in the speed of the two patients is identical.

Solution: Let us set up the null hypothesis.
Null Hypothesis: H_0: $\sigma_1^2 = \sigma_2^2$; variation in the speed of the two patients is identical.
Alternative Hypothesis: H_1: $\sigma_1^2 \neq \sigma_2^2$; variation in the speed of the two patients is not identical.

R-Code for F test
```
>x=c(2.7, 4.8, 3.6, 5.3, 5.1, 4., 2.9, 4.1, 5.1)
>y=c(4.3, 4.4, 4.6, 4.9, 5.2, 5.3, 4.9)
>Ftest=var.test(x,y,ratio=1,alternative="two.sided",conf.
level=0.95)
>Ftest
```

Results
```
F test to compare two variances
data: x and y
F = 6.4223, num df = 8, denomdf = 6, p-value = 0.03585
alternative hypothesis: true ratio of variances is not
equal to 1
95 percent confidence interval:
   1.146925 29.874810
sample estimates:
ratio of variances
      6.422348
```

Interpretation: The calculated value of F comes out to be 6.4223, and the corresponding p-value of the test is 0.03585. Since the p-value of the test is less than $0.05 = 1 - 0.95$ (1 − the confidence interval) of the test, we reject the null hypothesis and conclude that variation in the speed of the two patients is not identical.

Paired t-test

This test is used to compare the average of a sample of subjects in a before-after setting, such as the mean systolic blood pressure of the same group of patients before and after an exercise session or the average blood glucose level of a group of patients before and after lunch, etc.

(i) Assumptions
    a. The samples are of equal size.
    b. The observations correspond to the same sampling unit.
(ii) Hypothesis of the Test
    Null Hypothesis: H_0: There is no significant difference between the means.
    Alternative Hypothesis: H_1: The means of the two samples differ significantly.
(iii) Test Statistic

$$t = \frac{\bar{d}}{S_d / \sqrt{n}} \sim t \text{ distribution with } (n-1) \text{ df}$$

where $\bar{d} = \frac{\sum d_i}{n}$, $d_i = x_i - y_i$ and $S_d^2 = \frac{1}{n-1}\sum(d_i - \bar{d})^2$

(iv) *Reject H_0 if p-value of the test statistics is less than 0.05 (if tested for 5% level of significance). For any other level of significance, decision is to be taken accordingly* (Kale, 2005; Lehmann, 1986).

A researcher wants to find if summer holidays have an effect on the physical fitness of students. For this purpose, a fitness test is carried out once before and once after the holidays for 12 students. The scores of the 12 students are as follows:[7]
    Test whether summer holidays have an effect on the physical fitness of students.

Table 5.2 Physical fitness of students

Student:	1	2	3	4	5	6	7	8	9	10	11	12
Before:	36	38	39	47	46	51	32	42	45	49	36	38
After:	40	32	43	42	51	46	33	41	42	52	47	49

Solution: The null hypothesis of the test is as follows:
    H_0: There is no difference in the average physical fitness score of students before and after the summer holidays.

Alternative Hypothesis:

H_1: There is a significant difference in the average physical fitness score of students before and after the summer holidays.

R-Code

```
>x=c(36,38,39,47,46,51,32,42,45,49,36,38)
>y=c(40,32,43,42,51,46,33,41,42,52,47,49)
>ttest=t.test(x,y,paired=TRUE,alternative="two.sided",conf.
level=0.95)
>ttest
```

Results

```
Paired t-test
data: x and y
t = -0.93949, df = 11, p-value = 0.3677
alternative hypothesis: true mean difference is not equal to 0
95 percent confidence interval:
 -5.292681 2.126014
sample estimates:
mean difference
        -1.583333
```

Interpretation: The calculated value of t comes out to be -0.93949, and the corresponding p-value of the test is 0.3677. Since the p-value of the test is more than $0.05 = 1 - 0.95$ (1 – the confidence interval) of the test, we accept the null hypothesis and conclude that there is no significant difference in physical fitness of students before and after the summer holidays.

Non-Parametric Tests

In Section 4 of the chapter, non-parametric tests were introduced. In the following sections, discussion on the different non-parametric tests (Gibbons and Chakraborti, 2003) and their computation using the R environment is placed (Schmuller, 2017). But before that, merits, demerits, and terminologies concerning non-parametric tests are placed next.

Advantages of Non-Parametric Tests

The non-parametric tests have certain advantages over the parametric methods. Some of them are as follows:

- It is simple to understand.
- The calculations associated are relatively simple compared to parametric tests.
- Also, these tests can be used even when the actual measurements are not available but the ranks of the observations are given. Non-parametric methods can also be applied to data measured in nominal or ordinal scale.
- The non-parametric tests are based on very mild assumptions compared to parametric tests; thus, this test can be easily applied. Frequently, it is assumed that the

variables just come from a continuous distribution. The parametric tests are based on some strong assumptions and cannot provide proper results when the underlying assumptions are violated.

- In non-parametric methods, there is no restriction on the minimum size of the sample. Even with a small sample size, non-parametric methods are fairly powerful.

Disadvantages of Non-Parametric Tests

Some of the disadvantages commonly encountered by the non-parametric method can be as follows:

- Though the assumptions in non-parametric tests are less restrictive than parametric tests, the assumption of independence is as important in non-parametric tests as in the case of parametric tests.
- Though it is often claimed that the non-parametric tests are very simple computationally, this is not always true. Some non-parametric tests demand lots of calculations.
- In the case of estimation, parametric methods are more robust compared to non-parametric methods, as the estimates remain unbiased even when the underlying assumption of normality is violated.
- The parametric tests are more efficient compared to the non-parametric tests, as a parametric test requires a smaller sample size compared to a non-parametric test to achieve the same level of power.

Some Terms Associated with Non-Parametric Test

Run: A run is a sequence of symbols followed or preceded by other type of symbols or no symbols. For example, let us consider the following sequence:

MMMFFFFMFMMF

Here, we have six runs in all with three runs consisting of 'M' and three runs of 'F'. The number of runs in a sequence is taken as an indicator of randomness.

Ties: Often, while ranking the data in the case of non-parametric tests, we find two or more observations with the same value. In such a case, a tie is said to have occurred.

Nominal Scale of Measurement: The most elementary scale in measurement. This is the scale in which each subject is classified into one of the available categories. The categories are mutually exclusive.

The Ordinal Scale of Measurement: This measurement incorporates the classifying and labelling as done in the nominal scale, but in addition to that, it performs the task of arranging them in a proper order. In other words, the subjects are ranked based on the level of a particular attribute.

Contingency Table: A contingency table is a two-way table in which the columns are classified according to one criterion or attribute, and the rows are classified according to the other criterion or attribute. Thus, we get a number of cells, where the number in a particular cell represents the number of observations at one label of an attribute cross classified under another level of the second attribute.

Table 5.3 Contingency table

	A_1	A_2	...	A_i	...	A_r	Total
B_1	f_{11}	f_{12}	...	f_{1i}		f_1r	(B_1)
B_2	f_{21}	f_{22}	...	f_{2i}		f_{2r}	(B_2)
'	'	'	'	'	'	'	'
'	'	'	'	'	'	'	'
'	'	'	'	'	'	'	'
B_j	f_{j1}	f_{j2}	...	f_{ji}		f_{jr}	(B_j)
'	'	'	'	'	'	'	'
'	'	'	'	'	'	'	'
'	'	'	'	'	'	'	'
B_s	f_{s1}	f_{s2}	...	f_{si}		f_{sr}	(B_s)
Total	(A_1)	(A_2)	...	(A_i)	...	(A_r)	N

Chi-Square Test of Independence

The chi-square tests found its expression in the work of Pearson (1900). This is a non-parametric test used to test the independence of attributes. This is to check if the two attributes under consideration is independent of each other or not, based on their frequencies generally arranged in a two-way table. Let A and B be two attributes, where A is divided into r classes, A_1, A2, . . ., Ar, and B is divided into s classes, B_1, B2, . . ., Bs. The various categories under each of the attributes can be classified into a (r × s) two-way table commonly called the contingency table (Table 5.3).

The null hypothesis is as follows: Ho: The two attributes are independent of each other.

Where f_{ji} represents the number of cases possessing both the attributes A_i ($i = 1, 2, . . ., r$) and B_j ($j = 1, 2, . . ., s$) and N is the grand total.

Here, we want to test the null hypothesis.

H_0: The two attributes, A and B, are independent of each other.

The null hypothesis is tested against the alternative hypothesis.

H_1: The two attributes, A and B, are dependent on each other.

Assumptions

- The data is at nominal level of measurement and grouped into several categories.
- For applying the chi-square test, the frequencies in the various cells should be reasonably large, i.e., ≥ 5.
- The subjects in each of the group are randomly and independently selected.

The expected frequency of any cell under the hypothesis that the attributes A and B are independent is given by the following:

$$e_{ij} = \frac{\left(A_i\right) \times \left(B_j\right)}{N}$$

The test statistic is given by the following:

$$\chi^2 = \sum_{i=1}^{s} \sum_{j=1}^{r} \left(\frac{f_{ij} - e_{ij}}{e_{ij}}\right)^2 \sim \chi^2 \text{ variate with } (s - 1) \times (r - 1) \text{ degrees of freedom.}$$

The decision of accepting or rejecting the null hypothesis can be taken based on the p-value of the test. We *reject* H_0 if p-value of the test statistics is less than 0.05 (if tested for 5% level of significance). For any other level of significance, decision is to be taken accordingly.

In a study (Table 5.4), Sharkey et al.[8] found that in a total of 112 patients, 27 developed bradycardia.[9] Test if there is independence between the type of treatment (phenylephrine[10] or norepinephrine)[11] and bradycardia based on the observed frequencies using the χ^2 test. The data is as follows:

Table 5.4 Study of bradycardia

Bradycardia		Treatment groups		
		Phenylephrine	Norepinephrine	Total
	Yes	21	6	27
	No	35	50	85
	Total	56	56	112

Source: Sharkey et al.

Here, we are to test the following hypothesis:

H_0: The type of treatment is independent of the bradycardia status of the patients.

R-Code

```
> data = matrix(c(21,6,35,50),nrow=2,byrow=T,dimnames=
list("Bradycardia "=c("Yes","No")," Treatment Group" =
c("Phenylephrine ","Norepinephrine"))) # command to send
data to R
> data # to see if the data is properly received by R compiler
                  Treatment Group
  Bradycardia Phenylephrine   Norepinephrine
        Yes            21                6
        No             35               50

>chisq.test(data)


Pearson's Chi-squared test with Yates' continuity correction
data: data
X-squared = 9.5651, df = 1, p-value = 0.001983
```

Here, the p-value of the χ^2 test is 0.001983, which is < 0.05. This indicates that the null hypothesis is rejected. Thus, we may conclude that the type of treatment is related to the bradycardia status of the patients.

Chi-Square Test of Goodness of Fit

This is another non-parametric test based on chi-square, which is used to test if the observed frequencies are significantly different from the theoretical frequencies. In short, it is called testing the goodness of fit. The following is the null hypothesis:

H_0: The observed frequencies fit to the theoretical frequencies.

Assumptions

- The data is at nominal level of measurement and grouped into several categories.
- For applying the chi-square test, the frequencies in the various categories should be reasonably large, i.e., ≥ 5.
- The sum of the observed frequencies and the expected frequencies should be equal, i.e.,

$$\Sigma o_i = \Sigma e_i$$

The Test Statistic

Once the expected frequencies are computed, they are compared with the observed frequencies for which Pearson suggested the test statistic as follows:

$$\chi^2 = \sum_{i=1}^{k} \left(\frac{(o_i - e_i)}{e_i} \right)^2 \sim \chi^2 \text{ distribution with } k - 1 \text{ degrees of freedom.}$$

If the value of o_i and e_i of each category is closer to each other, then the calculated value of the χ^2 statistic will be small; otherwise, it will be large. The larger the value of χ^2, the more likely it is that o_i does not go with the expected frequencies leading to a small p-value and eventually rejecting the null hypothesis of goodness of fit.

We *reject H_0 if* p-value of the test statistics is less than 0.05 (if tested for 5% level of significance). For any other level of significance, decision is to be taken accordingly.

Illustration 16.1: A researcher tries to find out if cancer is more likely to be diagnosed in patients who are in a low-income category, based on socio-economic status (SES) quartiles. Thus, four SES are identified, viz. high, moderate, low, and very low. Data from the community sample of cancer patients are collected over a ten-year period. A total of 2,050 patients are identified. The number of patients of the high, moderate, low, and very low groups are 165, 283, 622, and 980, respectively. Apply chi-square test of goodness of fit at 1% level of significance to test if the cancer is equally prevalent across the different SES.

Here, we are to test the following null hypothesis:

H_0: The positive diagnostics of subjects with cancer is independent of their socio-economic status.
To be tested against the alternative hypothesis:
H_1: There exists a relation between the socio-economic status of the patients of being positively diagnosed with cancer.

R-Code

```
>chisq.test(c(165, 283,622,980), p=c(0.25, 0.25, 0.25, 0.25))
# If SES quarters are independent of cancer diagnostic pa-
    tients, then
# each of them shall have equal proportion i.e. 0.25

    Chi-squared test for given probabilities

    data: c(165, 283, 622, 980)
    X-squared = 788.24, df = 3, p-value < 2.2e-16
```

Conclusion: At 1% significance level, the data provide sufficient evidence (p-value $= 2.2 \times 10^{-16}$ less than 0.01) that the proportion of cancer patients in the different SES quarters are different from being equal.

Wilcoxon One-Sample Signed Rank Test (Non-Parametric Alternative to Student's t-Test)

Let a sample, $X_1, X_2, \ldots, X_n$, be a random sample drawn from a population function with cumulative distribution function $F(x)$. This test is used to check the hypothesis:

H_0: $F(\mu) = 0.5$ (i.e., μ is the average value of the dataset), tested against any one of the following alternatives

H_1: $F(\mu) \neq 0.5$ or H_1: $F(\mu) > 0.5$ or H_1: $F(\mu) < 0.5$

Assumptions

- $F(x)$ is the cumulative distribution function of the random variable X and is absolutely continuous.
- The density function $f(x)$ is symmetric about the median, i.e., $F(\mu - x) = 1 - F(x + \mu)$ and $f(\mu - x) = f(x + \mu)$.
- No two observations in the random sample are equal.

We *reject H_0 if* p-value of the test statistics is less than 0.05 (if tested for 5% level of significance). For any other level of significance, decision is to be taken accordingly.

Illustration 17.1: The hypochondriasis[12] score of a patient taken randomly on eight days are as follows:

30, 35, 45, 53, 47, 62, 21, 17, 38, 61, 42, and 47

Test if the median score of the patient is significantly higher than 30, which is an indicator of mild hypochondriasis.

Here, we are to test the null hypothesis:

H_0: The central value of the population from which the sample is drawn is not significantly different from a specified value, i.e., $\mu = 30$

To be tested against the alternative hypothesis:

H_1: $\mu > 30$

R-Code

```
> Score = c(30, 35, 45, 53, 47, 62, 21, 17, 38, 61,
42, 47)
>wilcox.test(Score,mu = 30, alternative = "greater",
exact = F)
Wilcoxon signed rank test with continuity correction
    data: Score
    V = 58, p-value = 0.01465
    alternative hypothesis: true location is greater than 30
```

Conclusion: At 5% significance level, the data provide sufficient evidence (p-value = 0.0146 less than 0.05) that the null hypothesis of the average equal to 30 is to be rejected and accept the alternative that the average hypochondriasis score is greater than 30, i.e., based on the data and corresponding test, one can say that the patient is having signs of mild hypochondriasis.[13]

Wilcoxon Two-Sample Rank Sum Test (Non-Parametric Alternative to the Two-Independent Sample t-Test)

Though the test was proposed by Wilcoxon in (1945), it was popularized by Sidney Siegel (1956) in his famous textbook on non-parametric inference. This is a non-parametric test used to check if the central values of the two populations from which the two samples are drawn differ significantly. The two samples are identified as X_1, $X_2, \ldots, X_n$ and $Y_1, Y_2, \ldots, Y_m$, where the sizes of the two samples, viz. n and m, are not necessarily equal.

Null Hypothesis: Ho: The central values of the two populations from which the samples are drawn do not differ significantly.

Assumptions

- The two samples are independent of one another.

We *reject H_0* if p-value of the test statistics is less than 0.05 (if tested for 5% level of significance). For any other level of significance, decision is to be taken accordingly.

Illustration 18.1: The WHO depression self-assessment tool is used for the self-assessment of depressive symptoms of a group of patients who are suspected to have become a victim of depression. The scores of the patients belonging to two categories, viz. those with previous history of depression and the other with cases of depression in the family, are as follows:

Category I: 14, 12, 9, 8, 7, 16, 18, 12
Category II: 5, 7, 9, 10, 14, 13, 12, 8, 6

Test if the depression scores of the two categories differ to an extent that we can tell one category is more depressed than the other.

Here, we are to test the null hypothesis:

H_0: The central values of the two categories of patients do not differ significantly.

To be tested against the two-tailed alternative:

H_1: The central values of the two categories of patients differ significantly.

R-Code
```
>cat1 = c(14,12,9,8,7,16,18, 12)
>cat2 = c(5, 7, 9, 10, 14, 13, 12, 8, 6)
>wilcox.test(cat1, cat2, mu = 0, alternative = "two.sided",
paired = F)
Wilcoxon rank sum test with continuity correction
data: cat1 and cat2
W = 50, p-value = 0.1917
alternative hypothesis: true location shift is not equal to 0[14]
```

Conclusion: As the p-value is > 0.05, we accept the null hypothesis and conclude that the central values of the depression score of the two categories of patients do not differ significantly.

Wilcoxon Matched Pair Signed Rank Test (Non-Parametric Alternative to Paired Sample t-Test)

The test was proposed by Wilcoxon in (1945). Here, we are to compare the average of two related populations in a before-after setup based on sample observations. The observations of a group of subjects before an event and of the same subjects after an event is available. We are to compare if their averages differ significantly. Here, the term matched pairs are generally two observations taken on the same item or subject for two different situations. Let us consider two samples, $X_1, X_2, \ldots, X_n$ and $Y_1, Y_2, \ldots, Y_n$, be obtained from the same set of subjects at two different situations. This test is used to check the hypothesis:

H_0: There is no shift in the average between the before-after samples.

To be tested against the alternative H_1: The two samples differ significantly.

Assumptions
- The distribution function of both the random samples is absolutely continuous.
- The random samples are independent of each other.

We *reject H_0 if p*-value of the test statistics is less than 0.05 (if tested for 5% level of significance). For any other level of significance, decision is to be taken accordingly.

After taking to a change in the lifestyle the fasting blood sugar levels of a group of seven patients were recorded (Table 5.5). Their fasting blood sugar levels recorded during their regular life when they reported to the clinic were available. Both these values for the seven patients are as follows:

Table 5.5 Fasting blood sugar levels

Patient number	Fasting blood sugar (mg/dl)	
	Before	After
1	220	140
2	240	140
3	160	153
4	235	136
5	227	172
6	159	149
7	231	137

Perform appropriate non-parametric test to find out if the change in lifestyle had significantly decreased the fasting blood sugar levels of the patients.

Here, we are to test the null-hypothesis:

H_0: There is no shift in the average fasting blood sugar level of the patients before-and after the change in lifestyle.

R-Code

```
>b4 = c(220,240,160,235,227,159,231)
>aft = c(140,140,153,136,172,149,137)
>wilcox.test(b4, aft, mu=0, alternative="less", paired=T, exact = F)
Wilcoxon signed rank test with continuity correction
data: b4 and aft
V = 28, p-value = 0.9926
alternative hypothesis: true location shift is not equal to 0
```

Interpretation: As the p-value is > 0.05, we accept the null-hypothesis and conclude that there is no shift in the average fasting blood sugar level of the patients before and after the change in lifestyle at 5% level of significance.

Run Test for Checking the Randomness of a Dataset

This test is used to check the randomness of a dataset using the theory of runs. It is used to check if a random sample, $X_1, X_2, \ldots, X_n$, can be considered as a random sample from a continuous probability distribution. A common assumption in many statistical processes is that the observations are independent of each other, i.e., random in nature. This test can be used to check the assumption.

Here, H_0: The observations are random in nature.

The null hypothesis is tested against the alternative that the observations are non-random.

Assumptions

The observations in the sample are obtained under similar conditions.

Working Procedure

Here, from the sample of the form $X_1, X_2, \ldots, X_n$, the median is calculated. The sample is then rewritten in such a way that each observation above the sample median is replaced by '+' and that below the sample median is replaced by '–'. The number of runs of '+' and '–' in this series are then counted. In case the dataset is randomly distributed, then there shall not be any pattern in it, and the number of runs shall be more. This is the basis of the test.

We *reject H_0 if p-*value of the test statistics is less than 0.05 (if tested for 5% level of significance). For any other level of significance, decision is to be taken accordingly.

Illustration 20.1: The level of total cholesterol of a particular patient measured in terms of mg/dL at an interval of two hours in a particular day are shown next. Test if the values are randomly distributed.

Total cholesterol values (mg/dL): 210, 288, 239, 197, 235, 280, 292, 240. 266, 260, 288, 310

Here, the null hypothesis is as follows:

H_0: The total cholesterol values of the patient are random in nature.

The procedure for performing the run test is not available in the base package in R. For this, we need to install a package called "randtest" in R.

R-Code[15]

```
>install.packages("randtests")
> library(randtests)
> x = c(210, 288, 239, 197, 235, 280, 292, 240, 266, 260,
288, 310)
>runs.test(x)
Runs Test
data: x
statistic = 0.60553, runs = 8, n1 = 6, n2 = 6, n = 12,
p-value = 0.5448
alternative hypothesis: nonrandomness
```

Interpretation: As the *p-*value is > 0.05, we accept the null hypothesis and conclude that the values in the sample are randomly distributed at 5% level of significance.

The Kolmogorov-Smirnov One-Sample Test

Two Russian statisticians, Kolmogorov and Smirnov, in 1933 developed distribution free techniques based on empirical distributions. These statistical procedures used the maximum vertical distance between the density functions and is used to decide if a random sample is from a pre-specified density function. The test is used to check if the sample comes from a specified probability distribution. The Kolmogorov-Smirnov one-sample test is used to check if the random sample under consideration is drawn from a population with specified cumulative distribution function $F_0(x)$. This test is used to check the hypothesis:

H_0: $F(x) = F_0(x)$ against the alternatives H_1: $F(x) \neq F_0(x)$.

Assumption

■ $X_1, X_2, \ldots, X_n$ is a random sample of size n drawn from a continuous population.

We *reject* H_0 *if* p-value of the test statistics is less than 0.05 (if tested for 5% level of significance) (Smirnov, 1948). For any other level of significance, decision is to be taken accordingly.

Illustration 21.1: A random sample of 14 primary hypertension (PH) patients was taken, and their total cholesterol (mg/dL) was recorded.
149.1, 220.8, 230.6, 207.2, 281.3, 176.7, 260.4, 297.1, 199.0, 246.3, 224.0, 155.5, 182.2, 179.6

For further statistical analysis, it is necessary to test if the data are normally distributed.
   Here, the Kolmogorov-Smirnov one-sample test is used to check if the random sample under consideration is drawn from a normal distribution.
   The null hypothesis is Ho: The data comes from a normal distribution.

   R-Code
```
> sample = c(149.1, 220.8, 230.6, 207.2, 281.3, 176.7, 260.4,
297.1, 199.0, 246.3, 224.0, 155.5, 182.2, 179.6) # to test the
data for normality
>ks.test(sample,"pnorm")
Exact one-sample Kolmogorov-Smirnov test
data: sample
D = 1, p-value < 2.2e-16
alternative hypothesis: two-sided
```

Interpretation: As the p-value is < 0.05, we reject the null hypothesis and conclude that the data does not come from a normal distribution at 5% level of significance.

For other distributions, one can use the following commands in lieu of 'pnorm':

beta – pbeta; binomial – pbinom; negative binomial – pnbinom;
chi-square – pchisq; uniform – punif; gamma – pgamma; exponential – pexp; Poisson – ppois

The Kolmogorov-Smirnov Two-Sample Test
This test is used to check if two random samples under consideration is drawn from the same distribution. Here, the test is performed based on the maximum distance between two empirical distribution functions computed based on the sample. Let $X_1, X_2, \ldots,$ X_n be a random sample of size n drawn from a continuous population with distribution function $F(.)$. Similarly, $Y_1, Y_2, \ldots, Ym$ is a random sample of size m drawn from a continuous population with distribution function $G(.)$. Then based on their empirical cumulative distribution functions, $F_n(x)$ and $G_m(y)$, the null hypothesis of the equality of the distribution functions, viz. $F(.)$ and $G(.)$, are tested, i.e., $H_0 \colon F(z) = G(z)$ $\forall z$, against the alternatives $H_1 \colon F(z) \neq G(z)$. The test statistic for the purpose is as follows:

$$D = Sup_{m,n} \left| F_n(z) - G_m(z) \right|$$

We *reject* H_0 *if* p-value of the test statistics is less than 0.05 (if tested for 5% level of significance). For any other level of significance, decision is to be taken accordingly.

Illustration 22.1: A random sample of 13 primary hypertension (PH) patients was taken, and each person's total cholesterol (measured in mg/dl) was recorded. Similarly, a random sample of 11 normotensive (NT) patients was taken, and their total cholesterol (measured in mg/dl) were also recorded. The following are the values of the datasets.[16]

PH: 220.8, 230.6, 207.2, 281.3, 176.7, 260.4, 297.1, 199.0, 246.3, 224.0, 155.5, 182.2, 179.6

NT: 120.1, 200, 210.9, 184.8, 267.4, 150.8, 244.1, 285, 175.7, 228.4, 203.6

Test at 5% level of significance if the total cholesterol measures of the PH group and NT group are identically distributed.

Here, the Kolmogorov-Smirnov two-sample test is used to check if the random samples under consideration is drawn from the same distribution.

The null hypothesis is that H_0: The two samples come from the same distribution

H_1: The distributions from which the two samples are drawn are not identical

```
> PH = c(220.8, 230.6, 207.2, 281.3, 176.7, 260.4, 297.1, 199.0,
246.3, 224.0, 155.5, 182.2, 179.6)
> NT = c(120.1, 200, 210.9, 184.8, 267.4, 150.8, 244.1, 285,
175.7, 228.4, 203.6)
>ks.test(PH, NT, alternative="two.sided", exact = F)
Asymptotic two-sample Kolmogorov-Smirnov test
data: PH and NT
D = 0.1958, p-value = 0.9763
alternative hypothesis: two-sided
```

Interpretation: As the p-value is > 0.05, we accept the null hypothesis and conclude that the two samples appear from the same distribution at 5% level of significance.

McNemar's Test
This test proposed by McNemar in (1947) is used when nominal data on two attributes are available in pairs and arranged in the form of a 2 × 2 contingency table (Table 5.6). The test is commonly applied in health sciences to compare the performance of a medical test to a reference test applied in the same group of patients. The purpose is to find out if the outcome of a given medical test varies significantly from a standard test if applied to the same group of patients. Roughly, speaking the null hypothesis is that the probability of a person tested positive with a particular disease remains same in both the reference test and the test under consideration.

Table 5.6 McNemar's test

		Second test	
		Positive	Negative
First Test	Positive	a	b
	Negative	c	d

Table 5.7 Flight from Guwahati to Delhi COVID-19 test

		Second test	
		Positive	Negative
First Test	Positive	18	4
	Negative	16	51

The test statistic for testing the null hypothesis is given by the following:

$\chi^2 = \frac{(b-c)^2}{b+c}$ which follows χ^2 distribution with 1 degree of freedom

We *reject* H_0 *if* p-value of the test statistics is less than 0.05 (if tested for 5% level of significance). For any other level of significance decision, is to be taken accordingly.

A flight comes to Guwahati from Delhi. The flight has 89 passengers. Just after reaching Guwahati, they were tested for COVID-19, and it was found that out of 89 passengers, 22 were found to be positive. Accordingly, all the passengers of the flight were taken to quarantine. After 15 days, all the passengers are retested. This time, out of the 22 previously infected, 4 were found to be negative, while others were all positive. But out of the 67 negatively tested patients in the first test, 16 of them are positive now (Table 5.7). Perform the appropriate test to find out if quarantine was responsible for the change in status.

The null hypothesis of the test is that there is no relation between the before and after outcome.

```
> data = matrix(c(18, 4, 16, 51), nrow = 2, byrow = T, dimnames =
list("First Test" = c("positive", "negative"),"Second Test" =
c("positive", "negative")))
> data
                    Second Test
          First Test positive negative
             positive     18       4
             negative     16      51
>mcnemar.test(data)
    McNemar's Chi-squared test with continuity correction
data: data
McNemar's chi-squared = 6.05, df = 1, p-value = 0.01391
```

Interpretation: As the p-value is < 0.05, we reject the null hypothesis and conclude that the outcome of the two tests differs significantly at 5% level of significance and so one can consider the quarantine responsible for the spread of the virus.

Conclusion

In this chapter, an attempt is made to explain some common parametric and non-parametric tests of statistical hypothesis testing with examples taken from health science. We started from the basic definitions and terminology, explained the rationale of the tests, the assumptions, working formula, datasets for computation, interpretation, and also provided the R codes for each of the tests. The chapter intentionally avoids deduction of the different test statistic, as that aspect shall weaken the basic purpose of the chapter.

Though the data considered in this chapter relates to health science, these tests can be extended to datasets from other fields as well. In a sense, the tests are universal and can be applied to any other domain of knowledge as well, provided the assumptions of the test and the purpose matches the requirements.

Obviously, several tests exist in both the parametric and non-parametric setup. The chapter picks up some common tests, while several others remined unsung. No chapter can claim its exhaustiveness in terms of statistical tests of inference, as there are so many of them. But the chapter provides a starting point. With the knowledge of these tests and their computation in the R environment, researchers can explore several other tests and their computation, which are not covered in this chapter.

Discussion Questions

- What are the key differences between parametric and non-parametric statistical methods?
- Why is it important to test for assumptions like normality before using parametric tests?
- Can non-parametric methods be used even when data meets parametric assumptions? Why or why not?
- How do the robustness and flexibility of non-parametric tests make them useful in real-world research?
- What are the trade-offs between statistical power and assumption flexibility when choosing between parametric and non-parametric methods?
- In what types of research scenarios might a non-parametric test be more appropriate?
- How does sample size affect the choice between parametric and non-parametric tests?
- Give examples of data that would violate parametric assumptions and how you would analyze it.
- Why might non-parametric tests be considered more conservative or less powerful than parametric tests?
- How can understanding both types of methods improve your overall statistical reasoning and research design?

Notes

1 Parameters refer to characteristics of the population, like population mean (μ), population SD (σ), etc. These are constants.
2 Any sample size less than 30 is considered a small sample.
3 Source of the question: https://mgcub.ac.in/pdf/material/202004281117017c7cf77413.pdf
4 Source of the question: https://brainly.com/question/33658418
5 Source of the question: https://www.assignmentexpert.com/homework-answers/mathematics/statistics-and-probability/question-231620
6 Source of the question: ERIC Notebook (Second Edition) Common Statistical Tests and Applications in Epidemiological Literature
7 Source of the question: https://www.chegg.com/homework-help/questions-and-answers/
8 Sharkey, A. M., Siddiqui, N., Downey, K., Xiang, Y. Y., Guevara, J., & Carvalho, J. C. (2019). Comparison of intermittent intravenous boluses of phenylephrine and norepinephrine to prevent and treat spinal-induced hypotension in cesarean deliveries: randomized controlled trial. *Anesthesia & Analgesia, 129*(5), 1312–1318.
9 This is a type of abnormal rhythm of the heart, which takes place when the heartbeat falls below 60 beats per minute.
10 Phenylephrine is in a class of medications that are used to reduce the swelling of blood vessels in the nasal passages.
11 Norepinephrine is a chemical messenger that transmits nerve signals between nerve cells, muscle cells, and gland cells.
12 Hypochondriasis is an anxiety disorder in which the patient develops an excessive fear that he/she may fall seriously ill.
13 Alternative = 'less' is used in R command for the alternative H_1: $F(\mu) < 0.5$, and alternative = 'two.tailed' is used in R command for the alternative H_1: $F(\mu) \neq 0.5$.
14 This statement of the alternative hypothesis appears in R as default. This is another way of saying that the central values in the two populations differ significantly.
15 For the first command, the user needs to be connected online. The package shall be downloaded, and once the unpacking of the package 'randtest' is over, only then can the next command be used.
16 Note that in the two-sample Kolmogorov-Smirnov test, the two samples may be equal or unequal in size.

References

Braun, W. J. and Murdoch, D. J., 2007. *A first course on statistical programming with R*, Cambridge University Press.

Das, K. K. and Bhattacharjee, D., 2008. *A treatise on statistical inference and distributions*, Asian Books, New Delhi.

Ferguson, T. S., 2014. *Mathematical statistics: A decision theoretic approach* (Vol. 1), Academic Press.

Gibbons, J. D. and Chakraborti, S., 2003. *Nonparametric statistical inference*, Marcel Dekker. Inc. 645pp.

Kale, B. K., 2005. *A first course on parametric inference*, Alpha Science Int'l Ltd.

Lehmann, E. L., 1986. *Testing statistical hypothesis*, John Wiley & Sons.

McNemar, Q., 1947. Note on the sampling error of the difference between correlated proportions or percentages. *Psychometrika, 12*(2), pp.153–157.

Pearson, K., 1900. X. On the criterion that a given system of deviations from the probable in the case of a correlated system of variables is such that it can be reasonably supposed to have arisen from random sampling. *The London, Edinburgh, and Dublin Philosophical Magazine and Journal of Science, 50*(302), pp.157–175.

Schmuller, J., 2017. *Statistical analysis with R for dummies*, John Wiley & Sons.

Siegel, Sidney., 1957. Nonparametric statistics for the behavioral sciences. *The Journal of Nervous and Mental Disease*, 125(3), p.497.

Smirnov, N., 1948. Table for estimating the goodness of fit of empirical distributions. *The Annals of Mathematical Statistics*, 19(2), pp.279–281.

Student, 1908. The probable error of a mean. *Biometrika*, pp.1–25.

Welch, B. L., 1947. The generalization of student's problem when several different population variances are involved. *Biometrika*, 34, pp. 28–35.

Wilcoxon, F., 1945. Individual comparisons by ranking methods. *Biometrics Bulletin*, 1(6), pp.80–83.

PART II

Regression Models

## CHAPTER 6

Regression Analysis Through Illustrations

Amirhossein Jalali and Santosh Kumar Sharma

Learning Outcomes

This chapter equips readers with the ability to understand and apply regression analysis for investigating relationships between variables in health research. Focusing on linear and logistic regression models, learners will explore how to make inferences and predictions from health data. They will gain practical skills in developing models, assessing assumptions, analyzing categorical predictors, and evaluating model performance. Additionally, learners will learn how to effectively communicate regression findings using tools such as nomograms, translating statistical results into meaningful insights for clinicians, policymakers, and other health professionals.

Introduction

The term *'regression'* literally means stepping back towards the average. Regression analysis was first developed by Sir Francis Galton in the 19th century as a statistical method used to investigate and model relationships between variables. Regression is now a popular tool that plays a key role in understanding relationships between variables, identifying risk factors and predicting an outcome of interest across a wide range of disciplines, including the social sciences, medicine, public health, and biomedical sciences. Nowadays, it is a fundamental tool for understanding patterns, discovering interesting information, and making informed decisions. For example, it can be used to assess the risk of cancer for men suspected of prostate cancer based on available risk factors such as age, family history of cancer, their digital rectal examination and prostate specific antigen test, or investigating the impact of factors (such as age, gender, income level, access to healthy food options, and physical activity) affecting obesity rates in a community to inform targeted interventions and policies.

Regression has two main purposes: 1. explaining the relationships between variables and 2. developing predictive models for predicting an unknown outcome of interest

DOI: 10.4324/9781032701004-8

based on available relevant data. In health science, regression is crucial to identify risk factors, predict patient outcomes, and understand biological functions.

There are two types of variables used in regression analysis: the *response variable* (also called a *dependent variable* or *outcome*), which is the main variable of interest and can be explained by other available information; and the *explanatory variable* (also called an *independent variable* or *predictor*), which is used to explain or predict variations in the response variable.

This chapter includes the following sections: *Association and correlation*, which explores the relationships between variables graphically using scatterplots, correlation coefficients, and interpreting associations. This provides a foundation for future sections. *Linear regression model*, which covers the principles of linear regression with a focus on explaining and formulating the relationship between variables, in particular, the methodology for estimating a straight line that best fits the observed data, including the theoretical basis, practical model development, and interpretation. This will be expanded to include relationships between multiple variables. *Logistic regression model*, which is a generalised version of linear regression models to explore the relationship between a binary outcome of interest and one or more independent variables. *Communicating a regression model*, which discusses the importance of clearly communicating regression model results in practice to different audiences. Practical tools for facilitating this communication are also discussed and illustrated.

NFHS-5 Case Study

The National Family Health Survey (NFHS-5) in India (IIPS/India and ICF Macro 2021) has been used in this chapter as a case study. The study population includes male and female participants aged 15–49 years who took a survey from 2019 to 2021 in Kerala, India. The Kerala Estate in India is in a relatively advanced epidemiological transition, and the increasing proportion of older adults and the adoption of sedentary lifestyles in Kerala is attributed to an increase in non-communicable diseases (Sarma et al. 2019; Sharma et al. 2022; Negi et al. 2022).

Kerala data is publicly available on the DHS website (IIPS/India and ICF Macro 2021), where various demographic and health-related risk factors were collected as part of this study. To simplify the examples, 500 randomly selected samples of Kerala data will be used as illustrations throughout this chapter.

We aim to investigate systolic blood pressure (SBP) and the risk of hypertension in this cohort and explain their variability relative to demographic and lifestyle variables, such as age, gender, diastolic blood pressure (DBP), body mass index (BMI), and alcohol consumption. Table 6.1 shows a summary of the characteristics of the participants in terms of the variables used in this chapter.

Association and Correlation

The relationship between two continuous variables is usually summarised graphically using a scatterplot or numerically using correlation coefficients. Typically, there is a variable of interest known as the outcome variable (Y), and the focus is on whether another continuous variable (X) can provide information about it. This is known as

Table 6.1 Characteristics of the 500 random participants from the NFHS-5 study

		Total	Hypertension	
		N = 500[1]	No, N = 434[1]	Yes, N = 66[1]
Age				
	15–24	137 (27%)	131 (30%)	6 (9.1%)
	25–34	121 (24%)	112 (26%)	9 (14%)
	35+	242 (48%)	191 (44%)	51 (77%)
Gender				
	Male	44 (8.8%)	38 (8.8%)	6 (9.1%)
	Female	456 (91.0%)	396 (91%)	60 (91%)
Body mass index (kg/m2)		23.5 (20.7, 26.3)	23.3 (20.5, 25.7)	25.2 (22.8, 27.7)
Alcohol consumption				
	No	495 (99.0%)	431 (99.3%)	64 (97.0%)
	Yes	5 (1.0%)	3 (0.7%)	2 (3.0%)
Systolic blood pressure (mmHg)		113.0 (103.5, 123.6)		
Diastolic blood pressure (mmHg)		76.5 (70.0, 82.5)		

[1] n (%); Median (IQR)

association, in which Y is plotted in the vertical direction in the scatterplot to illustrate how it changes as X (plotted on the x-axis) changes.

The relationship (or correlation) between two continuous variables is considered strong if there is a clear pattern between the variables. The pattern can be linear, where an imaginary straight line can roughly explain the pattern, or non-linear, where a more complex pattern can be described. In contrast, a weak relationship refers to cases where there may be some degree of relationship between the two variables, but they appear unconnected, which makes it difficult to determine any recognisable pattern.

For example, Figure 6.1 shows the relationship between two continuous variables in four different scenarios. Figure 6.1 (a) shows a strong positive relationship between two continuous variables, where an increase in one variable tends (on average) to be associated with an increase in another. Given that this relationship can be explained by a straight line, it is known as a linear relationship. The relationship between the two variables in Figure 6.1 (b) is still evident; however, it is not as strong as the previous one in Figure 6.1 (a). This is an example of a weak negative relationship, where an increase in one variable tends (on average) to be associated with a decrease in another variable. Figure 6.1 (c) shows no obvious relationship between the two variables simply because the points are scattered randomly around the horizontal line of zero, indicating that a change in one variable does not affect the other variable. Figure 6.1 (d) illustrates an example in which there is a clear relationship between two variables that cannot be explained by a straight line. This is usually referred to as a non-linear relationship, where the rate of increase or decrease does not remain constant, and the direction of the relationship may even change as it approaches specific points.

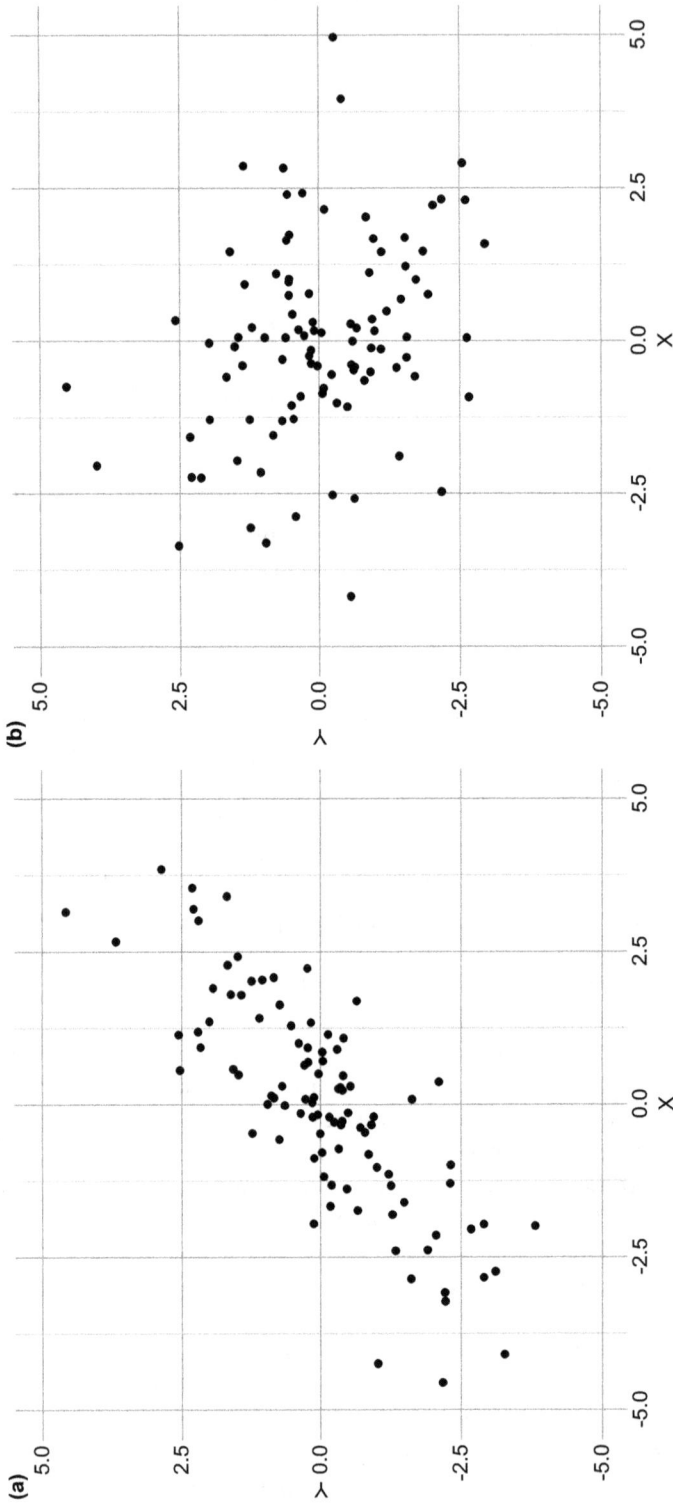

Figure 6.1 Four different types of relationships between two continuous variables: (a) a strong positive relationship, (b) a weak negative relationship, (c) no evident relationship, and (d) a non-linear relationship.

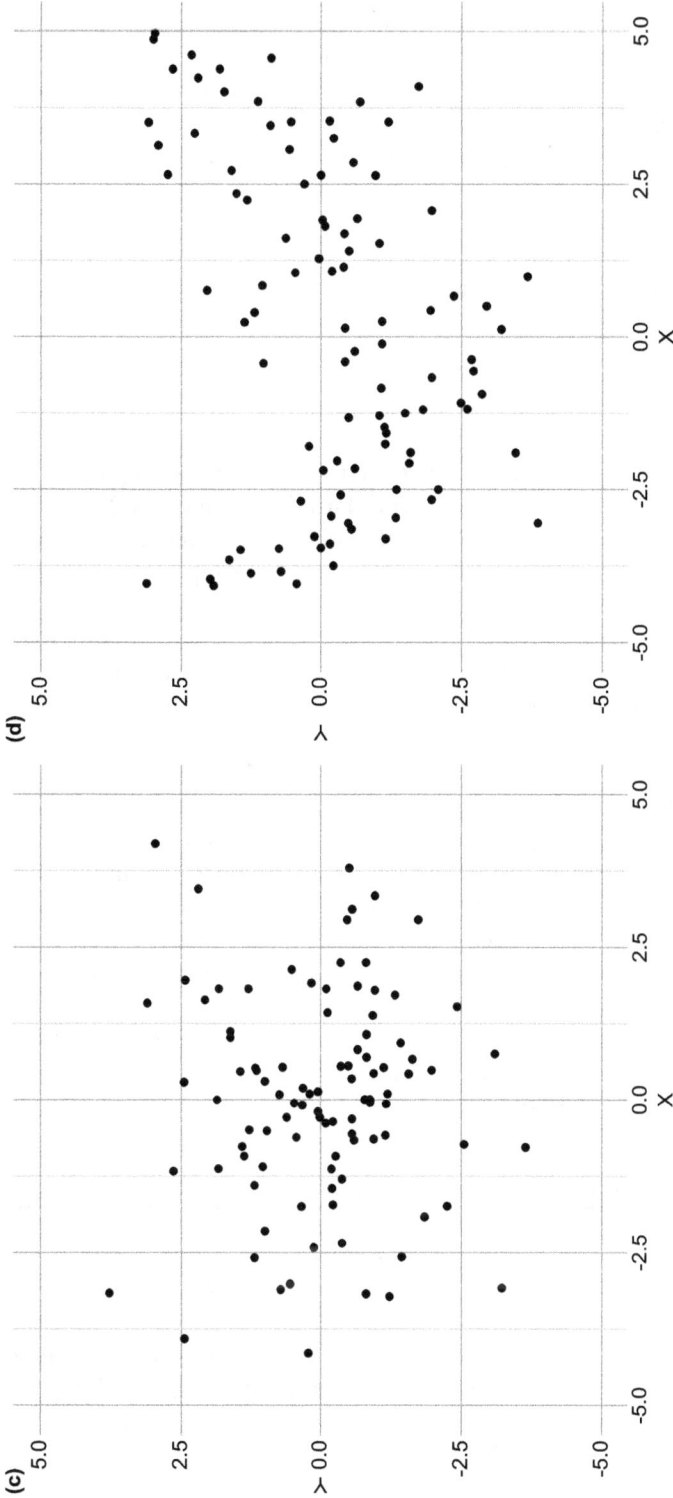

Figure 6.1 (Continued)

The *Pearson correlation coefficient* (denoted by r) is a numerical measure indicating the strength and direction of a linear relationship (or correlation) between two normally distributed continuous variables. A correlation coefficient ranges from –1 to +1, where 0 indicates no linear correlation between variables, and as the value deviates from zero, it indicates a higher degree of correlation between variables. A negative value indicates a negative linear correlation, whereas a positive one indicates a positive linear correlation. Therefore, a correlation coefficient provides an indication of whether and how two variables change with respect to each other.

The correlation coefficient between two variables, X and Y, is denoted by $r(X, Y)$ or simply r_{xy}, and it is defined as follows:

$$r_{xy} = \frac{Cov(X,Y)}{\sigma_X \sigma_Y} \tag{1}$$

where $Cov(X,Y)$ is the covariance between X and Y measuring the joint variability of two variables, and σ_X and σ_Y are the standard deviation of the X and Y variables.

The following (see Table 6.2) cut-off points for correlation coefficient values are recommended to determine the strength of a relationship in medical research (Hinkle, Wiersma, and Jurs 2003; Mukaka 2012).

As mentioned previously, the correlation coefficient is a measure of the strength of a linear relationship and cannot adequately reflect the strength of (even strong) non-linear patterns. An example of such a situation is seen in Figure 6.1 (d). In addition, it is important to note that the correlation coefficient is sensitive to outliers, making it more appropriate to use for data without outliers. In the presence of outliers, it is useful to estimate and compare correlations with and without outliers to see the impact the presence of outliers has on the value of the correlation coefficient.

In contrast to the Pearson correlation (i.e., formula 1), assuming variables are normally distributed, a *Spearman rank correlation* (commonly denoted by ρ) describes the monotonic relationship between two variables. Therefore, the Spearman correlation is relatively robust to outliers and can be used for non-normally distributed continuous data and ordinal data such as Likert scale variables (Schober et al. 2018).

Hypothesis tests can be used to investigate whether an estimated correlation coefficient shows a linear relationship between two variables, while taking sample size and estimation uncertainty into account.

Table 6.2. Correlation coefficient rule of thumb

Correlation coefficient (r)	Interpretation
0.9 to 1.0 (–0.9 to –1.0)	Very strong positive (negative) linear relationship
0.7 to 0.9 (–0.7 to –0.9)	Strong positive (negative) linear relationship
0.5 to 0.7 (–0.5 to –0.7)	Moderate positive (negative) linear relationship
0.3 to 0.5 (–0.3 to –0.5)	Weak positive (negative) linear relationship
0.0 to 0.3 (0.0 to –0.3)	Negligible linear relationship

The hypothesis test determines whether the unknown population correlation coefficient is zero ($H_0 : r = 0$), meaning there is no linear correlation, or there is a level of linear correlation between two continuous variables ($H_1 : r \neq 0$). The following t-test statistics follow the t-distribution with $n - 2$ degrees of freedom

$$t = r\sqrt{\frac{n-2}{1-r^2}} \tag{2}$$

Using statistical software (e.g., the cor.test()function in R), a *p*-value can be calculated, and a decision can be made. In the case of a very small *p*-value (usually defined as < 0.05), a linear relationship between two variables is detected, and its direction and strength can be determined depending on the value of the correlation coefficient.

Larger sample sizes generally provide more precise estimates of the population correlation coefficient, and there is a stronger likelihood of rejecting the hypothesis that the unknown correlation coefficient is equal to zero; however, this does not necessarily indicate the presence of a strong linear relationship. We also need to look at the magnitude of the estimated correlation coefficient to assess the strength of the correlation.

A final note is that a significant correlation between two variables may indicate an association but does not necessarily imply causation. Even in the case of identifying a highly significant and strong correlation, there could be unidentified variables that may confound the results (known as confounding variables). A causal relationship can only be determined in controlled study designs (e.g., randomized control trials), when subjects are randomly assigned to receive interventions.

Figure 6.2 summarises the distribution of systolic blood pressure and its variability across different age groups in the NFHS-5 case study. It can be seen that the age group '15–24 years old' and '25–34 years old' have almost similar medians and variability, but those in the age group '35 years old and above' have a higher median (about 10 mmHg) and slightly higher variability.

Initially, we will focus on quantifying the relationship between these two variables and investigating whether a change in diastolic blood pressure is associated with changes in systolic blood pressure. Later, we will take into account other relevant risk factors, such as age, sex, body mass index, and alcohol consumption, in order to explain the variation in systolic blood pressure in the context of Kerala, India.

A good way of describing a relationship between two variables, X and Y, is to visualise the variability of Y as X changes, examining the pattern of the (X, Y) points. In the scatterplot, we can observe how SBP values on the vertical axis are scattered for a given value on the x-axis.

Figure 6.3 illustrates a scatterplot of SBP (as the outcome to study on the vertical axis) and DBP (as the variable under consideration on the horizontal axis). We observe that the dots form an ellipse with the major axis pointing upwards towards the right, indicating that systolic blood pressure increases as the diastolic blood pressure increases.

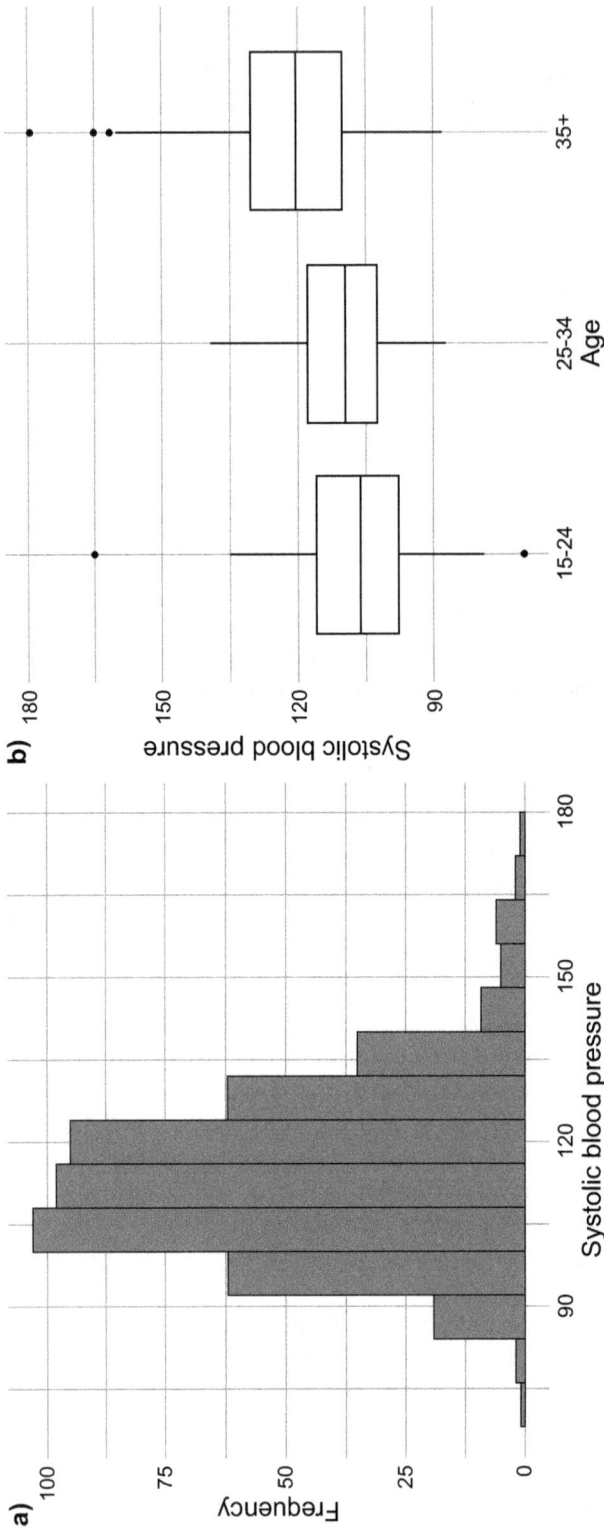

Figure 6.2 a) A distribution of systolic blood pressure and b) the distribution of systolic blood pressure across three age groups of 15 to 24, 25 to 34, and 35 years old and older.

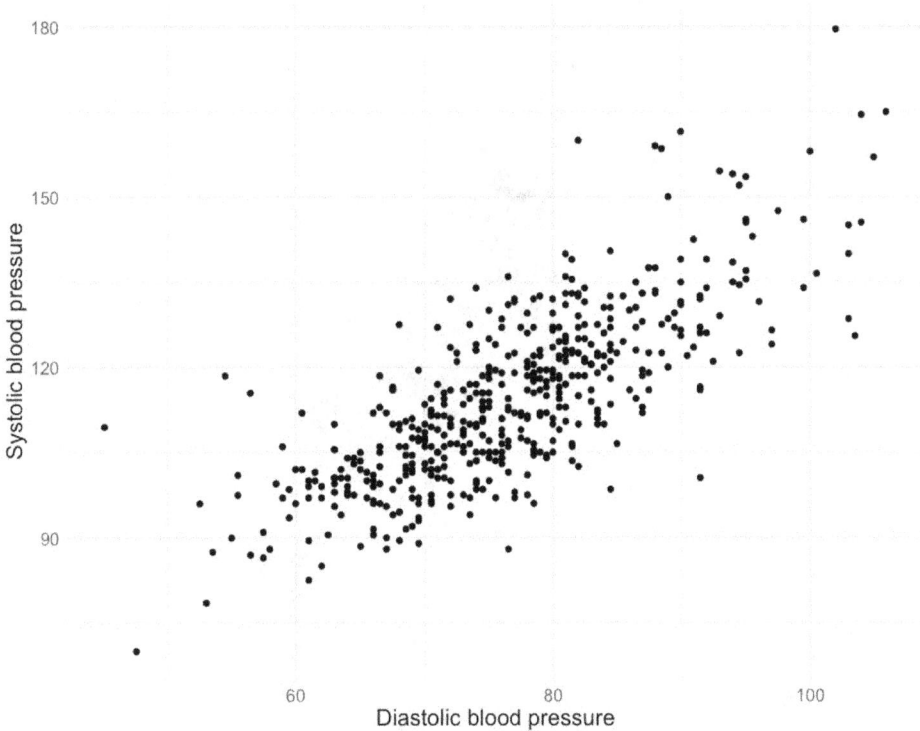

Figure 6.3 Scatterplot of systolic blood pressure and diastolic blood pressure.

The positive relationship between SBP and DBP can be examined separately for males and females. As shown in Figure 6.4, similar relationships exist for males and females, although the male sample size is relatively small, indicating considerable uncertainty.

The correlation coefficient between systolic blood pressure and diastolic blood pressure is estimated to be 0.81 for males and 0.77 for females. The p-values of < 0.001 are estimated for hypothesis tests to investigate whether the estimated correlation coefficients indicate significant linear relationships between systolic blood pressure and diastolic blood pressure among males and females.

Linear Regression Model

Once a reasonably moderate linear relationship has been identified between two variables (e.g., the relationship between systolic blood pressure and diastolic blood pressure in Figure 6.3), it would be helpful to summarise this relationship using a straight line. A straight line is a mathematical function representing the relationship between two variables, providing a summary of the variation of one variable relative to another.

A straight line is an appropriate means of summarising a linear relationship between two variables only when there is an underlying linear relationship.

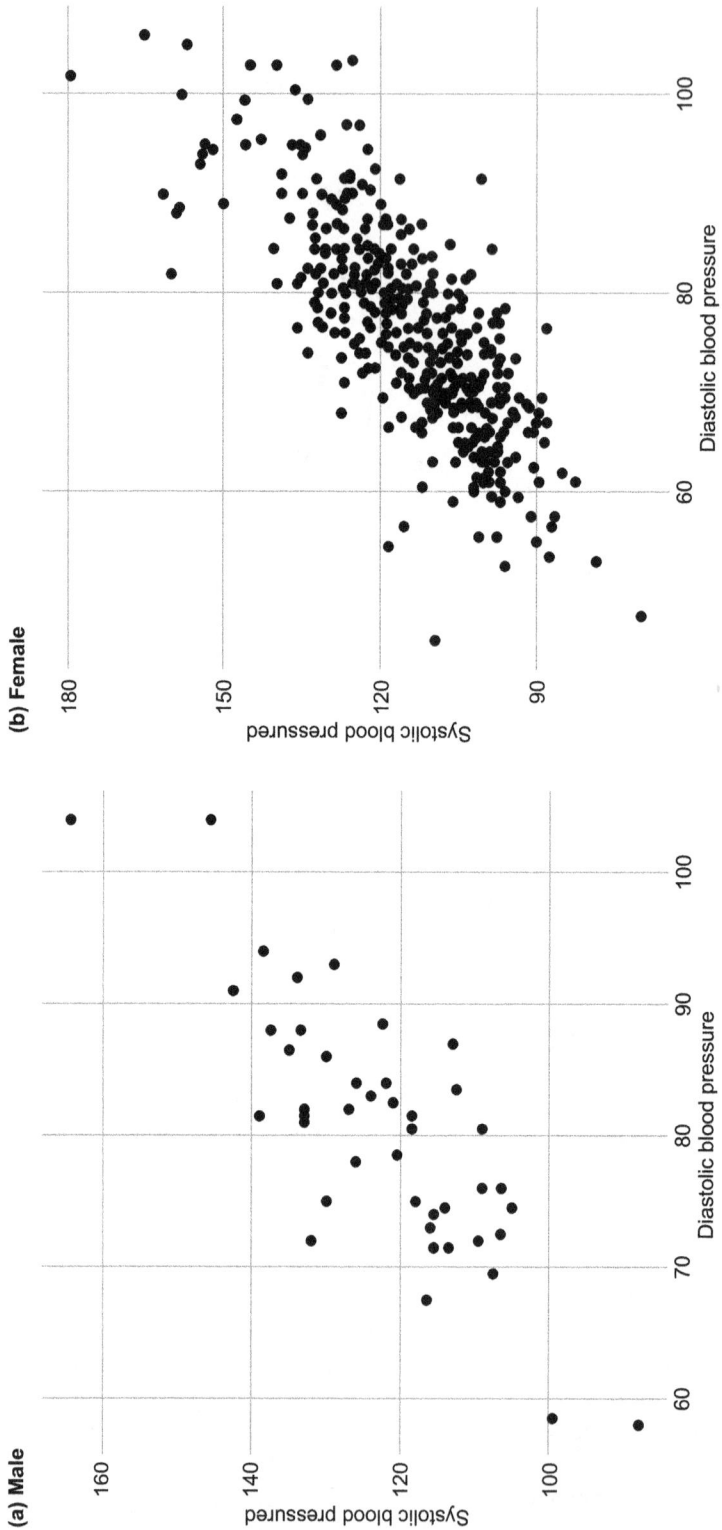

Figure 6.4 Scatterplot of systolic blood pressure and diastolic blood pressure for males (in a) and females (in b).

For a reasonably valid approximation, the scatterplot should satisfy the following conditions:

- **Linearity:** the scatterplot indicates a linear pattern among the data points.
- **Constant variability:** the variability of each variable remains relatively constant as another variable changes.
- **Independent observations:** observations are independent of each other, meaning that one observation does not affect the other. There should be, for example, no repeated observations in time or multiple measurements of the same subject.

In addition, the differences between observations and the fitted line should follow an approximately normal distribution. For relatively large sample sizes, it is generally acceptable if this distribution is reasonably symmetric. These assumptions provide a foundation for a class of methods known as regression, which form the basis of this chapter and will be further discussed in this section.

In the NFHS-5 study, it is reasonable to assume independent observations since each individual's data is measured independently, and no underlying structure, such as sequential observations, exists. In the scatterplot of SPB and DBP in Figure 6.3, there is an approximate linear pattern of data points, which is sufficient to explain the relationship between SPB and DBP using a straight line.

Figure 6.5 shows a straight line added to the scatterplot to summarise the relationship between SPB and DBP. This straight line also referred to as a regression line and includes two parameters:

- *slope*, which reflects the direction and magnitude of a relationship, and
- *intercept*, which determine the response variable when the explanatory variable is equal to zero, ensuring the estimate is unbiased.

For example, a positive slope estimated for the line in Figure 6.5 indicates a positive relationship between SPB and DBP variables, where an increase in DBP value is associated with an increase in SPB. In contrast, a negative slope would indicate a negative relationship between two variables. The magnitude of the slope indicates the level at which an increase in DBP is expected to suggest an increase in SPB.

The term regression generally refers to a set of statistical methods used to numerically explain the relationship between two or more variables through a mathematical equation. It provides a more informative way of summarising a relationship than through a visual representation, such as a scatterplot. We will initially focus on *linear regression models* as being the simplest regression type and the most commonly used across various research domains.

A linear regression model (Agresti 2015) can be described in the following general format:

$$\hat{Y} = a + bX + \varepsilon \tag{3}$$

where:
- X is the explanatory variable (which can be both numeric and categorical),
- Y is the observed response,

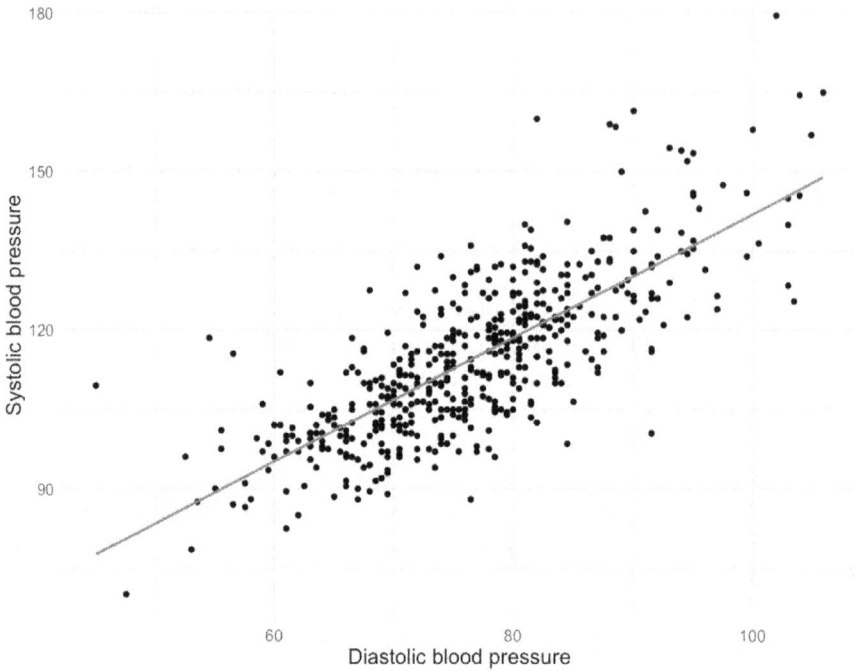

Figure 6.5 Scatterplot of systolic blood pressure and diastolic blood pressure with fitted straight line summarising the relationship between the two variables.

- a is a parameter known as intercept, representing the point where the line crosses the vertical axis (also the expected value of Y when the value of the explanatory variable is zero),
- b is a parameter known as slope; representing the angle or orientation of the line (reflecting the direction of the underlying relationship), and
- ε is the regression residual.

Fitting a regression model involves determining the regression parameters (slope and intercept) that best fit the data. A common approach known as the least squares method is to find optimal parameter values that minimise the difference between observed responses (y) and the estimated responses (denoted by $\hat{y}$) from the regression line (known as regression residuals, representing the random variability that cannot be explained by the explanatory variables). The least squares estimation and the related inferential procedures are limited to models in the form of (3), where the response variable is continuous and the residuals are assumed to be normally distributed.

The main variable of interest in the NFHS-5 study is systolic blood pressure as the response variable and diastolic blood pressure as the explanatory variable. Table 6.3 represents a summary of a regression model fitted to this dataset to describe the variability in SBP given the information in DBP.

Table 6.3 Linear regression of systolic blood pressure (mmHg) on diastolic blood pressure

	Coefficient	95% confidence interval	p-value
(Intercept)	24.99	18.46, 31.52	< 0.001
Diastolic blood pressure (mmHg)	1.17	1.08, 1.25	< 0.001
Sample size	500		
R²	0.598		

The regression parameters (or coefficients) are estimated using R software, with the intercept at 24.99 and the slope at 1.17. This means the estimated regression line between SBP and DBP can be expressed as follows:

$$\widehat{SBP} = 24.99 + (1.17 * DBP)$$

A slope of 1.17 is estimated for the effect of DBP on SPB, suggesting that for every one-unit increase in diastolic blood pressure, systolic blood pressure is expected to increase (on average) by 1.17 units (mmHg). The 95% confidence interval of 1.08 to 1.25 indicates that the estimated increase could be as low as 1.08 mmHg or as high as 1.25 mmHg. Overall, a p-value of less than 0.001 for slope suggests strong evidence against the null hypothesis that there is no effect of DBP on SBP.

A regression line represents the expected mean of the response variable for a given observation, and there is, of course, some degree of uncertainty associated with estimations. The residual provides a measure of the degree to which a line fits individual data points. Each residual, as indicated in Figure 6.6 (a), is simply represented by the vertical distance between the observation in the scatterplot and the predicted value on the regression line. Data points appear to be scattered randomly around the line, and residual variation remains roughly constant across different levels of DBP. In addition, the residual distribution in Figure 6.6 (b) shows an approximately normal distribution.

Most evaluation metrics for assessing whether the regression model fits the data well rely on the analysis of residuals. Two commonly used metrics for assessing regression fit and predictive accuracy of linear regression models are mean squared error (MSE) and R-squared (R2).

Mean squared error (MSE) measure (Wallach and Goffinet 1989) is the average of the squares of regression residuals, where the magnitude of each residual is taken into account. A lower MSE represents a closer match between the observed responses and the estimated responses, indicating better overall performance.

R-squared (R2) measure (Lewis-Beck and Skalaban 1990) is the proportion of variation in the response variable that is explained by the fitted regression line. R-squared ranges from 0 to 1, where a value closer to 1 suggests a better model fit to the data. With only one explanatory variable in the regression model, R-squared is simply calculated as the square of the correlation coefficient between the explanatory variable and the response variable. In the case of having several explanatory variables, it is quantified as the variation in the estimated responses ($\hat{Y}$) relative to the variation in the observed responses (Y).

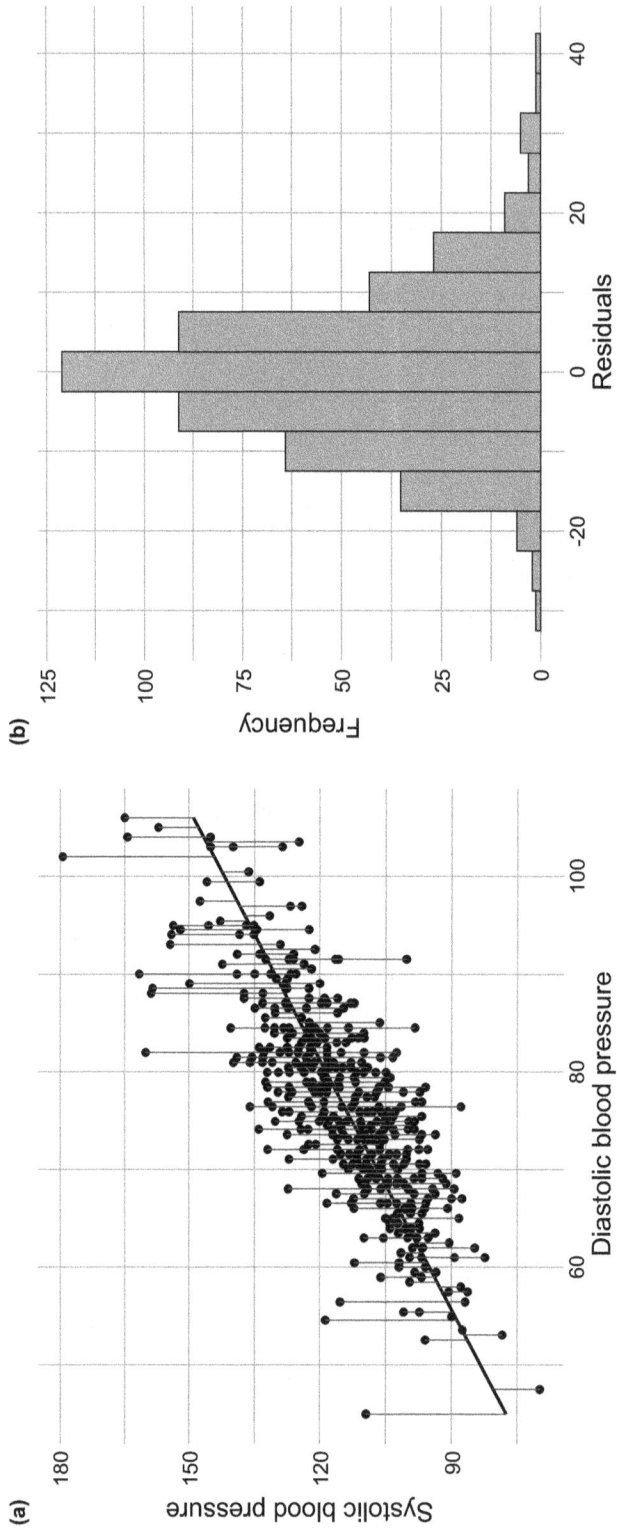

Figure 6.6 (a) Scatterplot of systolic blood pressure and diastolic blood pressure with fitted regression line and regression residuals displayed and (b) the distribution of the residuals.

The estimated R-squared of 0.598 in Table 6.3 indicates the fitted regression model can explain approximately 60% of systolic blood pressure variability. This implies that diastolic blood pressure alone can account for nearly two-thirds of the variability of systolic blood pressure.

MSE and R-squared are informative metrics for evaluating the performance of a regression model, in particular, when there are several explanatory variables. They provide an effective means of comparing two fitted models and identifying any additional goodness of fit as a result of incorporating any of the explanatory variables.

Multiple Linear Regression

A simple linear regression model allows us to explain a response variable based on a given explanatory variable. A limitation of such a model is that a single explanatory variable is rarely adequate for analyzing real-world behavior. This is a major disadvantage in the context of causal analysis. In many cases, there might be an interest to investigate associations between several explanatory variables and the response variable. A generalised version of linear regression, known as multiple linear regression, enables us to incorporate a combination of explanatory variables into a model for explaining the variation of a response variable.

Multiple linear regression (Madsen and Thyregod 2011) is expressed in the following format:

$$Y = a + b_1 X_1 + b_2 X_2 + b_3 X_3 + \ldots + b_n X_n + \varepsilon \tag{4}$$

where X_i s are the explanatory variables, a is the model intercept, b_i s are the regression coefficients, Y is the observed response (while $\hat{Y}$ denotes the expected value of the response variable based on given explanatory variables), and ε is the residual. Software packages that estimate regression coefficients of linear regression models (i.e., lm() function in R) also provide regression coefficient estimation for multiple regression models.

Before building a multiple linear regression model, the following assumptions need to be verified:

1. **Linearity**: there are linear relationships between the response variable and each continuous explanatory variable.
2. **Independence**: observations are independent of each other.
3. **Normality**: regression residuals, i.e., the differences between the observed response (Y) and the expected value of the response variable ($\hat{Y}$) are approximately normally distributed.
4. **Constant variability**: a constant variation of residuals is observed throughout the response variable.

In the NFHS-5 study, it is interesting to explore the impact of other explanatory factors on systolic blood pressure. R software (i.e., the lm() function in R) is used to estimate the regression coefficients, and Table 6.4 represents the summary of a multiple regression model for systolic blood pressure using several explanatory variables, such as body mass index (kg/m²), gender (male, female), age (15–24 years old, 25–34 years old, 35+ years old), and alcohol consumption (yes, no).

Using the estimated regression coefficients, the multiple regression model can be expressed as follows:

$$\widehat{SBP} = 33.68 + (1.06 * DBP) + (0.01 * BMI) + (-4.62 * Gender_{female})$$
$$+ (1.99 * Age_{25-34}) + (6.04 * Age_{\geq35}) + (2.42 * Alcohol_{yes})$$

The coefficient estimated as 1.06 for diastolic blood pressure appears to be slightly different from the slope estimated as 1.17 in Table 6.3, and this is the result of adjusting for the effect of other variables, such as BMI, gender, age, and alcohol consumption. The estimated coefficient suggests that, on average, for every one-unit increase in diastolic blood pressure, systolic blood pressure increases by 1.06 units, assuming other variables remain unchanged. The effect of a one-unit change in BMI is estimated at as small as a 0.01 mmHg change in SBP, which is not statistically significant (p > 0.90), indicating no relationship between the two variables.

For a categorical variable with two levels (such as gender with male and female levels), interpreting the coefficients is fairly straightforward, as it represents the average response when switching between the two categories. For example, the estimated −4.62 for $Gender_{female}$ suggests that females, on average, have 4.62 mmHg lower systolic blood pressure than males, assuming other variables are equal.

When categorical variables have more than two levels (such as age classified into '15 to 24 years old', '25 to 34 years old', and 'above 35 years old'), interpretation requires knowledge of which level is considered as the reference level. Here, the age group '15 to 24 years old' is defined as the reference group, and the effects of switching to the age group '25 to 34 years old' and 'above 35 years old' are estimated as 1.99 and 6.04, respectively. This indicates that those aged between 25 and 34 years old have systolic blood pressure that is 1.99 mmHg higher than those aged between 15 and 24 years old

Table 6.4 Multiple linear regression of systolic blood pressure on diastolic blood pressure and adjusted for age, gender, BMI, and alcohol consumption

	Coefficient	95% confidence interval	p-value
(Intercept)	33.68	25.76, 41.60	< 0.001
Diastolic blood pressure (mmHg)	1.06	0.98, 1.15	< 0.001
Age (15–24 years old)			
25–34 years old	1.99	−0.39, 4.37	0.100
35+ years old	6.04	3.85, 8.24	< 0.001
Gender (Male)			
Female	−4.62	−7.63, −1.60	0.003
Body mass index (kg/m²)	0.01	−0.20, 0.21	0.960
Alcohol consumption (No)			
Yes	2.42	−6.05, 10.90	0.600
Sample size	500		
Adjusted R²	0.626		

on average. A larger difference of 6.04 mmHg is expected when comparing the systolic blood pressure of those aged above 35 years old with those aged between 15 and 24 years old. The reference level for a categorical variable can be specified explicitly in the software (e.g., relevel() function in R) to facilitate meaningful interpretation.

Lastly, the effect of alcohol consumption on SBP compared to no alcohol consumption is calculated as 2.42 mmHg, which indicates that alcohol consumers have (on average) 2.42 mmHg higher systolic blood pressure. However, there is not enough evidence to support a significant relationship. In fact, the effect size could even be reversed due to the huge uncertainties involved (estimated confidence interval of –6.05 to 10.90).

Overall, the results suggest that diastolic blood pressure, gender, and age are significantly associated with systolic blood pressure, while BMI and alcohol consumption appear to not be associated with systolic blood pressure.

For assessing the goodness of fit of multiple linear regressions, and whether the inclusion of additional explanatory variables improves the fit of the model, a modified version of R-squared, known as adjusted R-squared, can be used.

Adjusted R-squared (Lewis-Beck and Skalaban 1990) is a commonly used metric for assessing the goodness of fit of multiple linear regressions and for determining whether the inclusion of additional explanatory variables improves the fit of the model. It is a modified version of the R-squared, taking into account the uncertainty arising from additional regression parameter estimation and has the same way of interpretation as the R-squared.

The adjusted R2 value of the fitted multiple regression model in Table 6.4 (i.e., 0.631) shows a slight improvement compared to the R2 value in Table 6.3 (i.e., 0.598). This indicates that the inclusion of age, gender, BMI, and alcohol consumption into the model may explain more of the variability in systolic blood pressure (i.e., 63.1%); however, most of the variation (i.e., 59.8%) is explained by just one variable, i.e., diastolic blood pressure.

Logistic Regression Model

A limitation of linear regression models is the assumption of a normally distributed response variable, and therefore normally distributed regression residuals. An extended family of regression models, known as the generalised linear models (GLM) (Dobson and Barnett 2018; McCullagh and Nelder 1989), are available to model response variables that are not continuous or cannot be considered normally distributed.

The generalised linear model has two components:

1. the probability distribution of the response variable; and
2. the equation (known as link function) connecting the mean of the response variable to a linear combination of the explanatory variables.

Logistic regression model is one of the special cases of GLM models for modeling a binary response variable, which, due to its simplicity, interpretability, and effectiveness, is widely used for risk assessment and decision-making processes across different domains.

In health and public health research, as in other fields, it is quite common to study a binary response variable, such as the presence or absence of a disease, such as cancer, whether a person has received a vaccine (yes or no), the presence or absence of side effects from a medication, whether a person has ceased smoking or not, or the presence or absence of a genetic mutation. All these variables have two possible conditions, and similar to multiple linear regression, it may be interesting to investigate the relationship between one or a set of explanatory variables with this binary response variable.

There are many measures to estimate the strength of the correlation between a binary variable and risk factors. One typical measure in medical research is formed from the ratio of odds among two groups. The odds of an event (Y) occurring is defined as the ratio between the probability of the event occurring (i.e., $p(Y)$) and the probability of it not occurring (i.e., $1 - p(Y)$). The $Odds = p(Y)/1 - p(Y)$. So the *odds ratio* (OR) is defined as the ratio between the odds of an event occurring in one group compared to another, as follows:

$$Odds\,ratio = \frac{odds(Y_1)}{odds(Y_2)} = \frac{\dfrac{p(Y_1)}{1 - p(Y_1)}}{\dfrac{p(Y_2)}{1 - p(Y_2)}} \tag{5}$$

Unlike linear regression models (see[4]) that estimate the mean response, logistic regression models quantify the probability that a binary response will occur using a logarithmic transformation of the odds of the response occurring (known as the logit link function). The logit link function ensures that the predicted probabilities fall within the range of 0 and 1.

Logistic regression has the following structure, where the explanatory variables $(X_i s)$ can be quantitative (numeric) or categorical variables:

$$\text{logit}\big[p(Y)\big] = \ln\left[\frac{p(Y)}{1 - p(Y)}\right] = a + b_1 X_1 + b_2 X_2 + \ldots + b_n X_n \tag{6}$$

where $p(Y)$ is the probability (equivalent to the expected proportion) of the condition of interest occurring given the explanatory variables, a is the model intercept, and b_i s are the regression coefficients representing the strength and direction of the relationship between the independent variables and the log odds of the binary outcome. Software packages (such as glm() function in R) are available to estimate regression coefficients for logistic regression models.

In the logistic regression model, the estimates of regression coefficients are typically interpreted in terms of odds ratios for the given explanatory variable compared to another, where the odds ratios are computed through the exponentiation of the regression coefficient. It can be used to determine whether a modifying risk factor has a particular impact on a binary outcome of interest. Since the odds ratio is a ratio of a measure for two different groups:

■ OR = 1 indicates no difference in the odds of event occurring between the two groups,

- OR > 1 indicates the odds of event occurring is higher in group 1 compared to group 2, and
- OR < 1 indicates the odds of event occurring is lower in group 1 compared to group 2.

Hypertension is another variable of interest in the NFHS-5 study, in which it would be interesting to explore how variables such as body mass index, sex, age, and alcohol consumption influence its prevalence. According to the WHO guidelines (World Health Organization 2011), hypertension can be diagnosed if systolic blood pressure is greater than 140 mmHg, diastolic blood pressure is greater than 90 mmHg, and/or an individual is currently using anti-hypertensive medication. Hypertension is coded as 'Yes' (presence of hypertension) and 'No' (absence of hypertension), which is a binary variable. The logistic regression model can be used to investigate its associations with selected explanatory variables, and a summary of the fitted logistic regression is shown in Table 6.5.

As already mentioned, the impact of explanatory variables is usually explained through the interpretation of odds ratios. In the case of categorical variables, the choice of reference level is particularly important, as it serves as a basis for comparing with the other categories. For example, as the reference level for gender is set as 'Male', the corresponding odds ratio for 'Female' indicates the odds of hypertension for females relative to males.

In Table 6.5, the odds ratio for females is estimated as 1.09, which indicates that the odds of hypertension among females are about 9% higher than in males. However, the estimated 95% confidence interval of (0.41, 3.59) is wide and contains 1, indicating a high degree of uncertainty in the odds ratio estimate, and the p-value is $0.9 > 0.05$. The estimated odds ratio of 1.38 (for '25–34 years old') suggests the odds of hypertension for those in the age group 25 to 34 years old are expected to be approximately 40% higher than those aged between 15 and 24 years old (as the reference level). Considering the 95% confidence interval for this estimate and the p-value of 0.6, this does not indicate a significant difference between the odds for two groups. Additionally, the odds of hypertension for those over 35 years old are expected to be more than four times the

Table 6.5 Logistic regression for risk of hypertension of systolic blood pressure on diastolic blood pressure and adjusted for age, gender, BMI, and alcohol consumption

	Odds ratio	95% confidence interval	p-value
(Intercept)	0.01	0.00, 0.06	< 0.001
Gender (Male)			
Female	1.09	0.41, 3.59	0.900
Age (15–24 years old)			
25–34 years old	1.38	0.47, 4.33	0.600
35+ years old	4.37	1.88, 12.0	0.002
Body mass index (kg/m²)	1.07	1.01, 1.14	0.031
Alcohol consumption (No)			
Yes	4.82	0.50, 38.0	0.140
Sample size	500		
Area under curve (AUC) = 0.7153			

odds for those aged between 15 and 24 years old, which indicates a significant difference between the two groups (p-value of 0.002). However, the wide confidence interval of 1.88 to 12.0 suggests that the estimated effect is not precise.

The interpretation of the continuous explanatory variables, on the other hand, is slightly different, where the odds ratio reflects the change in the odds of the event occurring for every unit increase in the explanatory variable. In the case of BMI, for example, the odds ratio is estimated to be 1.07 (see Table 6.5), which indicates that every one-unit increase in BMI is expected to increase the odds of hypertension by 7%.

Once a logistic regression model has been fitted, an evaluation of its performance is essential (Hosmer, Lemeshow, and Sturdivant 2013; Steyerberg et al. 2010). This includes evaluating the following:

- Model discrimination: quantifying how the model stratifies those at high risk from those at low risk, and
- Model calibration: assessing the degree of agreement between the estimated risk and its observed incidence rate.

Several methods are proposed to assess the calibration of a model, of which the Hosmer-Lemes how test (HL) is the most widely used. However, the HL test has been argued to have limited usefulness and low interpretability (Kramer and Zimmerman 2007; Paul, Pennell, and Lemeshow 2013; Nattino, Pennell, and Lemeshow 2020). Alternatively, a simple graphical assessment through the scatterplot of estimated risk and observed incidence is often recommended (Steyerberg et al. 2010).

One of the most widely used measures of discrimination is the area under the receiver operating characteristic (ROC) curve known as the AUC. *Area under the curve* (AUC) (Hanley and McNeil 1982) is a commonly used metric to assess the discriminant ability of a logistic regression model. AUC is an aggregate measure of model performance across all possible classification thresholds in logistic regression models or more generally in diagnostic tests. It evaluates the accuracy of the classification of individuals with and without the outcome of interest.

AUC ranges from 0 to 1, where a higher value indicates a more accurate classification of individuals with and without the outcome of interest. An AUC of 1 indicates an ideal classification, and an AUC of 0.5 indicates that the model is no better than a random guess. The higher the value of AUC, the more accurate the model is at discriminating subjects with and without the outcome of interest. An AUC value of between 0.7 and 0.9 is typically considered moderate, and greater than 0.9 is considered as high accuracy (Fischer, Bachmann, and Jaeschke 2003). The logistic regression model in Table 6.5 has an estimated AUC of 0.72, indicating a moderate accuracy of the model in distinguishing between people with and without hypertension.

Communicating a Regression Model

The importance of communicating statistical findings in an accurate and accessible manner that allows the target audience to use the results in practical settings has been discussed by several authors (Newell et al. 2014; Jalali et al. 2019; McCabe and Newell 2022). Once a regression model has been developed and a good fit has been verified, the question arises of how to communicate such a model in an informative and accessible manner, in particular, to convey the role of explanatory variables on the response. For example, there is an argument when summarising a logistic regression model that a summary expressing the probability of the outcome occurring is more informative than one based on the ratio of odds (Davies, Crombie, and Tavakoli 1998).

The standard way of communicating a regression model (as it has been used in Table 6.4 and Table 6.5) is the use of a model summary table, where the importance of explanatory variables is usually assessed by coefficients of the estimated odds ratios and *p*-values. However, some argue that this might not be the most informative way to present the results of a model and answer typical questions such as '*Which explanatory variable has the biggest effect on response?*' or '*How would the response variable affect by changes in modifiable risk factors?*' (Newell et al. 2014).

Since the *coefficient effects* are sensitive to the explanatory variables' scale (e.g., minutes, hours and years), and the *p-value* is sensitive to the sample size, assessing the variables' effect sizes may not be straightforward. Several tools have been proposed to facilitate this communication effectively. *Nomograms* (Banks 2006; Allcock 1962) are one such useful tool widely used in various disciplines and play a critical translational role.

A nomogram is simply a calculating tool for a mathematical function used since 1880. They can also be generated for a fitted regression model to facilitate the calculation of a point estimate of the response variable for a particular set of values of the explanatory variables. Nomograms are popular tools used in a variety of studies for risk stratification (Kattan 2003) to assist with clinical decision-making. Examples include the implementation of logistic regression models used for predicting the risk of prostate cancer to inform the need for prostate biopsy (Ankerst et al. 2014; Jalali et al. 2020).

Software such as the rms (Harrell Jr 2024) and DynNom (Jalali et al. 2022) R packages are available to create such nomograms for a developed regression model. Figure 6.7 shows a nomogram for calculating the risk of hypertension based on the logistic regression model fitted in Table 6.5.

The nomogram includes rulers for each explanatory variable, in addition to two rulers for calculating the total points contributing to the estimation of the response variable. The length of each ruler represents the magnitude of each variable's effect size on the response. For example, major contributions to the risk of hypertension are related to whether the subject is in the age group of '35 years old and above' and whether the subject consumes alcohol, which correspond to larger point differentials.

Nomograms also transform regression models into an easy-to-use graphical tool for predicting a response variable. To do this, the values/levels of explanatory variables need to be linked to their corresponding points, and a sum of the points is then mapped from the 'total points' to obtain the 'predicted value', which, in this case (see Figure 6.7), is a probability of hypertension. For example, see the dashed lines in Figure 6.7, which correspond to the points for a 28-year-old female with a BMI of 25 kg/m2 and who does not consume alcohol. These are 13 (Age = '25–34 years old'), 3 (Gender = 'Female'), 43 (BMI = 25), and 0 (Alcohol = 'No'), respectively. Therefore, a total point of 60 (see the solid line) is calculated, which is mapped to the predicted value of approximately 0.075, indicating a 7.5% risk of hypertension in such an individual. Similarly, a 40-year-old female, with a BMI of 25kg/m2 and who consumes alcohol, has an estimated 55% risk of hypertension.

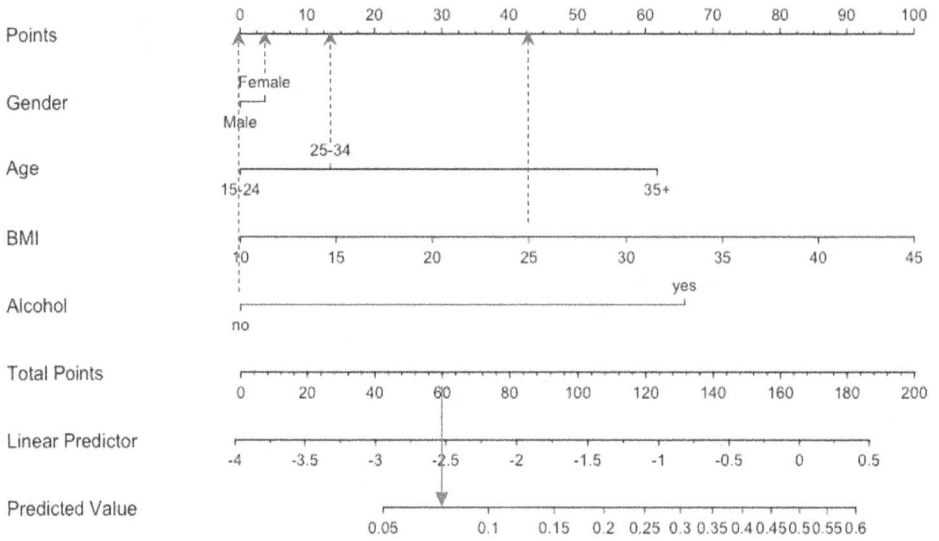

Figure 6.7 Nomograms created using the nomogram()R function in the rms package for calculating the probability of hypertension based on the logistic regression model fitted to the NFHS-5 data.

Static nomograms, such as Figure 6.7, are particularly useful in providing a visual representation of variable importance, represented by the size of their corresponding rulers. It is also a practical tool for using a fitted regression model to make predictions about the response variable. However, they do not communicate the degree of uncertainty associated with the prediction (e.g., confidence interval for prediction). As already discussed, there is a high degree of uncertainty associated with the estimated effect of alcohol consumption.

Recent developments include *dynamic nomograms* (Jalali et al. 2019), which provide a tool for regression models allowing users to interact with them to make predictions, where the associated uncertainty is incorporated in the form of confidence intervals. DynNom package (Jalali et al. 2022) in R generates dynamic nomograms as an interactive application, providing a graphical prediction tool for regression models that quantifies the expected response, along with relevant uncertainty, for a given set of explanatory variables.

Screenshots of a dynamic nomogram for calculating the risk of hypertension using the logistic regression model (in Table 6.5) are displayed in Figure 6.8. The developed application consists of a sidebar panel on the left for entering the values of explanatory variables and a right-hand panel to display the estimated (mean) response for any given set of explanatory values. Numeric explanatory variables appear as sliders (bounded by their observed ranges), and categorical explanatory variables appear as drop-down boxes (including their observed levels). Each error bar represents an estimation accompanied by a 95% confidence interval (quantifying the uncertainty around the estimation) for a given scenario.

Figure 6.8 (a) illustrates the app used to estimate the probability of hypertension with their corresponding 95% confidence intervals in the four scenarios shown in Figure 6.8 (b) in the 'Numerical Summary' tab. For example, the probability of hypertension for a

a)

Dynamic Nomogram

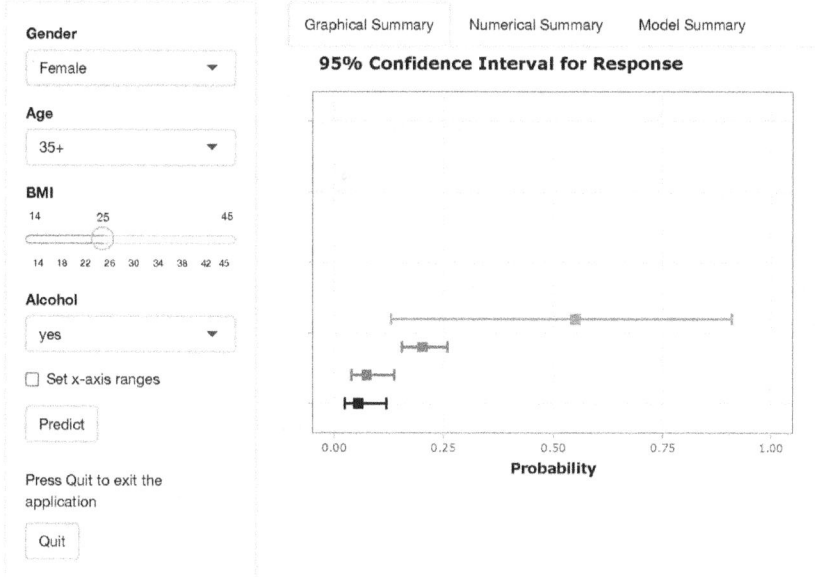

b)

Dynamic Nomogram

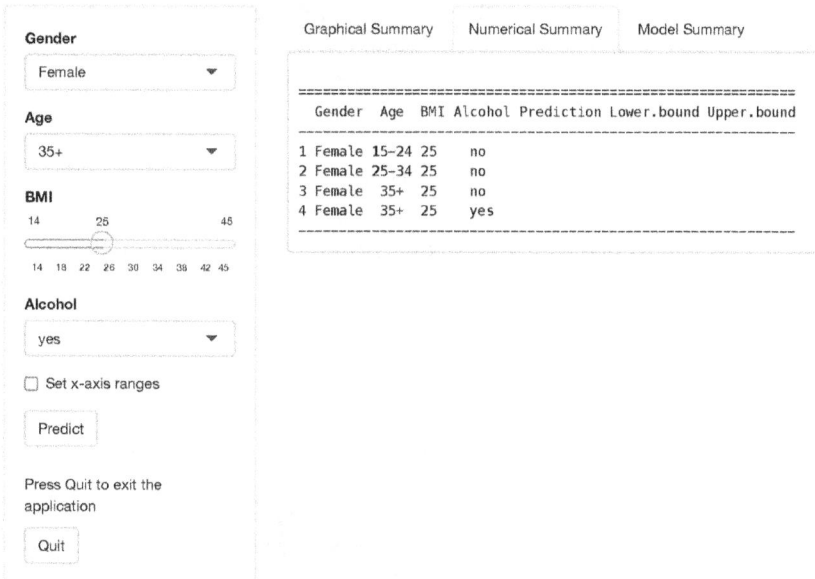

Figure 6.8 Screenshots of dynamic nomograms for the logistic regression model estimating the probability of hypertension based on the NFHS-5 data. (a) The 'Graphical Summary' tab. (b) The 'Numerical Summary' tab. The dynamic nomogram is published and accessible via a web-hosted application.

Source: Hypertension (2024)

28-year-old female with a BMI of 25 kg/m2 and no alcohol consumption is estimated as 0.074 with a 95% confidence interval of 0.039 to 0.137 (see the blue error bar in Figure 6.8 (a)). This indicates a relatively precise estimate in which the probability may be as low as 0.039 or as high as 0.137.

Similar to static nomograms, the variables' importance can be represented graphically through the assessment of the change in the predicted value. For example, the effect of age group changes is evident in error bars (which represent scenarios of a 15–24-year-old female with a BMI of 25kg/m² and no alcohol consumption, a 25–34 year old female with a BMI of 25 and no alcohol consumption, and a female above 34 years old with a BMI of 25 and no alcohol consumption, respectively). This is particularly useful for models containing modifiable risk factors. For example, there is a considerable effect of alcohol consumption on the probability of hypertension (for those above 34 years old, female with a BMI of 25), which is evident from the topmost error bar (alcohol consumption) and the second error bar from the top (no alcohol consumption). However, the very wide confidence interval of the topmost error bar shows a great deal of uncertainty, making it difficult to draw a confident conclusion about alcohol consumption.

The DNbuilder() function in R can be used to develop and publish a dynamic nomogram as a web application that will be accessible to the target audience of the model. The dynamic nomogram built for the Kerala NFHS-5 data based on the logistic regression model in Table 6.5 is available online at https://dynnom.shinyapps.io/hypertension/ (Hypertension 2024).

Conclusion

Regression analysis is a very powerful statistical technique widely used in various disciplines, including public health, medical research, and biomedical science, for explaining and formulating the relationship between variables. In this chapter, we discussed the principles of regression analysis and explored their application through a real-world case study the NFHS-5 study.

We explored common regression models, such as linear regression and logistic regression models. In addition, we discussed the importance of clearly communicating regression model results and illustrated practical tools that can facilitate this communication for nontechnical audiences.

Discussion Questions

■ How does regression analysis help explain relationships between risk factors and health outcomes?
■ What guides the choice between linear and logistic regression in a given study?
■ Why is it important to check assumptions in linear regression, and how do we interpret categorical variables within a model?
■ What role do model evaluation metrics play in assessing regression outputs?
■ Finally, how can tools like nomograms make complex statistical results more accessible to nonspecialist audiences in clinical and public health settings?

Acknowledgments
The authors sincerely appreciate Professor Ailish Hannigan for her time, thoughtful feedback, and support through the development of this book chapter.

References

Agresti, Alan. 2015. "Foundations of Linear and Generalized Linear Models | Wiley." https://www.wiley.com/en-ie/Foundation of+Linear+and+Generalized+Linear+Models-p-9781118730034.

Allcock, Harold John. 1962. The Nomogram: The Theory and Practical Construction of Computation Charts. Pitman.

Ankerst, Donna P., Josef Hoefler, Sebastian Bock, Phyllis J. Goodman, Andrew Vickers, Javier Hernandez, Lori J. Sokoll, et al. 2014. "Prostate Cancer Prevention Trial Risk Calculator 2.0 for the Prediction of Low- vs High-Grade Prostate Cancer." Urology 83 (6): 1362–8. https://doi.org/10.1016/j.urology.2014.02.035.

Banks, Jerry. 2006. "Nomograms." In Encyclopedia of Statistical Sciences. Wiley Online Library. https://doi.org/10.1002/0471667196.ess1795.pub2.

Davies, Huw Talfryn Oakley, Iain Kinloch Crombie, and Manouche Tavakoli. 1998. "When Can Odds Ratios Mislead?" BMJ: British Medical Journal 316 (7136): 989–91.

Dobson, Annette J., and Adrian G. Barnett. 2018. An Introduction to Generalized Linear Models. 4th ed. New York: Chapman and Hall/CRC. https://doi.org/10.1201/9781315182780.

Fischer, Joachim E., Lucas M. Bachmann, and Roman Jaeschke. 2003. "A Readers' Guide to the Interpretation of Diagnostic Test Properties: Clinical Example of Sepsis." Intensive Care Medicine 29 (7): 1043–51. https://doi.org/10.1007/s00134-003-1761-8.

Hanley, J. A., and B. J. McNeil. 1982. "The Meaning and Use of the Area under a Receiver Operating Characteristic (ROC) Curve." Radiology 143 (1): 29–36. https://doi.org/10.1148/radiology.143.1.7063747.

Harrell Jr, Frank E. 2024. "Rms: Regression Modeling Strategies." https://cran.r-project.org/web/packages/rms/index.html.

Hinkle, Dennis E., William Wiersma, and Stephen G. Jurs. 2003. Applied Statistics for the Behavioral Sciences. 5th ed. Boston, MA, [London]: Houghton Mifflin; [Hi Marketing] (distributor). http://catalog.hathitrust.org/api/volumes/oclc/50716608.html.

Hosmer, David W., Stanley Lemeshow, and Rodney X. Sturdivant. 2013. Applied Logistic Regression. 3rd ed. Wiley. https://www.wiley.com/en-ie/Applied+Logistic+Regression%2C+3rd+Edition-p-9780470582473.

Hypertension. 2024. "Dynamic Nomogram of Hypertension." https://dynnom.shinyapps.io/hypertension/.

IIPS/India, and ICF Macro. 2021. "National, State and Union Territory, and District Fact Sheets 2019–21 National Family Health Survey NFHS5 (English)." India: International Institute for Population Sciences. https://dhsprogram.com/publications/publication-OF43-Other-Fact-Sheets.cfm.

Jalali, Amirhossein, Alberto Alvarez-Iglesias, Davood Roshan, and John Newell. 2019. "Visualising Statistical Models Using Dynamic Nomograms." PLoS One 14 (11): e0225253. https://doi.org/10.1371/journal.pone.0225253.

Jalali, Amirhossein, Robert W. Foley, Robert M. Maweni, Keefe Murphy, Dara J. Lundon, Thomas Lynch, Richard Power, et al. 2020. "A Risk Calculator to Inform the Need for a Prostate Biopsy: A Rapid Access Clinic Cohort." BMC Medical Informatics and Decision Making 20 (July): 148. https://doi.org/10.1186/s12911-020-01174-2.

Jalali, Amirhossein, Davood Roshan, Alberto Alvarez-Iglesias, and John Newell. 2022. "DynNom: Visualising Statistical Models Using Dynamic Nomograms." https://cran.r-project.org/web/packages/DynNom/index.html.

Kattan, Michael W. 2003. "Nomograms Are Superior to Staging and Risk Grouping Systems for Identifying High-Risk Patients: Preoperative Application in Prostate Cancer." Current Opinion in Urology 13 (2): 111.

Kramer, Andrew A, and Jack E. Zimmerman. 2007. "Assessing the Calibration of Mortality Benchmarks in Critical Care: The Hosmer-Lemeshow Test Revisited." Assessing the Calibration of Mortality Benchmarks in Critical Care: The Hosmer-Lemeshow Test Revisited 35 (9): 2052–6.

Lewis-Beck, Michael S., and Andrew Skalaban. 1990. "The R-Squared: Some Straight Talk." Political Analysis 2 (January): 153–71. https://doi.org/10.1093/pan/2.1.153.

Madsen, Henrik, and Poul Thyregod. 2011. Introduction to General and Generalized Linear Models. Boca Raton: CRC Press. https://doi.org/10.1201/9781439891148.

McCabe, George P., and John Newell. 2022. "The Art of Translational Statistics." Stat 11 (1): e519. https://doi.org/10.1002/sta4.519.

McCullagh, P., and J. A. Nelder. 1989. Generalized Linear Models. Boston, MA: Springer US. https://doi.org/10.1007/978-1-4899-3242-6.

Mukaka, M. M. 2012. "A Guide to Appropriate Use of Correlation Coefficient in Medical Research." Malawi Medical Journal: The Journal of Medical Association of Malawi 24 (3): 69–71.

Nattino, Giovanni, Michael L. Pennell, and Stanley Lemeshow. 2020. "Assessing the Goodness of Fit of Logistic Regression Models in Large Samples: A Modification of the Hosmer-Lemeshow Test." Biometrics 76 (2): 549–60. https://doi.org/10.1111/biom.13249.

Negi, Jyotsna, Hari Sankar D., Arun B. Nair, and Devaki Nambiar. 2022. "Intersecting Sex-Related Inequalities in Self-Reported Testing for and Prevalence of Non-Communicable Disease (NCD) Risk Factors in Kerala." BMC Public Health 22 (1): 544. https://doi.org/10.1186/s12889-022-12956-w.

Newell, John, Jalali Amirhossein, Alberto Alvarez-Iglesias, Martin O'Donnell, and John Hinde. 2014. "Translational Statistics and Dynamic Nomograms." In, 73–74. Ireland.

Paul, Prabasaj, Michael L. Pennell, and Stanley Lemeshow. 2013. "Standardizing the Power of the Hosmer–Lemeshow Goodness of Fit Test in Large Data Sets." Statistics in Medicine 32 (1): 67–80. https://doi.org/10.1002/sim.5525.

Sarma, P. S., Rajeev Sadanandan, JissaVinodaThulaseedharan, Biju Soman, Kannan Srinivasan, R. P. Varma, Manju R. Nair, et al. 2019. "Prevalence of Risk Factors of Non-Communicable Diseases in Kerala, India: Results of a Cross-Sectional Study." BMJ Open 9 (11): e027880. https://doi.org/10.1136/bmjopen-2018-027880.

Schober, P., Boer, C., and Schwarte, L. A. 2018. "Correlation Coefficients: Appropriate Use and Interpretation." Anesthesia & Analgesia 126 (5), pp.1763–8.

Sharma, Santosh Kumar, Devaki Nambiar, Hari Sankar, Jaison Joseph, Surya Surendran, and Gloria Benny. 2022. "Decomposing Socioeconomic Inequality in Blood Pressure and Blood Glucose Testing: Evidence from Four Districts in Kerala, India." International Journal for Equity in Health 21 (1): 128. https://doi.org/10.1186/s12939-022-01737-x.

Steyerberg, Ewout W., Andrew J. Vickers, Nancy R. Cook, Thomas Gerds, Mithat Gonen, Nancy Obuchowski, Michael J. Pencina, and Michael W. Kattan. 2010. "Assessing the Performance of Prediction Models: A Framework for Traditional and Novel Measures." Epidemiology 21 (1): 128. https://doi.org/10.1097/EDE.0b013e3181c30fb2.

Wallach, D., and B. Goffinet. 1989. "Mean Squared Error of Prediction as a Criterion for Evaluating and Comparing System Models." Ecological Modelling 44 (3): 299–306. https://doi.org/10.1016/0304-3800(89)90035-5.

World Health Organization, Ala. 2011. "Global Status Report on Noncommunicable Diseases 2010." Geneva, Switzerland: World Health Organization. http://whqlibdoc.who.int/publications/2011/9789240686458_eng.pdf.

## CHAPTER 7

Statistical Model for Measuring Awareness About the Use of Pentavalent Vaccination Among Infants Through NFHS Data

Shainee Saha and Kishore Kumar Das

Learning Outcomes

Readers will understand the application of statistical methods to assess public health awareness, specifically regarding the pentavalent vaccine in India. They will gain experience in using NFHS-5 data to perform descriptive analysis, chi-square tests, and binary logistic regression. The chapter will help learners explore how demographic variables, such as education, religion, and ethnicity, influence vaccine awareness. Through this, they will appreciate the importance of data-driven insights in shaping health policy and targeting immunization programs effectively.

Introduction

Immunization is one of the most important public health interventions and a cost-effective strategy to control infectious diseases, especially in children. This immunization program in India was introduced in 1978 as Expanded Programme of Immunization (EPI), and then Universal Immunization Programme (UIP) was launched in 1985 (WHO/UNICEF, 2023). Then in phased manner, it was implemented to all districts in the country by 1989–1990. Immunization coverage rose from below 20% in the 1980s to nearly 61%, yet over one-third of children remain un-immunized (MoHFW, 2013).

Pentavalent vaccine (Bairwa et al., 2012; Agarwal, 2016; Karami et al., 2017) is a combination of vaccines which protects against five killer diseases, viz., diphtheria, pertussis, tetanus, hepatitis B, and *Hemophilus influenza* type B (Hib) (MoHFW, 2012). This has been introduced in almost all GAVI eligible countries by 2011 (WHO/UNICEF, 2023). After initial controversies, India has introduced the pentavalent vaccine initially in two states, viz., Kerala and Tamil Nadu, through a routine immunization program in December 2011. At present, the pentavalent vaccine has been expanded to all 36 states/UTs. It is recommended that the children of the mother administer three doses of pentavalent vaccines. The first dose is administered at 6 weeks of age, the second dose at 10 weeks of age, and the third dose at 14 weeks of age (Bairwa et al., 2012; MoHFW, 2012; Agarwal, 2016).

Vaccines are the world's safest method to protect life of the children from life-threatening diseases. The objective of the study is to understand the socio-demographic factors responsible for the awareness of the pentavalent vaccines (Sack et al., 2003; Tipayamongkholgul et al., 2005; MoHFW 2012, 2013; Last, 1995).

The awareness of immunization with pentavalent vaccines has been analyzed using data from the National Family Health Survey round 5 (NFHS-5), a comprehensive survey conducted in India during 2019–2020 (NFHS, 2021). The National Family survey is a series of survey conducted by the Ministry of Health and Family Welfare (MoHFW), Government of India, in collaboration with the International Institute for Population Science (IIPS), Mumbai. The NFHS aims to provide reliable and up-to-date information on various aspects of health and family welfare in India. It collects data on a wide range of indicators related to health, nutrition, population, and family welfare, among others. The survey covers a representative sample of household across all states and union territories of India. It provides the latest data on various indicators related to health, nutrition, family planning, maternal and child health, and other important factors affecting the well-being of individuals and families in India. It covers broad range of topics, such as fertility, contraceptives use, maternal and child health, nutrition, women's empowerment, domestic violence, and healthcare utilization. It is worth noting that the NFHS surveys are conducted periodically, and each round provides updated data to monitor progress and changes in various health and social indicators over time (NFHS, 2021).

To explore the objectives of the study, the methodologies have been used are descriptive statistics, Pearson's chi-square test of independence, and logistic regression (Agresti, 1990; Smith and Mckenna, 2013; Tabachnick and Fidell, 2013; Osborne 2015; Pituch and Stevens, 2016; Hox, 1995; Pituch and Stevens, 2016; Smith and McKenna, 2013; McCullagh and Nelder, 1989; Hosmer and Lemeshow, 1989).

The objectives of the paper are to study the relationship between the pentavalent vaccines with the socio-demographic variables, viz., education level, religion, and ethnicity; and the awareness of the pentavalent vaccines among the people will be analyzed considering the covariates education level, religion, and ethnicity.

Material and Methods

Data Source

NFHS-5 refer to the National Family Health Survey 5, which is a large-scale survey conducted in India (NFHS, 2021). The National Family survey is a series of survey conducted by the Ministry of Health and Family Welfare, Government of India, in collaboration with the International Institute for Population Science (IIPS, 1998–1999), Mumbai (NFHS, 2021).

NFHS-5 is the fifth round of the survey, which was conducted between 2019 and 2020. It provides the latest data on various indicators related to health, nutrition, family planning, maternal and child health, and other important factors affecting the well-being of individuals and families in India (NFHS, 2021).

Immunizing children against vaccine preventable diseases can greatly reduce childhood morbidity and mortality. Information on vaccination coverage was collected from the child's health card and direct reporting from the mother. Coverage of all basic vaccinations among children aged 12–23 months was assessed based on whether they had received specific vaccines at any time before the survey (according to a vaccination card or the mother's report). The pentavalent vaccination of children has been considered in this survey.

Methodology

The methodology used to analyze the awareness of the use of pentavalent vaccine, considering some socio-demographic data of NHFS-5 dataset, are *descriptive statistics*, *chi-square test for independence*, and *binary logistic regression model* (Menard, 1995; McCullagh and Nelder, 1989; Agresti 1990; Hosmer and Lemeshow, 1989; Smith and Mckenna 2013; Tabachnick and Fidell 2013; Osborne 2015; Pituch and Stevens 2016; Hox, 1995; Pituch and Stevens, 2016; Kleinbaum, 1998).

Binary logistic regression models will be used to study the awareness of the pentavalent vaccinations as *not vaccinated* (0) and *vaccinated* (1). The variables educational level, religion, and ethnicity are considered as covariates.

Binary logistic regression is a statistical model used to predict the probability of a binary outcome variable based on one or more predictor variables. It is a type of regression analysis commonly used when the dependent variables are dichotomous, meaning it can take only two possible values (e.g., yes/no, success/failure, true/false).

The formula for the logistic function is as follows:

$$p = \frac{1}{(1 + \exp(-z))},$$

where p is the probability of the event occurring, e is the base of the natural logarithm (approximately 2.718), and z is a linear combination of the predictor variables.

The linear combination of the predictor variables in logistic regression is represented as follows:

$$z = \beta_0 + \beta_1 x_1 + \beta_2 x_2 + \cdots + \beta_p x_p,$$

where $\beta_0, \beta_1, \beta_2, \ldots, \beta_p$ are the regression coefficients for each predictor variable, and $x_1, x_2, x_3, \ldots, x_p$ are the corresponding values of the predictor variables.

Binary logistic regression is commonly used in various fields, including medicine, social sciences, marketing, and finance, for predicting outcomes, such as disease presence, voting behavior, and credit default.

The *descriptive statistics* refers to the branch of statistics that involves summarizing, organizing, and describing the main features or characteristics of a dataset or sample. It focuses on providing a concise and meaningful summary of the data, allowing for easier interpretation and understanding.

The *chi-square test for independence* is a statistical test used to determine whether there is a significant association between two categorical variables. It assesses whether the observed frequencies of the contingency table are significantly different from the expected frequencies under the assumption of independence.

The formula for the chi-square test statistics in the case of independence (also known as Pearson's chi-square test) is as follows:

$$\chi^2 = \sum_{i,j} \frac{(O_{ij} - E_{ij})^2}{E_{ij}},$$

where χ^2 represents the chi-square test statistic and O_{ij} and E_{ij} represent the observed frequency and the expected frequency in the ith row and jth column of the contingency table, respectively.

To calculate the expected frequency E_{ij}, you can use the following formula:

$$E_{ij} = (\text{row total}*\text{column total}) / \text{grand total}$$

After calculating the chi-square test statistics, we can compare it to the critical value from the chi-square distribution table with $(r-1)*(c-1)$ degrees of freedom, where r is the number of rows and c is the number of columns in the contingency table.

If the chi-square test statistics exceed the critical value or the p-value is less than the chosen significance level, it suggests evidence of a significant association between the variables. On the other hand, if the chi-square test statistics is below the critical value or the p-value is greater than the chosen significance level, it suggests no significant association between the variable.

Results and Discussion

Descriptive Statistics and Chi-Square Test for Independence

Three doses of the pentavalent vaccine have been recommended for immunization of the children. The Table 7.1 compare the three doses of the awareness of the reported pentavalent vaccinations. The frequency distribution of awareness of the reported received pentavalent 1, 2, and 3 vaccines is given next.

It is clear from Table 7.1 that not vaccinated about the received pentavalent 1 vaccine is 17.6%, received pentavalent 2 vaccine is 23.2%, and received pentavalent 3 vaccine is 29.7%. It shows an indication that the awareness about reported received pentavalent is decreasing. To study the awareness of the reported received pentavalent vaccine among the people, a few socio-demographic variables, viz., educational level, religion, and

Table 7.1 Awareness of the reported received pentavalent 1, 2, and 3 vaccines

Category of the received pentavalent	Received pentavalent 1 Count (Percent)	Received pentavalent 2 Count (Percent)	Received pentavalent 3 Count (Percent)
Not vaccinated	23,208 (17.6%)	30,502 (23.2%)	39,109 (29.7%)
Vaccinated	108,324 (82.4%)	101,030 (76.8%)	92,423 (70.3%)

ethnicity, are considered. The reported received pentavalent vaccines are the categorical variables considered as the dependent variables. The socio-demographic variables, viz., educational level, religion, and ethnicity, are the categorical variables and considered as the independent variables. From Table 7.2, it is seen that the pentavalent vaccines with the socio-demographic variables are not independent since they are found to be significant. Alternatively, one can choose the independent variables (covariates) considering the scores from the binary logistics models.

Table 7.2 Relationship of the received pentavalent vaccines with the socio-demographic characteristics

Variables	Received pentavalent vaccine 1			Pearson chi-square	Sig.
	Not vaccinated	Vaccinated	Total		
Educational level	23208	108324	131532	344.233	<.001
No Education	5543	20706	26249		
Primary	3035	12904	15939		
Secondary	11485	57949	69434		
Higher	3145	16765	19910		
Religion	23208	108324	131532	821.999	<.001
Hindu	15651	81242	96893		
Muslim	3919	15056	18975		
Christian	2703	7662	10365		
Sikh	314	2002	2316		
Buddhist/Neo-Buddhist	272	991	1263		
Others	349	1371	1720		
Ethnicity	23102	107786	130888	506.894	<.001
Caste	17301	87726	105027		
Tribe	4461	15431	19892		
No Caste/Tribe	1340	4629	5969		
	Received pentavalent vaccine 2				
Educational level	30502	101030	131532	411.919	<.001
No Education	7194	19055	26249		
Primary	3953	11986	15939		
Secondary	15206	54228	69434		
Higher	4149	15761	19910		
Religion	30502	101030	131532	831.720	<.001
Hindu	20761	76132	96893		
Muslim	5156	13819	18975		
Christian	3334	7031	10365		
Sikh	472	1844	2316		
Buddhist/Neo-Buddhist	335	928	1263		
Others	444	1276	1720		

(Continued)

Table 7.2 (Continued)

Variables	Received pentavalent vaccine 1			Pearson chi-square	Sig.
	Not vaccinated	Vaccinated	Total		
Ethnicity	30348	100540	130888	458.243	<.001
Caste	23051	81976	105027		
Tribe	5631	14261	19892		
No Caste/Tribe	1666	4303	5969		
	Received pentavalent vaccine 3				
Educational level	39109	92423	131532	477.491	<.001
No Education	9060	17189	26249		
Primary	5089	10850	15939		
Secondary	19621	49813	69434		
Higher	5339	14571	19910		
Religion	39109	92423	131532	798.823	<.001
Hindu	26971	69922	96893		
Muslim	6482	12493	18975		
Christian	4053	6312	10365		
Sikh	634	1682	2316		
Buddhist/Neo-Buddhist	396	867	1263		
Others	573	1147	1740		
Ethnicity	38917	91971	130888	392.535	<.001
Caste	29926	75101	105027		
Tribe	6956	12936	19892		
No Caste/Tribe	2035	3934	5969		

Binary Logistic Regression

Binary logistic regression will be studied considering pentavalent 1, 2, and 3 vaccines as the dependent variables and educational level, religion, and ethnicity as the independent variables. The following tables illustrated the awareness of the reported pentavalent vaccines using the binary logistic regression models.

In the dependent variable, *Not vaccinated* is the reference category for received pentavalent vaccines. Among the independent variables, *No education* is the reference category for educational level, *Hindu* for religion, and *Caste* for ethnicity.

From Table 7.3, it is seen that, in terms of educational level, among people with awareness of the pentavalent vaccine, those with higher education were 1.373 times more likely to be aware than those with no education. People with secondary education were 1.356 times more aware than those without education, and people with primary education were 1.181 times more aware than those without education.

In religion, Sikh people are 1.171 times more aware about the pentavalent vaccines than the Hindu people. Other than people belonging to the Sikh religious group, all are less aware than Hindu people, i.e., Muslim people are 21.2% less likely to be aware than the Hindu people. Christians are 39.5% less likely to be aware than the Hindu people. Buddhists/Neo-Buddhists are 25.3% less likely to be aware than the Hindu people.

Table 7.3 Results of the binary logistic regression model predicting the responses of uses of the pentavalent vaccine 1

Variables		B	Sig.	Exp(B)	95% C.I. for Exp(B)	
					Lower	Upper
Educational level	No Education	Reference Category				
	Primary	.166	<.001	1.181	1.123	1.241
	Secondary	.305	<.001	1.356	1.308	1.407
	Higher	.317	<.001	1.373	1.307	1.442
Religion	Hindu	Reference Category				
	Muslim	−.239	<.001	.788	.755	.821
	Christian	−.502	<.001	.605	.570	.642
	Sikh	.158	.010	1.171	1.039	1.321
	Buddhist/Neo-Buddhist	−.292	<.001	.747	.651	.856
	Others	−.181	.004	.835	.738	.943
Ethnicity	Caste	Reference Category				
	Tribe	−.151	<.001	.860	.819	.902
	No Caste/Tribe	−.259	<.001	.772	.722	.825
Constant		1.440	<.001	4.223		

In ethnicity, tribe people are 14% less likely to be aware about the pentavalent vaccine than the case people, and no caste/tribe people are 22.8% less likely aware to be than the caste people.

From Table 7.4, it is seen that in the educational level, the people belonging to higher education are 37.8% more likely to be aware than people with no education. People with secondary education are 34.8% more likely to be aware than those without education, and those with primary education are 18.1% more aware than uneducated individuals.

In religion, Sikh people are 1.9% aware about the pentavalent vaccines than the Hindu people. Other than people belonging the Sikh religious group, all are less aware than the Hindu people, i.e., Muslim people are 23.1% less likely to be aware than the Hindu people. Christians are 36.8% less likely to be aware than the Hindu people. Buddhists/Neo-Buddhists are 19.9% less aware than the Hindu people.

In ethnicity, tribe people are 12.9% less likely to be aware about the pentavalent vaccine than the caste people, and no caste/tribe people are 17% less likely to be aware than the caste people.

From Table 7.5, it is seen that in the educational level, the people belonging to higher education are 38.9% more likely aware than the people having no education. People with secondary education are 33.7% more aware than those with no education, and those with primary education are 15.4% more aware than those without any education.

In religion, all people belonging to other than Hindu religion are less aware about the pentavalent vaccines than the Hindu people. The Muslim people are 22.4% less likely to be aware than the Hindu people. Christians are 35.2% less likely to be aware than the Hindu people. The people belonging to Sikh religious groups are 1.5% less to be aware than the Hindu people, Buddhist/Neo-Buddhist are 11.9% less likely to

Table 7.4 Results of the binary logistic regression model predicting the responses of uses of the pentavalent vaccine 2

Variables		B	Sig.	Exp(B)	95% C.I. for Exp(B)	
					Lower	Upper
Educational level	No Education	Reference Category				
	Primary	.166	<.001	1.181	1.128	1.236
	Secondary	.299	<.001	1.348	1.304	1.393
	Higher	.321	<.001	1.378	1.318	1.441
Religion	Hindu	Reference Category				
	Muslim	-.263	<.001	.769	.740	.798
	Christian	-.459	<.001	.632	.598	.668
	Sikh	.018	.725	1.019	.919	1.129
	Buddhist/Neo-Buddhist	-.222	.001	.801	.705	.910
	Others	-.154	.007	.857	.766	.959
Ethnicity	Caste	Reference Category				
	Tribe	-.138	<.001	.871	.833	.910
	No Caste/Tribe	-.186	<.001	.830	.781	.883
Constant		1.092	<.001	2.979		

Table 7.5 Results of the binary logistic regression model predicting the responses of uses of the pentavalent vaccine 3

Variables		B	Sig.	Exp(B)	95% C.I. for Exp(B)	
					Lower	Upper
Educational level	No Education	Reference Category				
	Primary	.143	<.001	1.154	1.106	1.203
	Secondary	.290	<.001	1.337	1.296	1.379
	Higher	.328	<.001	1.389	1.333	1.447
Religion	Hindu	Reference Category				
	Muslim	-.254	<.001	.776	.749	.804
	Christian	-.435	<.001	.648	.615	.682
	Sikh	-.015	.752	.985	.898	1.081
	Buddhist/Neo-Buddhist	-.127	.041	.881	.780	.995
	Others	-.184	.001	.832	.749	.923
Ethnicity	Caste	Reference Category				
	Tribe	-.109	<.001	.896	.860	.934
	No Caste/Tribe	-.132	<.001	.876	.827	.929
Constant		.745	<.001	2.107		

be aware than the Hindu people, and other religious people are 12.4% less likely to be aware than the Hindu people.

In ethnicity, tribe people are 10.4% less likely to be aware about the pentavalent vaccine than the caste people, and no caste/tribe people are 12.4% less likely to be aware than the caste people.

Conclusion

It is clear from the study that the awareness about the pentavalent vaccines seems to be either lacking or needs to work with the censored data. It reflects reluctance among the mothers not to take the full course of the pentavalent vaccine and shows reluctance not to take the full course among the educated and not educated people, the religious people, and ethnic groups. This has finally been examined using binary logistic regression. A regression model has been used to predict the responses regarding the uptake of pentavalent vaccines. To increase awareness about the pentavalent vaccines, there should be more intervention programs, viz., campaign programs, etc. about the benefit of pentavalent vaccines.

Discussion Questions

- How do education, religion, and ethnicity impact awareness of the pentavalent vaccine in India?
- Why is it important to analyze vaccination awareness using large-scale datasets like NFHS-5?
- What insights can chi-square tests and logistic regression provide in understanding public health behaviors?
- How can the government use these findings to improve immunization outreach?
- Lastly, what are the challenges in translating statistical findings into effective health interventions?

References

Agarwal, Anil Kumar (2016 July–December) 'Pentavalent' -shot the challenge, *Journal of Immunology and Immunopathology*, 18(2), 105–110.

Agresti, A. (1990) *Categorical Data Analysis*. Wiley, New York.

Bairwa, Mohan, Pilania, Manju, Rajput, Meena, Khanna, Pardeep, Kumar, Neelam, Nagar, Mukesh, Chawla, Sumit and Sharma, Pt B. D. (2012 September) Pentavalent vaccine: A major breakthrough in India's universal immunization programme, *Human Vaccines & Immunotherapeutics*, 8(9), 1314–1316.

Hosmer, D. W. and Lemeshow, S. (1989) *Applied Logistic Regression*. Wiley, New York.

Hox, J. J. (1995) *Applied Multilevel Analysis*. TT-Publikaties, Amsterdam.

International Institute for Population Sciences (IIPS) (1998–99) *National Family Health Survey*. Bombay.

Karami, Manoochehr, Ameri, Pegah, Bathaei, Jalal, Berangi, Zeinab, Pashaei, Tahereh, Zahiri, Ali, Zahraei, Seyed Mohsen, Erfani, Hussein and Ponnet, Koen (2017) Adverse events following immunization with pentavalent vaccine: Experiences of newly introduced vaccine in Iran, *BMC Immunology*, 18(1), 42.

Kleinbaum, David G. (1998) *Logistic Regression: A Self-Learning Text*. Springer, USA.

Last, J. M. (1995) *A Dictionary of Epidemiology*. 3rd Edition. New York, Oxford University Press.

McCullagh, P. M. and Nelder, J. A. (1989) *Generalized Linear Models*. 2nd Edition. Chapman & Hall/CRC, New York.

Menard, S. (1995) *Applied Logistic Regression Analysis*. Sage, Thousand Oaks.

MoHFW (2012) *Pentavalent Vaccine: Guide for Health Workers with Answers to Frequently Asked Questions*. Ministry of Health and Family Welfare, Government of India.

MoHFW. (2013) *Operational Guidelines: Introduction of Haemophilies Influenzae b (H2b) as Pentavalent Vaccine in Universal Immunization Program of India*. Ministry of Health and Family Welfare, New Delhi.

NFHS (2021) *Compendium of Fact Sheets.* MoHFW, India.

Osborne, J. W. (2015) *Best Practices in Logistic Regression.* Sage, Los Angeles.

Pituch, K. A. and Stevens, J. A. (2016) *Applied Multivariate Statistics for the Social Sciences.* 6th Edition, Routledge, New York.

Sack, R. B., Siddique, A. K., Longini, I. M. Jr., Nizam, A. and Yunus, M. (2003 January 1) A 4-year study of the epidemiology of Vibrio cholera in four rural areas of Bangladesh, *Journal of Infectious Diseases*, 187(1), 96–101.

Smith, T. J. and McKenna, C. M. (2013) A comparison of logistic regression pseudo R^2 indices, *Multiple Linear Regression Viewpoints*, 39(2), 17–26.

Tabachnick, B. G. and Fidell, L. S. (2013) *Using Multivariate Statistics.* 6th Edition. Pearson, New York.

Tipayamongkholgul, M., Podhipak, A., Chearskul S. and Sunakorn P. (2005 January) Factors associated with the development of tuberculosis in BCG immunized children, *Southeast Asian Journal of Tropical Medicine and Public Health*, 36(1), 145–150.

WHO and UNICEF (2023) Progress and challenges with achieving universal immunization coverage, WHO/UNICEF.

## CHAPTER 8

Addressing Confounding in Health Science Research

Ahmed Hossain

Learning Outcomes

Learners will understand the concept of confounding and its critical role in distorting causal relationships in health research. They will gain knowledge of identifying and adjusting for confounders using both traditional and modern statistical techniques, including randomization, stratification, and machine learning methods like LASSO and Ridge regression. The use of directed acyclic graphs (DAGs) will be introduced as a visual aid to conceptualize causal pathways and identify potential confounding variables. Learners will also explore the importance of biological plausibility in assessing true causal effects and learn to avoid common pitfalls in confounding control and data interpretation.

Introduction

Confounding is a widespread challenge in epidemiological research that can significantly distort the findings of studies investigating cause-and-effect relationships (Ali et al., 2021a; Jager et al., 2008). It occurs when a third variable, unrelated to the exposure of interest, affects both the exposure and the outcome, resulting in a misleading association between them. To minimize the impact of confounding and ensure accurate causal inference, researchers must diligently identify and control for potential confounding variables. Failing to account for confounding often occurs due to improper statistical analyses and data aggregation across multiple studies. This emphasizes the pressing need to develop and implement effective control strategies to mitigate the impact of confounding variables in health science research.

Establishing a causal relationship between independent and dependent variables requires careful research design and analysis. Correlation does not imply causation. For example, a study may find a strong association between employment opportunities and mental health symptoms, but this does not necessarily mean that employment causes mental health issues (Hossain et al., 2021). Understanding the distinction between

DOI: 10.4324/9781032701004-10

independent and dependent variables is crucial for interpreting research findings in health and other fields. Addressing these challenges ensures the validity and reliability of research findings, which can have significant implications for clinical practice and policymaking.

Researchers employ various strategies throughout the study design and analysis phases to minimize the influence of confounding variables. One key approach is randomization, particularly in clinical trials, where participants are randomly assigned to different intervention groups (VanderWeele, 2019). This method helps distribute confounders evenly among the groups, reducing their potential impact. Another strategy is stratification, which involves dividing the study population into subgroups based on the confounding variable and analyzing these subgroups separately (Ali et al., 2021b). Matching is also a valuable technique where participants with similar confounding characteristics are paired in different study groups to control for those variables (Islam et al., 2021).

Multivariate statistical methods, such as regression analysis, are extensively used to adjust for multiple confounders simultaneously (Ali et al., 2020a; Chowdhury et al., 2022; Ali et al., 2020b; Hossain et al., 2020a). These techniques allow researchers to isolate the effect of the independent variable on the dependent variable while accounting for the influence of confounders. Sensitivity analysis can also assess the robustness of study findings to potential confounding. Outcome regression is an innovative way to control confounding variables by building a statistical model that predicts the outcome variable while accounting for the influence of confounding variables. Standardization involves transforming the data to make the confounding variables comparable across groups.

Implementing control strategies requires careful planning and a thorough understanding of the research context. Researchers must identify potential confounders during the study design phase and select appropriate methods to control them. Transparent reporting of confounder control is crucial for replication and validation. Traditional methods like randomization, matching, and stratification are effective, but newer techniques like latent variable modeling and machine learning offer more nuanced approaches. Directed acyclic graphs can also depict relationships between variables, facilitating unbiased causal effect estimation.

Recent methodological innovations provide promising new strategies for addressing confounding in complex observational studies. As outlined by Hossain (2025), integrating machine learning with causal graph frameworks offers a dual approach: causal graphs visually map confounding structures, while machine learning enables dynamic adjustment for multiple interacting factors. This combined methodology is especially valuable for multifactorial outcomes, such as sleep disturbance, where lifestyle, psychological, and environmental influences interact non-linearly. Future research should leverage such frameworks to elucidate complex causal pathways and enhance the robustness of epidemiological findings.

Addressing confounding is vital for the integrity of health science research. By employing robust control strategies, researchers can enhance the accuracy of their findings, contributing to more effective health interventions and policies. As health science evolves, ongoing efforts to refine methodologies will be essential in advancing our understanding of complex health phenomena and improving public health outcomes. This article discussed a few techniques to control confounding variables in multivariable data.

Definition of Confounding Variables

A confounding variable, also known as a confounder, plays a pivotal role in epidemiological studies, influencing the association between the independent variable (the factor under investigation) and the dependent variable (the disease or outcome of interest) (Jager et al., 2008; Schober and Vetter, 2020). This additional factor is correlated with the disease and the independent variable, potentially introducing distortion or masking the true effects of the primary variable on the disease being studied (Skelly et al., 2012). Confounding factors in a study are not restricted to variables directly impacting the exposure and outcome; they can exhibit diverse relationships with the exposure and outcome. Such as the following:

1. A confounder can influence the exposure and the outcome directly.
2. It can affect the exposure and be influenced by another factor that affects the outcome.
3. Alternatively, it can affect the outcome and be influenced by another factor that affects the exposure.

The article 'On the Definition of a Confounder' by VanderWeele and Robinson (2014) clarifies the concept of confounding and introduces the term 'surrogate confounder.' For example, one study of caffeine intake and heart disease risk failed to consider physical activity, a known confounder. Since individuals who exercise regularly tend to consume more caffeine and have a lower heart disease risk, physical activity serves as a surrogate confounder in the study. However, using physical activity level as a surrogate for the unmeasured confounder may not fully address the confounding effect, leading to potential bias in the study results.

To illustrate a confounding variable, as shown in Figure 8.1, consider a hypothetical scenario where a researcher investigates the association between *coffee consumption* and *heart disease*. The initial hypothesis suggests that coffee drinkers might have a higher prevalence of heart disease than coffee non-drinkers. However, a confounding variable like *smoking* could distort the relationship. It is observed that coffee drinkers in the study also tend to smoke more cigarettes than coffee non-drinkers. Consequently, smoking becomes a confounding variable in this analysis, creating ambiguity about whether the increased heart disease risk is genuinely associated with coffee consumption or if it is attributable to the confounding variable of smoking.

This situation underscores the complexity of untangling causation in epidemiological studies, especially without experimental designs. Due to various constraints like technical, ethical, or financial considerations, researchers often rely on observational

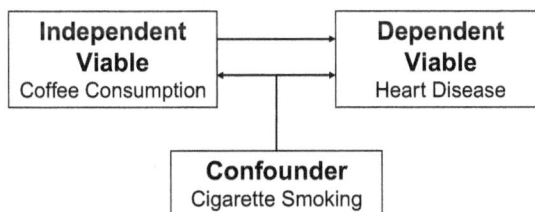

Figure 8.1 Example of a confounding variable.

studies in public health. Understanding and accounting for confounding variables are critical in these studies to draw accurate and meaningful conclusions about causal relationships. It is essential to conduct meticulous epidemiological studies, carefully considering potential confounders, to inform the development of effective preventive measures in public health.

Here are some more examples of confounding variables:

1. While smoking is strongly associated with ischemic heart disease, income level can be a confounder. High-income individuals might have better access to healthcare and healthier lifestyles, leading to lower heart disease rates, even if there is a positive association between income level and smoking.
2. Research exploring the impact of exercise on depression could be confounded by social support, as individuals with more substantial social support are more likely to exercise and have lower depression rates. Social support provides encouragement, motivation, and positive reinforcement, which can help individuals initiate and maintain regular exercise routines.
3. Studies investigating the link between diet and lung cancer risk may face confounding from smoking, as smokers are more likely to have an unhealthy diet and a higher risk of lung cancer. Smoking is associated with other unhealthy lifestyle behaviors, such as poor diet, alcohol consumption, and sedentary lifestyle; these factors may confound the association between diet and lung cancer risk.

Effect of Confounding Variables in Health Research

Confounding variables pose a significant challenge in health research by influencing independent and dependent variables, potentially distorting the observed relationships, and leading to false or misleading results (Grimes and Schulz, 2002). Upward and downward confounding refer to the direction of bias that occurs when an extraneous variable is not adequately controlled for in a study (Chowdhury et al., 2022).

Upward confounding: Upward confounding occurs when a positively associated confounding variable overestimates the effect of the exposure on the outcome, leading to an inflated observed association (Schuster et al., 2023). In other words, the observed association between the exposure and the outcome appears stronger than it is because the confounding variable artificially inflates the effect size. Failure to account for the confounder leads to overestimating the true association between the exposure and the outcome.

Downward confounding: Downward confounding arises when a negatively associated confounding variable underestimates the impact of the exposure on the outcome, resulting in a weakened observed association (Liu et al., 2020). Failure to adequately address this confounder can obscure or underestimate the true relationship between the exposure and the outcome.

In epidemiology, when discussing the relationship between exposure and outcome, some factors are considered 'on the causal pathway.' This means these factors are intermediate steps through which the exposure leads to the outcome. Adjusting for these factors in statistical analyses could remove the effect of interest because they are part of the sequence of events linking the exposure and outcome. To illustrate with an example, let's consider smoking as an exposure and lung cancer as the outcome variable. If we view chronic cough as an intermediate step along the causal pathway between smoking and lung cancer, adjusting for chronic cough in the analysis could potentially obscure the genuine association between smoking and lung cancer. This is because chronic cough is influenced by smoking and, consequently, plays a role in the development of lung cancer.

In summary, when some factors are part of the causal pathway, adjusting for them in statistical analyses may not be appropriate, as it can alter the relationship between exposure and outcome interpretation.

Statistical Models

New techniques like latent variable modeling with negative controls, inverse probability of treatment weighting (IPTW), and g-estimation offer more flexibility in applying standardization for confounding control (Gustavson et al., 2022). The method introduces a latent variable to represent unobserved confounding factors. It assumes that these factors affect both the exposure and the negative control (a variable unrelated to the outcome) to the same degree.

Machine learning techniques like LASSO, ridge regression, and random forests are pivotal in identifying confounding variables and mitigating bias, especially in large healthcare datasets, where unmeasured confounding may exist (Benasseur et al., 2022). The article also noted that hybrid methods, combining traditional techniques like stepwise regression, directed acyclic graphs, and knowledge-based approaches with machine learning, showed promising results. By employing these diverse strategies, researchers can enhance the reliability and robustness of their findings in health science research.

Identifying Confounders by Causal Graphs

Causal graphs, also known as directed acyclic graphs (DAGs), visually represent the causal relationships between variables in each system or phenomenon. In evaluating potential confounding bias and other biases in epidemiological studies, causal graphs are a gold standard tool (Tennant et al., 2021). By visually mapping out the relationships between variables, including exposure, outcome, and potential confounders, causal graphs allow researchers to assess the likelihood of confounding and other biases affecting their study results.

Researchers can use causal graphs to identify variables that may act as confounders, mediators, or moderators in the relationship between the exposure and outcome of interest. By including these variables in their analyses or adjusting for them appropriately, researchers can control for potential sources of bias and obtain more accurate estimates of the true causal effect. However, DAGs don't usually show how variables might influence each other indirectly (interactions). This is because they focus on the overall structure of relationships, not the specific details of how strong or curved those relationships might be.

We investigated a hypothetical DAG to adjust potential confounders in investigating the relationship between smoking and ischemic heart disease. This figure was constructed through DAGitty (http://www.dagitty.net/dags.html#) and is given in Figure 8.2. This graphical method depicts hypothesized causal relationships and deduces the statistical associations implied by these causal relationships. We consider two potential confounders: income level and age. The minimally sufficient adjustment set combines the fewest nodes that are ancestors of both the exposure and outcome. These 'adjusted variables' are then introduced into the multivariate modeling as potential confounders. In this example, minimal sufficient adjustment contains income level in the model for estimating the total effect of smoking on ischemic heart disease.

In this conceptual diagram, Figure 8.2, each circle represents an individual exposure ('node') of theoretical relevance to this hypothesis; each node is interconnected by directional arrows ('edges') that represent theoretical associations based on the researchers' assessment of a priori literature and determination of biological plausibility. Smoking was the main exposure of interest (green node with black border), and heart disease (blue node with black border) was the outcome of interest. In this instance, all the other exposures ('nodes') are theoretically causally associated with (i.e., ancestors of) both the exposure and the outcome.

Identifying Confounders Using the Change of an Effect Size

Historically, researchers used the change in estimate method to identify confounders by observing how the effect size of an exposure changes when potential confounders

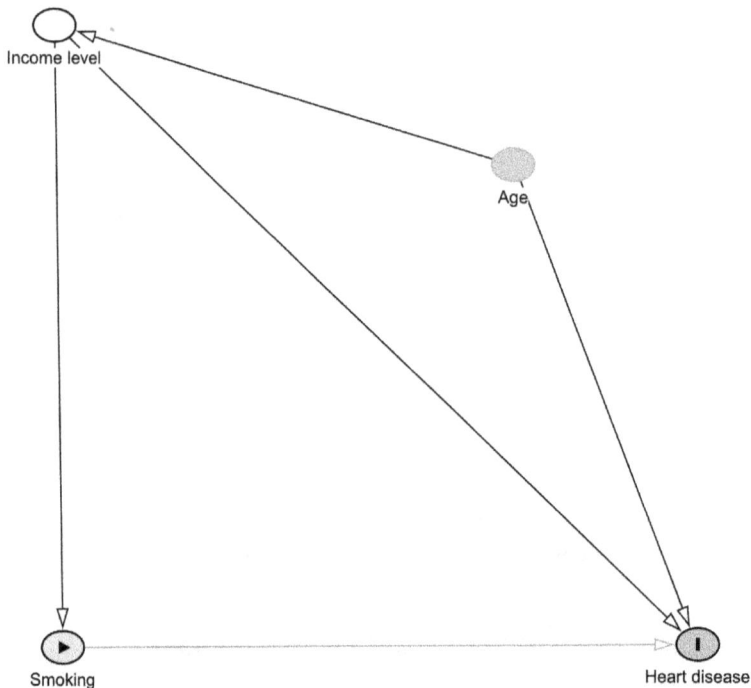

Figure 8.2 DAG demonstrating causal relationships and potential biasing pathways affecting the association between smoking and heart disease (produced using DAGitty V.2.3 software).

are adjusted for in the analysis. If the effect size changed substantially, it was considered evidence of confounding (Skelly et al., 2012; Farmer and Lawrenson, 2004). Calculating odds ratios in the context of confounding variables involves examining how the association between an exposure and an outcome changes when considering the influence of a third variable. The odds ratio (OR) is a statistical measure used in epidemiology and other research fields to assess the strength and direction of association between two categorical variables. It is commonly employed in case-control studies and logistic regression analyses. The odds ratio is calculated as the odds of an event occurring in one group to the odds of the same event occurring in another group. Here are a few examples illustrating the impact of confounding variables on odds ratios:

Example 1: Consider a scenario where a research study explores the link between smoking (exposure) and ischemic heart disease (outcome). However, age emerges as a potential confounding variable since older individuals are more likely to both smoke and develop ischemic heart disease. Odds ratios are calculated with and without considering age to ascertain whether age acts as a confounding variable.

- *Without considering age,* the odds of developing lung cancer among smokers are compared to the odds among non-smokers. Let's assume the calculated value is 5.0, signifying that smoking is associated with a fivefold increase in the risk of lung cancer.
- *After considering age,* a logistic regression model is applied, incorporating age as a variable. The resulting adjusted odds ratio is determined to be 3.0.

If the odds ratio decreases after adjusting for age, this signals that age plays a confounding role, influencing the association between smoking and lung cancer. In this context, the reduction from 5.0 to 3.0 indicates that age was indeed a confounding variable impacting the observed relationship between smoking and lung cancer.

Example 2: Suppose research explores the association between regular exercise (exposure) and obesity (outcome). Socio-economic status (SES) is a confounding variable, as it is linked to both exercise habits and obesity. To investigate whether age is a confounding variable, we must calculate the odds ratio with and without considering the SES variable.

- *Without considering SES,* the odds of experiencing obesity among those who exercise regularly are compared to those who don't exercise regularly. Let's assume the calculated value is 0.7, indicating that regular exercise is associated with a 30% reduction in the risk of weight gain.
- *After considering SES,* we applied a logistic regression model with SES adjustment and found that the odds ratio was 1.2.

If the odds ratio undergoes a significant change after adjusting for SES, it implies that SES functions as a confounding variable affecting the association between exercise and obesity. In this context, a substantial change in the odds ratio from 0.7 to 1.2 suggests that SES was confounding, influencing the observed relationship between exercise and obesity.

However, researchers are advised against relying on the change in estimate method to identify confounders, especially when dealing with non-collapsible measures like the odds ratio. Non-collapsible measures can introduce bias in estimating the association due to inconsistent effects of confounder adjustment across different strata. Hence, alternative methods or approaches are recommended for identifying and adjusting for confounding in statistical analyses.

Confounder Control: Elimination vs. Inclusion

Controlling for confounders in research is crucial to ensure meaningful conclusions from the data (Bradbury et al., 2012). Two main approaches exist: elimination and inclusion. Both have strengths and weaknesses, so choosing the right one depends on specific study and data.

Confounder Elimination

The method excludes or restricts individuals with confounding characteristics from the analysis (Lipsitch et al., 2010). For example, in studying the relationship between smoking and developing lung cancer, it is possible to eliminate individuals who are older adults, which could affect the development of lung cancer. It is simple to implement and reduces potential confounding bias. In another hypothetical study examining the association between smoking and ischemic heart disease in community adults, age could act as a confounder. Implementing restrictions to control age-related confounding during the study design is a straightforward approach. This might involve limiting the study to adults aged 60 years and older. While restriction can partially address confounding by age, it may limit the generalizability of study findings to other groups.

However, it can lead to smaller sample sizes, reducing generalizability and power. Moreover, it may not eliminate all relevant confounders, potentially missing important effects.

Confounder Inclusion

The method includes adding confounding variables as predictors in your statistical model (Hossain et al., 2020b). For example, in the exercise and weight loss study, we may include variables like income level and access to healthy food alongside exercise in the regression analysis.

The multivariable regression analysis can control for multiple confounders simultaneously, potentially revealing more nuanced relationships (Schneeweiss et al., 2017; Hajian-Tilaki, 2012). Moreover, a latent variable strategy with negative controls helps account for hidden factors affecting exposure and outcome, leading to more accurate estimates of how prenatal factors influence outcomes (Gustavson et al., 2022).

Another example is in a clinical trial testing the effectiveness of a new drug; if researchers suspect that age may confound the results, they could control it by including age as an independent variable. Participants might be divided into different age groups, and the impact of the drug could be assessed within each age group separately. This way, the potential influence of age on the results is explicitly considered.

One strength of this method lies in its ability to maintain larger sample sizes, enhancing generalizability and statistical power. However, its successful application necessitates the careful selection of relevant confounders. Additionally, this method demands more intricate analysis, potentially requiring advanced statistical techniques.

Conclusion

Understanding confounding is essential for accurate causal inference. Researchers must rigorously design and analyze studies by defining confounding, employing control mechanisms, and linking it to exchangeability and collapsibility. Identifying and adjusting for confounding variables is critical, ensuring they meet adjustment criteria without introducing bias. Beyond correlation with exposure, assessing their true impact on outcomes is vital to avoid spurious associations. Biological mechanisms and sensitivity analyses can enhance the stability of results under different adjustment strategies. Careful control of confounding in epidemiological studies ensures accurate exposure-outcome estimates. Directed acyclic graphs (DAGs) are valuable tools for visualizing variable relationships, identifying confounders, and improving causal effect estimates. While traditional methods like randomization and stratification remain useful, newer approaches like latent variable modeling with negative controls offer advanced flexibility in addressing confounding.

Discussion Questions

- Why is it important to distinguish between correlation and causation in health research, and how does confounding complicate this distinction?
- How can tools like DAGs improve our understanding of potential confounders in a study?
- What are the advantages and limitations of traditional methods, like matching or stratification, compared to newer approaches, such as LASSO or machine learning models?
- How can overlooking confounding variables affect health policy and clinical recommendations?
- Finally, in what ways can researchers ensure robust confounder control when analyzing complex health data?

References

Ali, M., Ahsan, G. U., & Hossain, A. (2020a). Prevalence and associated occupational factors of low back pain among the bank employees in Dhaka city. Journal of occupational health, 62(1), e12131. https://doi.org/10.1002/1348-9585.12131

Ali, M., Ahsan, G. U., Khan, R., Khan, H. R., & Hossain, A. (2020b). Immediate impact of stay-at-home orders to control COVID-19 transmission on mental well-being in Bangladeshi adults: Patterns, explanations, and future directions. BMC research notes, 13(1), 494. https://doi.org/10.1186/s13104-020-05345-2

Ali, M., Uddin, Z., & Hossain, A. (2021a). Economic stressors and mental health symptoms among Bangladeshi rehabilitation professionals: A cross-sectional study amid COVID-19 pandemic. Heliyon, 7(4), e06715. https://doi.org/10.1016/j.heliyon.2021.e06715

Ali, M., Uddin, Z., & Hossain, A. (2021b). Combined effect of vitamin D supplementation and physiotherapy on reducing pain among adult patients with musculoskeletal disorders: A quasi-experimental clinical trial. Frontiers in nutrition, 8, 717473. https://doi.org/10.3389/fnut.2021.717473

Benasseur, I., Talbot, D., Durand, M., Holbrook, A., Matteau, A., Potter, B. J., Renoux, C., Schnitzer, M. E., Tarride, J. É., & Guertin, J. R. (2022). A comparison of confounder selection and adjustment methods for estimating causal effects using large healthcare databases. Pharmacoepidemiology and drug safety, 31(4), 424–433. https://doi.org/10.1002/pds.5403

Bradbury, B. D., Gilbertson, D. T., Brookhart, M. A., & Kilpatrick, R. D. (2012). Confounding and control of confounding in nonexperimental studies of medications in patients with CKD. Advances in chronic kidney disease, 19(1), 19–26. https://doi.org/10.1053/j.ackd.2012.01.001

Chowdhury, S. R., Kabir, H., Mazumder, S., Akter, N., Chowdhury, M. R., & Hossain, A. (2022). Workplace violence, bullying, burnout, job satisfaction and their correlation with depression among Bangladeshi nurses: A cross-sectional survey during the COVID-19 pandemic. PLoS one, 17(9), e0274965. https://doi.org/10.1371/journal.pone.0274965

Farmer, R. Lawrenson, R. (2004). Lecture notes in epidemiology and public health medicine, pp. 67–68. Blackwell Publishing.

Grimes, D. A., & Schulz, K. F. (2002). Bias and causal associations in observational research. Lancet (London, England), 359(9302), 248–252. https://doi.org/10.1016/S0140-6736(02)07451-2

Gustavson, K., Davey Smith, G., & Eilertsen, E. M. (2022). Handling unobserved confounding in the relation between prenatal risk factors and child outcomes: A latent variable strategy. European journal of epidemiology, 37(5), 477–494. https://doi.org/10.1007/s10654-022-00857-6

Hajian-Tilaki, K. (2012). Methodological issues of confounding in analytical epidemiologic studies. Caspian journal of internal medicine, Summer, 3(3), 488–95. PMID: 24009920; PMCID: PMC3755849.

Hossain, A. (2025). Utilizing machine learning and causal graph approaches to address confounding factors in health science research: A scoping review. F1000Research, 14, 129.

Hossain, A., Baten, R. B. A., Sultana, Z. Z., Rahman, T., Adnan, M. A., Hossain, M., Khan, T. A., & Uddin, M. K. (2021). Predisplacement abuse and postdisplacement factors associated with mental health symptoms after forced migration among rohingya refugees in Bangladesh. JAMA network open, 4(3), e211801. https://doi.org/10.1001/jamanetworkopen.2021.1801

Hossain, A., Hossain, S. A., Fatema, A. N., Wahab, A., Alam, M. M., Islam, M. N., Hossain, M. Z., & Ahsan, G. U. (2020a). Age and gender-specific antibiotic resistance patterns among Bangladeshi patients with urinary tract infection caused by Escherichia coli. Heliyon, 6(6), e04161. https://doi.org/10.1016/j.heliyon.2020.e04161

Hossain, A., Niroula, B., Duwal, S., Ahmed, S., & Kibria, M. G. (2020b). Maternal profiles and social determinants of severe acute malnutrition among children under-five years of age: A case-control study in Nepal. Heliyon, 6(5), e03849. https://doi.org/10.1016/j.heliyon.2020.e03849

Islam, M., Sultana, Z. Z., Iqbal, A., Ali, M., & Hossain, A. (2021). Effect of in-house crowding on childhood hospital admissions for acute respiratory infection: A matched case-control study in Bangladesh. International journal of infectious diseases. IJID: Official publication of the international society for infectious diseases, 105, 639–645. https://doi.org/10.1016/j.ijid.2021.03.002

Jager, K. J., Zoccali, C., Macleod, A., & Dekker, F. W. (2008). Confounding: What it is and how to deal with it. Kidney international, 73(3), 256–260. https://doi.org/10.1038/sj.ki.5002650

Lipsitch, M., TchetgenTchetgen, E., & Cohen, T. (2010). Negative controls: A tool for detecting confounding and bias in observational studies. Epidemiology (Cambridge, MA.), 21(3), 383–388. https://doi.org/10.1097/EDE.0b013e3181d61eeb

Liu, L., Hou, L., Yu, Y., Liu, X., Sun, X., Yang, F., Wang, Q., Jing, M., Xu, Y., Li, H., & Xue, F. (2020). A novel method for controlling unobserved confounding using double confounders. BMC medical research methodology, 20(1), 195. https://doi.org/10.1186/s12874-020-01049-0

Schober, P., & Vetter, T. R. (2020). Confounding in observational research. Anesthesia and analgesia, 130(3), 635. https://doi.org/10.1213/ANE.0000000000004627

Schneeweiss, S., Eddings, W., Glynn, R. J., Patorno, E., Rassen, J., & Franklin, J. M. (2017). Variable selection for confounding adjustment in high-dimensional covariate spaces when analyzing healthcare databases. Epidemiology (Cambridge, MA), 28(2), 237–248. https://doi.org/10.1097/EDE.0000000000000581

Schuster, N. A., Rijnhart, J. J. M., Bosman, L. C., Twisk, J. W. R., Klausch, T., & Heymans, M. W. (2023). Misspecification of confounder-exposure and confounder-outcome associations leads to bias in effect estimates. BMC medical research methodology, 23(1), 11. https://doi.org/10.1186/s12874-022-01817-0

Skelly, A. C., Dettori, J. R., & Brodt E. D. (2012 February). Assessing bias: The importance of considering confounding. Evidence based spine xare Journal, 3(1), 9–12. https://doi.org/10.1055/s-0031-1298595. PMID: 23236300; PMCID: PMC3503514.

Tennant, P. W. G., Murray, E. J., Arnold, K. F., Berrie, L., Fox, M. P., Gadd, S. C., Harrison, W. J., Keeble, C., Ranker, L. R., Textor, J., Tomova, G. D., Gilthorpe, M. S., & Ellison, G. T. H. (2021). Use of Airected Acyclic Graphs (DAGs) to identify confounders in applied health research: Review and recommendations. International journal of epidemiology, 50(2), 620–632. https://doi.org/10.1093/ije/dyaa213

VanderWeele, T. J. (2019). Principles of confounder selection. European journal of epidemiology, 34(3), 211–219. https://doi.org/10.1007/s10654-019-00494-6

VanderWeele, T. J., & Robinson, W. R. (2014). On the causal interpretation of race in regressions adjusting for confounding and mediating variables. Epidemiology (Cambridge, MA), 25(4), 473–484. https://doi.org/10.1097/EDE.0000000000000105

PART III

Survival Analysis, Meta-Analysis and Systematic Reviews

Survival Analysis of Factors Associated with Progression of Cervical Cancer Patients

Mukesh Kumar and Kamalesh Kumar Patel

Learning Outcomes

Learners will understand how survival analysis is applied in clinical research to study time-to-event data, particularly in assessing disease progression and mortality. Using the GSE44001 dataset of 300 cervical cancer patients, they will explore the impact of clinical factors, like cancer stage and tumor diameter, on patient survival. They will gain hands-on experience with both semi-parametric and parametric models and learn to interpret hazard ratios and survival probabilities. The study reinforces the importance of early diagnosis and highlights the predictive value of tumor characteristics in treatment planning and prognosis for cervical cancer patients.

Introduction

Cervical cancer (CerC) develops in the tissue of the cervix, which is caused by the human papillomavirus. CerC is the fourth most common cancer in women globally. Although CerC rates are going down significantly in some well-developed nations of the world, it is still a global concern due to minimal access to better health facilities in several countries of the world (Bray *et al.,* 2018). CerC is a significant public health issue, where it remains responsible for cancer deaths of women. The effect of tumor diameter on the survival of CerC patients has been extensively studied, and several reports have suggested that larger tumor size is linked with worse outcomes of life (Kim *et al.,* 2023). A study conducted in Seoul, Korea, investigated the relationship between tumor diameter and survival in CerC patients. The study analyzed data from 691 patients of CeC between 2009 and 2013 and underwent surgery as their primary treatment (Hwang *et al.,* 2020). Tumor diameter has been identified as an important clinical factor in cancers, including CerC. One study by Kim found that patients with a tumor larger than 4 cm had significantly worse overall survival rates than those with smaller tumor (Park *et al.,* 2011). Another study by Park found that tumor size was an independent predictor of lifetime in early-stage CerC patients (Shin *et al.*, 2008). In addition to tumor diameter, other factors such as age, stage at diagnosis, and comorbidities have also been found to impact on survival rates in CerC patients. A study by Lee et al. found that older age and comorbidities were associated with worse survival outcomes (Kumar *et al.*, 2020). Survival analysis, an extensively used inferential statistical technique, has been carried out in this study in which we have come up with different survival analysis techniques, viz. non-parametric (NP) techniques, semi-parametric (SP) techniques, and parametric techniques (Royston *et al.*, 2011). While carrying out survival analysis, one faces many challenges, like selection of statistical model, method of estimation for the parameter of selected model, and most relevantly, using the clinical information suitably in further analysis for getting results that should be realistic, reliable, and can be easily interpreted (Saroj *et al.*, 2021). Thus, analysis of clinical data using statistical techniques can surely help us in identifying determinants and extracting useful vital information, which is needed at every stage of the development of treatment strategies. Clinical data, being different in nature from other types of data, requires special techniques for its analysis (Kleinbaum *et al.*, 2012). Furthermore, we have compared different techniques and models as well to infer which one is logically appropriate on the basis of evidences produced from used clinical data. In survival analysis, the Kaplan-Meier (KM) plot is based on probability of survival, and it is estimated by product limit formula. If the values of all dependent variables are zero, then the Cox model equals the baseline hazard function. Another leading assumption of the Cox model is that the baseline hazard function is unspecified, so it is called the SP model. When the outcome of an event follows a specific distribution with unknown parameters, it is called a parametric survival model (Gardiner, 2010).

In other words, those models have any specific functional form of models, called parametric models. There are various parametric models, such as log-normal, Weibull, exponential, etc. It is not easy to fit appropriate parametric models by using goodness of fit as a parametric model. Besides that, if we are not sure which parametric model will be appropriate in this situation, the Cox model is the reliable choice. The Cox model and the logistic model are alternative approaches, based on different assumptions: the Cox model is used for survival times and accounts for censoring, whereas the logistic model is based on binary outcomes (0,1) and does not consider survival times or censoring. A dataset with a total of 300 CerC patients with variables – stage (IA2, IB1, IB2, and IIA), tumor diameter (in mm), disease free survival (in months), and progression (main event of interest) – has been analyzed. This study is designed for the analysis of clinical factors, which gives an initial information about the presence of CerC and the prediction of risk and survival time of patients. Based on this classification, KM curve is drawn for predicting the patient's survival time. For survival analysis, we have used statistical methods to evaluate the clinical parameters. Further, the overall survival of patients has been observed based on clinical parameters.

Material and Methods
Data Source
The current study was done on early CerC patients, those treated by revolutionary medical procedures with adjuvant treatments at the SMC, University School of Medicine,

Seoul, Korea, from January 2002 to September 2008. The GSE44001 dataset comprises 300 patients of CerC with their parameters: stages (IA2, IB1, IB2, and IIA), disease-free survival (DFS), and progression information. The non-parametric (KM estimation), semi-parametric (Lin and Yang additive hazard model), and Cox and parametric (Accelerated failure time) models have been applied in survival analysis based on well-known and popular distributions, such as Weibull, exponential, log-normal, log-logistic, etc., to analyze clinical factors. Overall survival has been calculated based on significant factor tumor diameters into different categories (Lin *et al.*, 2002, 1995).

Basic Terminology

Survival Time: It shows the time period from a defined initial point (such as diagnosis, treatment initiation, or onset of a condition) until the occurrence of a specified event, often the death of a patient or the failure of a treatment. It is a key measure in survival analysis, which studies the time until an event occurs (e.g., patient death, body part failure).

Kaplan-Meier (KM) Curves: A KM curve is a statistical tool used to compute the survival probability over time. It provides a visual representation of the survival function, showing the proportion of patients surviving for a duration after a getting treatment or intervention. KM curves are used to show that survival probabilities for different patient groups.

Hazard Ratio (HR): The HR is the exponentiated coefficient of a predictor $exp(\beta_i)$. It represents the relative risk of the event occurring for a one-unit increase in the predictor variable. It describes the risk of experiencing the event at a given time. $exp(\beta_i)$ quantifies the proportional change in the HR for a one-unit increase in X_i, with respect to other covariates constant. HR > 1 shows an increased risk of the event, HR < 1 shows a decreased risk of the event, and HR = 1 shows that the predictor has no effect on the event risk.

Akaike Information Criterion (AIC): To check whether a model is a best fit or not, we prefer to use an AIC criterion for clinical data. The AIC was firstly given by Hirotugu Akaike in 1974. It gives the AIC value based on the number of parameters and the maximum value of the model's likelihood function. The model that provides the minimum AIC value is considered as the bet-fitted model *[7]*. The AIC value is computed by the following:

$$AIC = 2k - 2\ln\left(\hat{L}\right)$$

Where,
  k = Number of estimated parameters
  L = Maximum value of likelihood function for a given model

P-value: A *p*-value has a minimum probability of rejecting the null hypothesis. It is a statistical measure to determine the power of a hypothesis test. Specifically, it shows how likely the observed data would occur when the null hypothesis is considered as true. *P*-value assesses the null hypothesis, i.e., covariate has no effect.

Intercept: It refers to the value where a line or curve intersects the y-axis in a graph. It shows the projected value of the variable (Y) as dependent when all independent variables (X) (predictors)are equal to zero.

Confidence interval: A confidence interval (CI) is a range in which the value of the estimate lies. This value is derived from the sample data, such as a mean or proportion. It is a way of expressing uncertainty in an estimate and is widely used in statistical analysis.

Dependent Variable (Survival Time)

The dependent variable in the Cox model is survival time, which refers to the duration until a specific event occurs. This event could be time until death or recovery in medical research or time until equipment failure in engineering studies or time until relapse in clinical trials. Survival time can be either fully observed (event occurs) or censored (if the event has not occurred by the end of the study or the subject is lost to follow-up). The model is primarily interested in how different factors affect the likelihood of the event occurring over time.

Independent Variables (Predictors)

The independent variables in the survival model are the predictor variables (also known as covariates or risk factors). These can be quantitative: numerical values such as age, cholesterol levels, or blood pressure. Categorical: non-numerical categories like gender, treatment groups, or disease stages.

Methods of Survival Analysis
Some survival methods are discussed in the following sections:

Non-parametric (NP) Method

Kaplan-Meier (KM) Estimation Method
The Kaplan-Meier (KM) estimation model is a non-parametric survival method. It estimates the survival function from time-to-event data. It is commonly employed in medical research and other fields to understand the probability of survival over time. There are several key components of the KM model. The dependent variable in the KM model is survival time, which refers to the duration until a specific event occurs. This event could be death or disease onset in medical studies, equipment failure in reliability engineering, or relapse or recovery in clinical trials. Survival time can be either fully observed when the event occurs or censored. The independent variable in the KM model is an event indicator, which specifies whether the event of interest has occurred for each individual. This indicator takes two values: 1: Event occurred (e.g., death or failure) and 0: Event is censored (e.g., the individual is still alive or event has not happened).

Let $(t_1, t_2, ..., t_k)$ be the ordered survival times, $(m_1, m_2, ..., m_p)$ be the no. of events (counted) at distinct point of time as failure time, and $R(t_i)$ be the total no. of patients who have survived at least to lifetime (t_i). $R(t_i)$ is called the risk set and considered as base for computing survival probabilities. Thus, the survival probability is computed as follows:

$$S(t_k) = \Pi\left[\left(R(t_i) - m_k\right) / R(t_k)\right]$$

An alternative approach to estimate the survival probabilities by the product of conditional probabilities terms. It is estimated by the given formula:

$$S(t_k) = \Pi S(t_{k-1}) * P(T > t_k / T \geq t_k)$$

This non-parametric method is used to compute the survival curve on the basis of the stages of patients. The KM survival curve is a step function that decreases over time, with steps occurring at each event time.

Semi-Parametric (SP) Method

Ling-Yang Additive Hazard Model

The semi-parametric statistical regression model based on the assumption that its hazard function is expressed that additive of baseline hazard and linear combination of the covariates. The mathematically form of the model is considered as follows:

$$\varphi(t \mid x(t)) = \varphi_0(t) + \sum_{j=1}^{P} \varphi(t)X_j$$

Where X_j are the covariates and $\varphi_0(t)$ is the baseline hazard.
(Kumar *et al.*, 2020; Royston *et al.*, 2011)

$\sum_{j=1}^{P} \varphi(t)X_j$ is the linear combination of covariate X_j with their regression coefficients $\varphi(t)$.

If the proportionality assumption is violated, the results obtained may be misleading. In this case, this method gives better results. This method shows that each covariate has an additive effect on the hazard rate at each time point. But in the Cox model, all covariates are associated in the multivariate effect. This method is useful in medical statistics, epidemiology, and in other problems related to time-to-event data (Lin *et al.*, 1995; Kaplan *et al.*, 1958; Scheike *et al.*, 2002; Cox, 1972)

Cox Proportional Hazard Model (Cox Model)

Also known as Cox regression, this is a widely used statistical method for time-to-event analysis as a semi-parametric model. It examines the relationship between the timing of an event (such as disease onset or equipment failure) and one or more independent variables (predictors). The flexibility of the Cox model provides significant advantages in fields like medical research, epidemiology, and others. Introduced by Dr. David R. Cox in 1972, this regression model is specifically designed for analyzing survival data, enabling researchers to assess how different factors influence patient survival time (Wei, 1992). It also explores the association between the time to event data (e.g., death, disease progression) and one or more independent variables. These variables help determine the hazard function, which is the risk of the event occurring at a given time, assuming it has not occurred yet. The Cox model is described as follows:

$$\frac{h(t)}{h_0(t)} = \exp(\beta_1 x_1 + \beta_2 x_2 + \ldots + \beta_p x_p)$$

where $h(t)$ hazard function and $h_0(t)$ baseline hazard function with $(\beta_1, \beta_2, \ldots, \beta_p)$ regression coefficients that quantify the effect of each predictor on the hazard. $X_1, X_2, \ldots, X_p$ are the independent variables. The hazard function $h(t)$ provides the instant rate at which the event occurs at time t, given that the event has not yet occurred. The Cox model assumes that this hazard is related to the covariates through a log-linear relationship. The key assumption of the Cox model is that the hazard ratio between individuals remain constant over time (i.e., the effect of a predictor on the hazard is proportional and does not change over time). It is an unspecified function of time, which means the model does not assume any particular distribution for the baseline hazard, making the Cox model semi-parametric (Singh *et al.*, 2023; Yagi *et al.*, 2019).

In summary, the Cox model is a flexible tool for analyzing survival data, with survival time as the dependent variable and multiple predictors (independent variables) influencing the hazard rate of the event occurring over time. The model's key strength lies in estimating the hazard ratios for each predictor while assuming that their effect remains proportional over time.

Parametric method

This method consists a specific form of probability model or distribution. This method used to prediction of parameters by estimators. There are various parametric models, such as linear regression, logistic regression, Gaussian distribution, exponential distribution, etc.

The exponential distribution with mean lifetime σ is given in this form:

$$f(t, \mu) = \frac{1}{\mu} \exp\left(\frac{-y}{\mu}\right) \quad t \geq 0, \mu \geq 0$$

The Weibull distribution model is considered as follows:

$$f(t, \mu, \beta) = \frac{\beta}{\mu} t^{\beta-1} \exp\left(\frac{-t^{\beta}}{\mu}\right) \quad t > 0, \mu > 0, \beta > 0$$

The log-normal distribution model is considered as follows:

$$f(t, \mu, \beta^2) = \frac{1}{t\beta\sqrt{2\pi}} \exp\left(\frac{lnt - \mu)}{2\beta^2}\right) \quad t\varepsilon(0, \infty), \mu > 0, \beta > 0$$

The log-logistic distribution model is considered as follows:

$$f(t, \alpha, \beta) = \left(\frac{\beta}{\alpha}\right)\left(\frac{t}{\alpha}\right)^{\beta-1} \bigg/ \left[1 + \left(\frac{t}{\alpha}\right)^{\beta}\right]^2 \quad t, \alpha, \beta > 0$$

The earlier given lifetime models are fitted by using the R software.

Accelerated Failure Time (AFT) Model

This model describes how covariates accelerate or decelerate over the survival time. The AFT model's assumption is that the effect of covariates multiplies with the concerning time T. This model allows to estimate the outcome of predictor variables on lifetime data. A random time-to-event T_i, an AFT model, shows the relationship between covariates and log-transformed survival:

$$Y_i = \mu + \beta_1 X_1 + \beta_2 X_2 + \ldots + \beta_p X_p + \sigma \varepsilon_i$$

Where $X_1, X_2, \ldots, X_p$ is the predictor variables with the regression coefficients vector. $\beta = (\beta_1, \beta_2, \ldots, \beta_p) \varepsilon_i$ is the unexplained variation (residual) in the log-transformed survival times, and it follows normal distribution $(0, \sigma^2)$, where μ and σ are intercept and scale parameters, respectively (Kaplan et al., 1958; Horn et al., 2007).

Generally, different distributions are used in the AFT models, such as exponential distribution (constant hazard over time), Weibull distribution (increasing or decreasing hazard over time), log-normal (log of survival time, which follows normal distribution), and log-logistic (hazard shows distribution with heavier tail) (Dizaji et al., 2020).

Overall Survival

The overall survival has been calculated to show the pattern of survival graphically. In this section, we have seen the outcome of tumor diameter on the survival of CerC patients. The tumor diameter is categorized into three categories (0–3.0), (3.1–4.0), and (4.1 and above) in mm, respectively. It helps to predict the survival of patients based on tumor diameter.

Results

Stage and tumor diameter showed a significant impact on the survival of patients. Patients in stage IB2 experienced the lowest survival, while patients of stage IA2 and stage IB1, collectively, had experienced the highest survival. The result that patients of stage IB2 are experiencing more survival than patients of stage IIA seems controversial due to the fact that that number of patients having the event progression is least in stage IIA (see **Figure 9.1**).

The other method which has been widely used for estimating hazard rate is the SP Cox model to simultaneously find the effect of several factors on survival and adjusting for the confounding effects of the other variables. This model makes parametric postulates about the result of covariates on the hazard but no assumption regarding the nature of hazard function itself and, as such, is a robust statistical technique. Both univariate and multivariate analyses were performed. Further, a negative estimated coefficient implies that for change in stage from IA2 and IB1 collectively to stage IB2 (see Figure 9.2), patient's survival gets shortened by 67% ($e^{-1.108} = 0.33$), while on controlling the factor stage, a negative estimated coefficient of tumor diameter implies that for unit increment in tumor size, the patient's survival gets shortened by 28% ($e^{-0.332} = 0.72$). For the Ling-Yang additive hazard model, only the

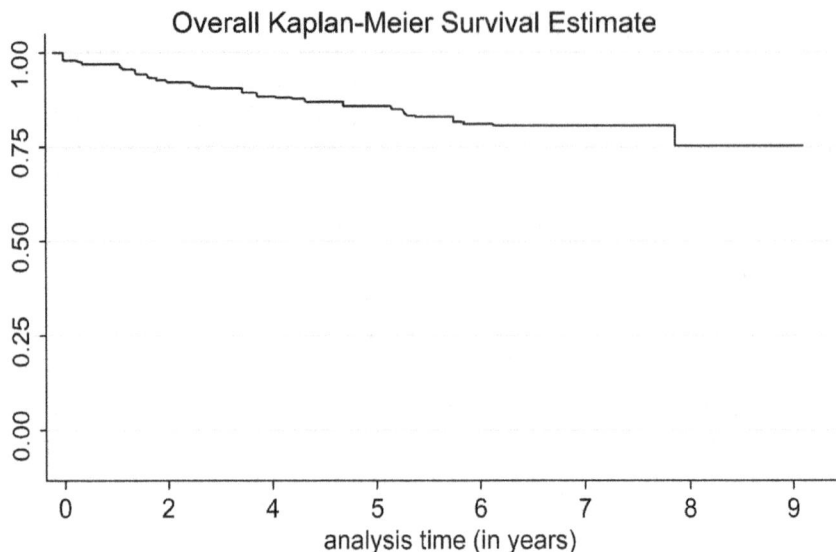

Figure 9.1 Estimate of survival probabilities stage-wise.

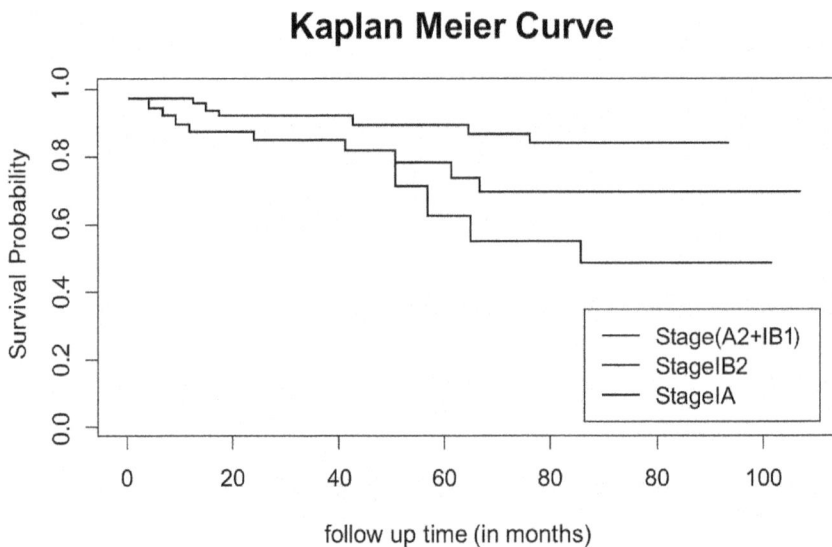

Figure 9.2 Survival curve by the tumor diameter of the patients.

tumor diameter was found to be responsible for the patient's survival with a constant effect (see Table 9.1).

From this model, the constant effect of tumor diameter on a patient's DFS is estimated at 0.0009, showing that for a unit increase in tumor diameter, on average, 9 in every 10,000 patients will have an increased risk of progression. As evident from the KM curve and p-value obtained by the log-rank test, patients in stages IA2 and IB1 have the highest survival followed by patients in stage IIA, which have been followed by the lowest survival of patients in stage IB2, and a significant difference in survival

Table 9.1 Lin and Ying additive hazard model

Lin and Ying's additive hazard model

Covariates	β	Robust SE	SE(β)	Z value	p-value	Lower 2.5%	Upper 97.5%
Tumor diameter	0.0009	0.000295	0.000319	3.130	0.001	0.000267	0.00152
Stage IB2	0.0047	0.002730	0.002860	1.710	0.090	−0.000730	0.01010
Stage IIA	0.0010	0.001520	0.001540	0.690	0.490	−0.001970	0.00407

Table 9.2 Table of univariate and multivariate analysis using Cox proportional hazard model

Univariate analysis using Cox model

covariates	β	Exp(β)	SE(β)	Z value	p-value	Lower 0.95(HR)	Upper 0.95(HR)
Tumor diameter	0.3234	1.3818	0.0752	4.3020	0.000017	1.1920	1.601
Stage IB2	1.4254	4.1595	0.3996	3.5670	0.000361	1.9007	9.103
Stage IIA	0.7953	2.2150	0.4160	1.9120	0.055893	0.9802	5.005

Multivariate analysis using Cox model

Covariates	β	Exp(β)	SE(β)	Z value	p-value	Lower 0.95(HR)	Upper 0.95(HR)
Tumor diameter	0.2539	1.2890	0.0816	3.1130	0.00185	1.0986	1.5120
Stage IB2	0.9988	2.7150	0.4324	2.3100	0.02090	1.1633	6.3370
Stage IIA	0.4085	1.5046	0.4398	0.9290	0.35299	0.6354	3.5630

In case of stage analysis, stage IA2 + IB1 has been taken as a reference stage.

exists between patients in stage IB2 and stage IA2 + IB1, collectively (see Figure 11.1). In the case of univariate analysis, a very low p-value implied a highly significant association of tumor diameter and DFS of patients, while for the covariate stage, the low p-value for the variable stage IB2 shows a significant association in an increase of HR (4.15 times) for patients belonging to this stage as compared to patients in stage IA2 + IB1, collectively. For the multivariate analysis, tumor diameter was found to be significantly associated with the patient's DFS adjusting for the variables stage IB2 and stage IIA. For adjusting tumor diameter, stage IB2 was found to be significantly associated with an increase (2.72 times) in HR as compared to patients in stage IA2+ IB1 (see Table 9.2).

For both the Cox and AFT models, no significant difference was observed between patients in stage IA2 + IB1, collectively, and stage IIA regarding their impact on the patient's survival, which indicates a kind of similarity between SP and parametric methods. The performance of various AFT models in multivariate analysis has been compared. Based on the low AIC value, the log-normal model was found to be the best-fitting model shown (see Table 9.3). Then we performed a multivariate, analysis-based, log-normal AFT model (see Table 9.4).

Table 9.3 Performance of various AFT models in multivariate analysis

Models	p-value	Log-likelihood	AIC Value
Weibull	0.00011	−253.5	517.0611
Exponential	0.00010	−253.5	515.0632
Log-logistic	0.00011	−253.2	516.5000
Log-normal	0.00019	−252.5	515.0356

Table 9.4 Multivariate analysis of variables using log-normal AFT model*

Models	β	SE(β)	p-value	C.I.
Intercept	7.406	0.631	0.000	6.1700–8.6421
Stage IB2	−1.108	0.530	0.040	−2.1468−−0.0688
Stage IIA	−0.462	0.495	0.350	−1.4332−−0.5086
Tumor diameter	−0.332	0.115	0.004	−0.5582−−0.1064

*In case of stage analysis, stage IA2 + IB1 has been taken as a reference stage.

The survival of patients has been observed that increasing the size of tumor diameter has a higher risk of death. The risk of death was higher, 2.92 and 2.35, among patients who had a tumor diameter of 4.1 and above and 3.1–4.0 mm (HR = 2.92; 95% CI: 1.35–6.31; HR = 2.35; 95% CI: 1.05–5.26), respectively, compared to tumor size (0–3.0 mm) (see Table 9.5). The overall survival of patients presented (see Figure 9.2). Thetumor diameter is divided into three categories based on tumor diameter: 0–3.0 mm, 3.1–4.0 mm, and 4.1 mm and above. The results show that tumor diameter is significantly associated with survival in CerC patients. Patients with smaller tumor (0–3.0 mm) had the best survival rate, with 92.5% of patients alive and only 7.5% deceased. Patients with larger tumor (4.1 mm and above) had the worst survival rate, with only 77.1% of patients alive and 23.0% deceased. The HR (see Table 9.5) indicates the relative risk of death for patients with each tumor diameter category, with patients in the 0–3.0 mm category serving as the reference group (HR = 1.00).

Patients with tumor in the 3.1–4.0 mm category had a HR of 2.35 (p < 0.05), indicating that they were 2.35 times more likely to die compared to patients with smaller tumor. Patients with tumors in the 4.1 mm and above category had a HR of 2.92 (p < 0.01), indicating that they were 2.92 times more likely to die compared to patients with smaller tumors. The confidence interval (C.I.) suggests that the hazard ratios are statistically significant and precise, with little chance of bias or error. The overall survival has been observed based on tumor diameter for one, two, five, and seven years, respectively (see Table 9.5). The survival probabilities have been obtained 0.952, 0.910, 0.846, and 0.838 for one, two, five, and seven years, respectively (see Table 9.6). It is observed that the survival probabilities decrease when tumor diameter increases in patients.

Discussion

As evident from the evidences produced through our analysis, both stage and tumor diameter have great impact on patients' survival. The result that patients of stage

Table 9.5 Results of Cox regression model of cervical cancer patients by selected indicators (N = 300)

Indicator	Alive		Death		p-value	Total	Hazard ratio	95% C.I.
	N	%	N	%				
Tumor diameter (in mm)								
0–3.0 mm	160	92.5	13	7.5	0.004	173	1.00	[1.00, 1.00]
3.1–4.0 mm	55	83.3	11	16.7		66	2.35*	[1.05, 5.26]
4.1 mm and above	47	77.1	14	23.0		61	2.92**	[1.35, 6.31]
Total	262	87.3	38	12.7		300		

Note: * p < 0.05, ** p < 0.01; C.I.: Confidence interval

Table 9.6 Results of the observed survival of cervical cancer patients by selected indicators

Indicators	Observed survival			
	One year	Three years	Five years	Seven years
Tumor diameter (in mm)				
0–3.0 mm	0.970	0.945	0.904	0.904
3.1–4.0 mm	0.936	0.846	0.804	0.804
4.1 mm and above	0.917	0.881	0.721	0.666
Overall survival	0.952	0.910	0.846	0.838

IB2 are experiencing more survival than patients of stage IIA seems illogical due to the fact that number of patients having the event progression is least in stage IIA. Only tumor diameter was found to be significant in case of Ling-Yang additive hazard model. This might happen due to the reason that patients in stage IB2 and stage IIA are too less in comparison to stage IA2 and stage IB1, collectively, and since effects are acting additively, more number of patients may be needed to obtain a fruitful result. Additive models can be well interpreted than multiplicative models in case of continuous explanatory variables (Madadizadeh *et al.*, 2017; Lim *et al.*, 2011; Xie *et al.*, 2013). This paper deals with the applications and illustration of statistical methods on CerC data. Findings of the study show that both stage and tumor diameter have a great impact on a patient's survival. Parametric, SP, and NP methods have been used for analysis purpose. Although the parametric methods are based on the assumption that a patient's survival time followed a specified distribution, both the Cox and AFT models have resulted in similarities between them due to statistical evidence produced from our data. Proportionality assumptions in the case of the Cox model must be the satisfied failing of which it is more appropriate to use the weighted Cox or stratified Cox model. In univariate and multivariate analysis for the variable stage, tumor diameter was performed. Performance of various AFT models in multivariate analysis has checked through AIC value and found that log-normal distribution was the best fit. It has also shown that the increasing size of tumor diameter has a higher risk of mortality. The outcomes of the performed study are stable with previous research findings, which are showing that tumor size is an important prognostic factor in cervical cancer (Hernán *et al.*, 2005; Swindell, 2009; Alam *et al.*, 2022; Tabatabaei *et al.*, 2022; Singh *et al.*, 2023; Yagi *et al.*, 2019, Tshewang *et al.*, 2021, Rajput *et al.*, 2020). A meta-analysis of 21 studies involving over 10,000 cervical cancer patients found that larger tumor size was associated with poorer survival outcomes, with each 1 cm increase in tumor size resulting in a 22% increase in the hazard of death (Hwang *et al.*, 2020). Similarly, another study of 234 cervical cancer patients found that tumor size was an independent predictor of survival, with larger tumors being associated with poorer outcomes (Shin *et al.*, 2008). The current study also has several strengths that support the validity of the findings. First, the study included a large sample size of 300 cervical cancer patients, which explore the statistical methods for analysis. Second, the study used rigorous statistical methods, including Cox regression analysis, to assess the impact of tumor diameter on survival while controlling for other relevant clinical variables.

Conclusion

Application of parametric models to clinical data is a great challenge for researchers due to the robustness of well-known semi-parametric Cox model. Overall, we have concluded that stage and tumor diameter are both significant factors for a CerC patient's survival. The current study aims to provide significant factors for screening, early diagnosis, and prognosis, as well as new therapeutic targets associated with CerC through statistical methods. By implementing targeted policies and programs, policymakers can help to improve the overall health outcomes of their populations and reduce the burden of cervical cancer in their communities.

Discussion Questions

- How does survival analysis help in understanding disease progression and treatment outcomes in cervical cancer?
- What does the study suggest about the role of tumor diameter and cancer stage in predicting patient survival?
- How can hazard ratios and confidence intervals guide clinical decisions?
- What are the strengths and limitations of using parametric vs. semi-parametric models in survival analysis?
- Lastly, how can early screening and diagnosis contribute to better outcomes in managing cervical cancer, and what policy or public health strategies could support this?

Acknowledgments

Authors are very thankful to editors, reviewers and the publisher for their comments to improve the quality of this chapter. I also acknowledge the program organized by the International Centre for Theoretical Sciences (ICTS) for participating in the program Machine Learning for Health and Disease (code: ICTS/mlhd2023/7).

References

Alam, T.F., Rahman, M.S. and Bari, W., 2022. On estimation for accelerated failure time models with small or rare event survival data. *BMC medical research methodology*, 22(1), p.169.

Bray, F., Ferlay, J., Soerjomataram, I., Siegel, R.L., Torre, L.A. and Jemal, A., 2018. Global cancer statistics 2018: GLOBOCAN estimates of incidence and mortality worldwide for 36 cancers in 185 countries. *CA: A cancer journal for clinicians*, 68(6), pp.394–424.

Cox, D.R., 1972. Regression models and life-tables. *Journal of the royal statistical society: Series B (methodological)*, 34(2), pp.187–202.

Dizaji, P.A., Farahani, M.V., Sheikhaliyan, A. and Biglarian, A., 2020. Application of additive hazards models for analyzing survival of breast cancer patients. *Journal of research in medical sciences*, 25(1), p.99.

Gardiner, J.C., 2010. Survival analysis: Overview of parametric, nonparametric and semiparametric approaches and new developments. In *SAS global forum* (Vol. 252). Cary, NC: SAS Institute, Inc.

Hernán, M.A., Cole, S.R., Margolick, J., Cohen, M. and Robins, J.M., 2005. Structural accelerated failure time models for survival analysis in studies with time-varying treatments. *Pharmacoepidemiology and drug safety*, 14(7), pp.477–491.

Horn, L.C., Fischer, U., Raptis, G., Bilek, K. and Hentschel, B., 2007. Tumor size is of prognostic value in surgically treated FIGO stage II cervical cancer. *Gynecologic oncology*, 107(2), pp.310–315.

Hwang, W.Y., Kim, J.H., Suh, D.H., Kim, K., No, J.H. and Kim, Y.B., 2020. The upper limit of optimal tumor size in patients with FIGO 2018 stage IB2 cervical cancer undergoing radical hysterectomy. *International journal of gynecological cancer*, 30(7), pp.975–980.

Kaplan, E.L. and Meier, P., 1958. Nonparametric estimation from incomplete observations. *Journal of the American statistical association*, 53(282), pp.457–481.

Kim, Y., Kang, G.H. and Kim, H., 2023. Prognostic significance of heterologous component in carcinosarcoma of the gynecologic organs: A systematic review and meta-analysis. *Journal of gynecologic oncology*, 34(6), p.e73.

Kleinbaum, D.G., Klein, M., Kleinbaum, D.G. and Klein, M., 2012. Recurrent event survival analysis. *Survival analysis: A self-learning text*, pp.363–423.

Kumar, M., Sonker, P.K., Saroj, A., Jain, A., Bhattacharjee, A. and Saroj, R.K., 2020. Parametric survival analysis using R: Illustration with lung cancer data. *Cancer reports*, 3(4), p.e1210.

Kumar, M., Sonker, P.K., Saroj, A., Jain, A., Bhattacharjee, A. and Saroj, R.K., 2020. Parametric survival analysis using R: Illustration with lung cancer data. *Cancer reports*, 3(4), p.e1210.

Lim, H.J. and Zhang, X., 2011. Additive and multiplicative hazards modeling for recurrent event data analysis. *BMC medical research methodology*, 11, pp.1–12.

Lin, D.Y. and Ying, Z., 1995. Semiparametric inference for the accelerated life model with time-dependent covariates. *Journal of statistical planning and inference*, 44(1), pp.47–63.

Madadizadeh, F., Ghanbarnejad, A., Ghavami, V., Bandamiri, M.Z. and Mohammadianpanah, M., 2017. Applying additive hazards models for analyzing survival in patients with colorectal cancer in Fars Province, Southern Iran. *Asian Pacific journal of cancer prevention: APJCP*, 18(4), p.1077.

Park, J.Y., Kim, D.Y., Kim, J.H., Kim, Y.M., Kim, Y.T. and Nam, J.H., 2011. Outcomes after radical hysterectomy according to tumor size divided by 2-cm interval in patients with early cervical cancer. *Annals of oncology*, 22(1), pp.59–67.

Rajput, M., Kumar, M., Kumari, M., Bhattacharjee, A. and Awasthi, A.A., 2020. Identification of key genes and construction of regulatory network for the progression of cervical cancer. *Gene reports*, 21, p.100965.

Royston, P. and Lambert, P.C., 2011. *Flexible parametric survival analysis using Stata: Beyond the Cox model* (Vol. 347). College Station, TX: Stata press.

Saroj, R.K., Murthy, K.N., Kumar, M., Bhattacharjee, A. and Patel, K.K., 2021. Bayesian competing risk analysis: An application to nasopharyngeal carcinoma patients data. *Computational and systems oncology*, 1(1), p.e1006.

Scheike, T.H. and Zhang, M.J., 2002. An additive–multiplicative Cox–Aalen regression model. *Scandinavian journal of statistics*, 29(1), pp.75–88.

Shin, D.W., Nam, J.H., Kwon, Y.C., Park, S.Y., Bae, D.S., Park, C.T., Cho, C.H., Lee, J.M., Park, S.M. and Yun, Y.H., 2008. Comorbidity in disease-free survivors of cervical cancer compared with the general female population. *Oncology*, 74(3–4), pp.207–215.

Singh, D., Vignat, J., Lorenzoni, V., Eslahi, M., Ginsburg, O., Lauby-Secretan, B., Arbyn, M., Basu, P., Bray, F. and Vaccarella, S., 2023. Global estimates of incidence and mortality of cervical cancer in 2020: A baseline analysis of the WHO global cervical cancer elimination initiative. *The lancet global health*, 11(2), pp.e197–e206.

Swindell, William R., 2009. Accelerated failure time models provide a useful statistical framework for aging research. *Experimental gerontology*, 44(3), pp.190–200.

Tabatabaei, F.S., Saeedian, A., Azimi, A., Kolahdouzan, K., Esmati, E. and Safaei, A.M., 2022. Evaluation of survival rate and associated factors in patients with cervical cancer: A retrospective cohort study. *Journal of research in health sciences*, 22(2), p.e00552.

Tshewang, U., Satiracoo, P. and Lenbury, Y., 2021. Survival analysis of cervical cancer patients: A case study of Bhutan. *Asian Pacific journal of cancer prevention: APJCP*, 22(9), p.2987.

Wei, L.J., 1992. The accelerated failure time model: A useful alternative to the Cox regression model in survival analysis. *Statistics in medicine*, 11(14–15), pp.1871–1879.

Xie, X., Strickler, H.D. and Xue, X., 2013. Additive hazard regression models: An application to the natural history of human papillomavirus. *Computational and mathematical methods in medicine*, 2013(1), p.796270.

Yagi, A., Ueda, Y., Kakuda, M., Tanaka, Y., Ikeda, S., Matsuzaki, S., Kobayashi, E., Morishima, T., Miyashiro, I., Fukui, K. and Ito, Y., 2019. Epidemiologic and clinical analysis of cervical cancer using data from the population-based Osaka cancer registry. *Cancer research*, 79(6), pp.1252–1259.

Systematic Review and Meta-Analysis

Unveiling Evidence in Health Research

Divya Jain, Prabudh Goel and Anjan Kumar Dhua

Learning Outcomes

Readers will understand the structured process and significance of systematic reviews and meta-analyses in evidence-based medicine. They will become familiar with using the PICO framework to formulate research questions, conducting comprehensive literature searches, registering protocols, and selecting studies systematically. The chapter will develop their ability to assess study quality using tools like the Cochrane Risk of Bias Tool and extract and synthesize data effectively. Additionally, learners will gain practical knowledge of meta-analysis techniques, including fixed and random effects models, heterogeneity assessment, and graphical tools, like forest and funnel plots, promoting transparency and robust research synthesis.

Introduction

Systematic reviews and meta-analyses are cornerstone methodologies in health research designed to synthesize existing evidence on a particular topic systematically and objectively (Akobeng 2005). Unlike traditional narrative reviews, which provide a qualitative summary based on the author's discretion, systematic reviews follow a rigorous and predefined protocol to minimize bias, ensuring a comprehensive aggregation of relevant literature. Meta-analyses extend this by quantitatively combining results from individual studies, offering a powerful tool to estimate the overall effect size or outcome of interest. Thus, they play a pivotal role in evidence-based medicine and healthcare decision-making.

Role in Evidence-Based Medicine

These methodologies are integral to evidence-based medicine, providing clinicians, policymakers, and researchers with high-quality evidence that informs clinical guidelines,

DOI: 10.4324/9781032701004-13

policy decisions, and future research directions. By aggregating data from multiple studies, they can reveal trends and evidence that individual studies may not be powerful enough to detect, thereby enhancing the reliability of healthcare interventions. In contrast to narrative reviews, systematic reviews and meta-analyses are characterized by their structured approach, including predefined eligibility criteria, an exhaustive search strategy, and explicit methods for data extraction and analysis. This systematic approach reduces the risk of bias and enhances the reproducibility and reliability of the findings.

Section 1: Foundations of Systematic Reviews

Objectives and Prerequisites

The primary objective of a systematic review is to answer a specific research question by collecting and summarizing all empirical evidence that fits pre-specified eligibility criteria. Essential prerequisites include a well-defined research question, clear inclusion and exclusion criteria, and a comprehensive literature search strategy.

PICO Framework

The PICO (population, intervention, comparison, outcome) framework is fundamental in formulating research questions for systematic reviews, ensuring that they are specific and focused. This framework helps identify a study's key components, which are essential for literature searches and study selection. Before understanding the PICO framework, a brief background of the disease in question is provided to assimilate the illustration easily.

Biliary atresia is a rare paediatric liver disorder characterized by the obstruction or absence of bile ducts, leading to liver accumulation. This condition typically presents within the first few weeks of life and can rapidly progress to liver fibrosis and cirrhosis if left untreated. The etiology of biliary atresia remains unclear, though it is believed to involve a combination of genetic, infectious, and immune-mediated factors (Hartley, Davenport, and Kelly 2009).

Clinical Manifestations and Diagnosis

The clinical presentation of biliary atresia includes persistent jaundice, dark urine, pale stools, and hepatomegaly. Early diagnosis is critical for managing the disease and improving outcomes.

Kasai Procedure: The Standard Surgical Operation

The Kasai portoenterostomy, or Kasai procedure, is the standard surgical treatment for biliary atresia offered as soon as possible before 90 days of life to achieve acceptable outcomes.

The Role of Steroids in Post-Kasai Management

The use of adjuvant therapies, such as steroids, in the postoperative management of biliary atresia has been a subject of considerable interest. Steroids are proposed to reduce inflammation and fibrosis, potentially improving bile flow and liver function after the

Kasai procedure. However, the efficacy and optimal regimen of steroid therapy in this context remain areas of ongoing research and debate.

With this background, an illustrative research question for conducting a systematic review and meta-analysis on the effectiveness of postoperative steroid use in patients with biliary atresia undergoing Kasai portoenterostomy could be framed using the PICO (population, intervention, comparison, outcome) framework as follows:

Research Question: *In infants with biliary atresia less than 90 days old undergoing Kasai portoenterostomy, does the use of postoperative steroids, compared to no steroids, improve jaundice clearance at 6 and 12 months post-operation?*

PICO Framework:

Population (P): Infants diagnosed with biliary atresia who are less than 90 days old undergoing Kasai portoenterostomy.

Intervention (I): Postoperative administration of steroids.

Comparison (C): No use of steroids postoperatively or the use of a placebo.

Outcomes (O): Jaundice clearance at 6 months and 12 months after the operation, which can be measured by normal bilirubin levels or the absence of clinically evident jaundice.

Protocol Development and Registration

Developing and registering a protocol, for instance, in PROSPERO, is crucial for ensuring transparency and preventing reporting bias. The protocol outlines the review's rationale, hypothesis, and planned methods, serving as a roadmap for conducting the review. Researchers are advised to submit this document to the principal investigator (PI) for review before making it available on registry websites.

Section 2: Conducting a Systematic Review

Literature Search Strategies

An exhaustive literature search is the backbone of a systematic review, requiring detailed planning to identify all relevant studies. It involves several steps:

Database Selection: Identify the most relevant electronic databases tailored to the health research topic. Common databases include PubMed, Embase, Cochrane Library, and Web of Science.

Search Term Development: We need to create a list of keywords and medical subject headings (MeSH) terms related to the PICO elements and then combine these terms using Boolean operators (AND, OR, NOT) to refine the search.

An illustrative search strategy for the research question illustrated (see PICO earlier) in PubMed involves identifying key concepts from your research question and translating them into searchable keywords and medical subject headings (Meshy) terms. Your research question focuses on the use of steroids after the Kasai procedure in patients with biliary atresia. Here's how one can develop a structured search strategy:

Step 1: Identify Key Concepts

Our main concepts are as follows: biliary atresia, Kasai procedure, and steroids

Step 2: Generate Keywords and MeSH Terms

We have to list all relevant keywords and MeSH terms for each concept. MeSH terms are standardized terms used in PubMed to index articles and ensure consistent retrieval of information.

Concept 1: Biliary Atresia

Keywords: Biliary Atresia, Neonatal Cholestasis

MeSH Term: "Biliary Atresia" [MeSH]

Concept 2: Kasai Procedure

Keywords: Kasai Procedure, Portoenterostomy, Hepatoportoenterostomy

MeSH Term: "Portoenterostomy, Hepatic" [MeSH]

Concept 3: Steroids

Keywords: Steroids, Corticosteroids, Prednisolone, Prednisone

MeSH Term: "Steroids" [MeSH], "Adrenal Cortex Hormones" [MeSH]

Step 3: Combine Keywords and MeSH Terms Using Boolean Operators

We need to use Boolean operators (AND, OR, NOT) to combine your search terms. "OR" broadens your search by including any of the terms listed, while "AND" narrows your search by requiring the presence of terms from different concepts.

Illustrative Search Strategy

("Biliary Atresia" [MeSH] OR Biliary Atresia OR Neonatal Cholestasis) AND ("Portoenterostomy, Hepatic" [MeSH] OR Kasai Procedure OR Portoen-terostomy OR Hepatoportoenterostomy) AND ("Steroids" [MeSH] OR "Adrenal Cortex Hormones" [MeSH] OR Steroids OR Corticosteroids OR Prednisolone OR Prednisone)

Step 4: Apply Filters

We need to consider applying filters to refine our search further, such as age (e.g., Child: birth – 18 years), article type (e.g., clinical trials, reviews), language (e.g., English), and publication date (e.g., last five years).

Search Execution

We have to perform the search across all selected databases. AMSTAR (A Measurement Tool to Assess Systematic Reviews) recommends the usage of at least two databases (Beverley et al. 2017). Document the search strategy, including the search date, any limits applied, and the number of results to be included in the final publication.

Supplemental Searches

Search for unpublished studies, gray literature, and hand-search key journals and con-ference proceedings to minimize publication bias. Additionally, forward snowballing (citation tracking) and backward snowballing (citation searching) are done to comple-ment database searches, ensuring a more exhaustive review of the literature and provid-ing a deeper understanding of the research landscape surrounding a topic

Screening and Selection

Screening studies based on predefined inclusion and exclusion criteria ensures that only relevant studies are included in the review (Figure 10.1). This process typically involves a two-stage screening (title/abstract and full text) by two independent reviewers to minimize bias, as illustrated next:

Initial Screening: Review titles and abstracts against the inclusion and exclusion criteria. Two independent reviewers usually do this to ensure reliability.

Full-Text Screening: Obtain and review the full text of articles that pass the initial screening. Apply the same inclusion and exclusion criteria.

Resolution of Discrepancies: Any reviewer disagreements are resolved through discussion or consultation with a third reviewer.

Data Extraction and Quality Assessment

Data extraction is a critical phase in conducting a systematic review, as it involves collecting pertinent information from each study in a standardized, systematic, and

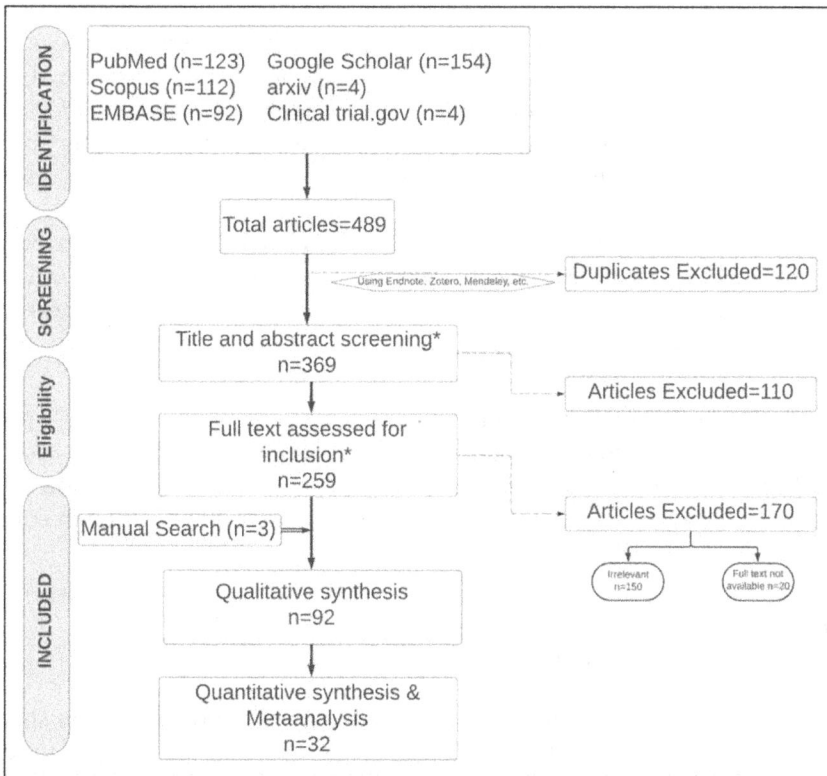

Figure 10.1 Flowchart shows the process of screening and selecting articles as an illustrative example. (Note: steps with a "*" are typically done by two independent reviewers, as explained before.)

reproducible manner. The purpose is to gather sufficient detail to facilitate data synthesis and to allow for reproducibility of the findings by others. The form should be specifically tailored to capture all relevant information that aligns with the research question and objectives of the systematic review. The points to consider are as follows:

Designing the Form:
The form should be comprehensive and designed to capture all necessary information to answer the research question. It should be laid out logically, aligning with the structure of the studies being reviewed.

Key Components:
Bibliographic Details: Author names, publication year, journal name, etc.
Study Characteristics: Study design, sample size, duration, setting, etc.
Participant Demographics: Age, gender, ethnicity, disease status, etc.
Intervention and Comparator Details: Dose, frequency, duration, control conditions, etc.
Outcomes: Primary and secondary outcomes, time points measured, units of measurement, etc.

Electronic Forms:
Utilizing electronic forms can facilitate the extraction process and reduce manual errors. Software like Microsoft Excel, REDCap, or Google Forms can be used to create customizable forms. It is important to *pilot the data extraction form* before full-scale data extraction begins. It is essential that during piloting the form, one should do the following:

Test the Form: We should select a small number of studies to test the data extraction form. This process helps identify any issues with the form's design or content.
Revise: Based on the pilot test, we may have to revise the form to ensure it efficiently captures all relevant data.

Conducting the Data Extraction
The actual data extraction can commence once the form has been tested and finalized. Two reviewers should independently extract data using the form to reduce bias and errors. Any discrepancies should be resolved through consensus or arbitration by a third reviewer.

Quality Control in Data Extraction
To ensure the quality of the data extraction process:

Consistency Checks: Regular checks for consistency across reviewers should be conducted. It is important to calibrate reviewers' understanding of the extraction items regularly.
Audit Trails: Maintaining an audit trail of the data extracted, including notes on any decisions or deviations from the protocol, is crucial for transparency.

Training and Standardization: Training sessions for reviewers prior to the start of data extraction can be beneficial.

Regular meetings to discuss challenges and resolve uncertainties can help maintain the quality and consistency of the data extracted.

Assessing the Quality and Risk of Bias and Generation of Visualization Charts

Assessing the quality of studies is essential in systematic reviews to ensure the credibility of findings. High-quality studies strengthen the evidence base, while low-quality studies may introduce bias and affect the overall conclusions of the review.

Risk of Bias Assessment

The risk of bias assessment evaluates the extent to which a study's design and execution may have compromised the validity of its results. This assessment is crucial, as biases can lead to an overestimation or underestimation of the true effect of an intervention.

Tools for Quality and Bias Assessment

Cochrane Risk of Bias Tool
The Cochrane Collaboration's tool for assessing the risk of bias is widely used in systematic reviews. It focuses on the following domains:
Selection Bias: Related to the randomization process.
Performance Bias: Related to blinding of participants and personnel.
Detection Bias: Pertains to blinding of outcome assessment.
Attrition Bias: Involves incomplete outcome data.
Reporting Bias: Concerns selective reporting of outcomes.
Other Bias: Includes any other potential sources of bias not covered by the earlier categories.

Newcastle-Ottawa Scale (NOS)
For non-randomized studies, the NOS is often employed. It assesses studies based on three broad perspectives:

Selection of Study Groups
Comparability of Groups
Ascertainment of Either the Exposure or Outcome of Interest

Visualization of Quality and Risk of Bias
Bar Graphs

Bar graphs are simple visual representations used to display the number of studies with low, unclear, or high risk of bias in each domain. They provide a quick overview of the overall risk of bias in the included studies (Figure 10.2).

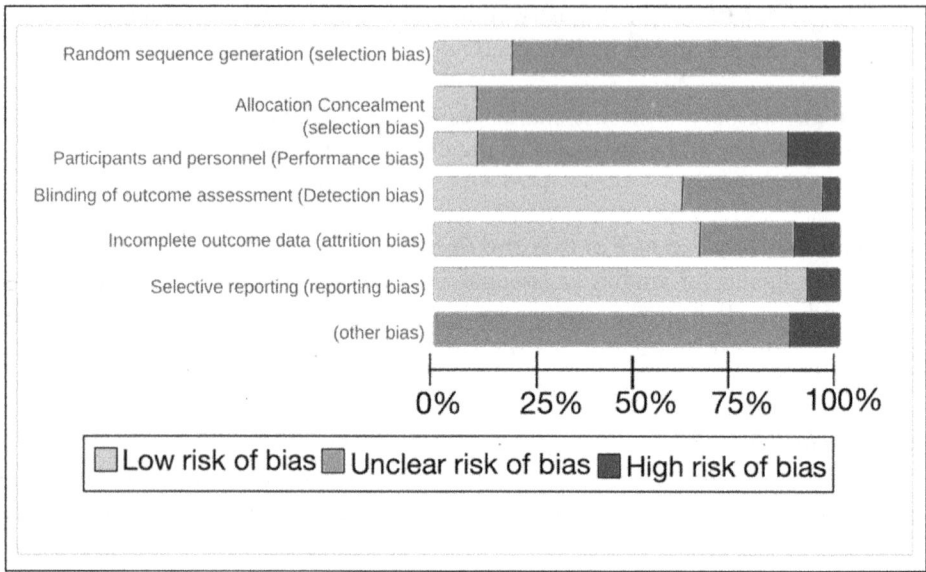

Figure 10.2 Illustrating a bar graph as a visualization tool to examine the risk of bias of studies included in a particular review.

Traffic Light Plots

Also known as "risk of bias summary figures", these plots use colours (green, yellow, red) to represent low, unclear, and high risk of bias, respectively (Figure 10.3). A row represents each study, and each domain by a column, creating a matrix that allows for rapid visual assessment.

Funnel Plots

Funnel plots are used to visually assess publication bias. The plot should look like a pyramid or a symmetrical inverted funnel, as seen in Figure 10.4. They plot the treatment effects from individual studies against a measure of study size. An asymmetrical plot suggests potential publication bias.

The various characteristics of the plot and its interpretation are as follows:

Vertical Axis (Precision): Precision, usually the inverse of the standard error (SE), is plotted on the vertical axis. Studies with higher precision (usually larger studies) are expected to be closer to the top of the plot, while those with lower precision (smaller studies) appear towards the bottom.

Horizontal Axis (Effect Size): The estimated effect size from each study is plotted on the horizontal axis. The true effect is assumed to be at the top of the funnel, with the highest precision.

Asymmetrical Funnel Shape: The funnel shape should be symmetrical in the absence of publication bias. This means that studies are distributed evenly on both sides of the effect size representing the true effect.

	D1	D2	D3	D4	D4	D5	D6	D7	Overall
Study AA, 2020	⊕	⊕	⊕	⊕	⊕	⊕	⊕	⊕	⊕
Study AB, 2020	⊕	⊖	⊕	⊕	⊕	⊕	⊕	⊕	⊕
Study AA, 2021	⊕	⊕	⊕	⊖	⊕	⊕	⊕	⊕	⊕
Study AB, 2021	⊕	⊖	⊕	⊕	⊕	⊕	⊕	⊕	⊕
Study AA, 2022	⊗	⊕	⊕	⊕	⊕	⊕	⊕	⊗	⊗
Study AB, 2022	⊖	⊕	⊕	⊕	⊕	⊕	⊕	⊕	⊖
Study AA, 2023	⊕	⊕	⊕	⊕	⊕	⊕	⊕	⊕	⊕
Study AB, 2023	⊕	⊕	⊕	⊖	⊕	⊕	⊕	⊕	⊖
Study AA, 2016	⊕	⊕	⊕	⊖	⊕	⊕	⊕	⊕	⊖
Study AB, 2014	⊗	⊗	⊕	⊖	⊕	⊗	⊕	⊖	⊗
Study AA, 2001	⊕	⊕	⊕	⊕	⊕	⊕	⊕	⊕	⊕
Study AB, 2009	⊕	⊕	⊖	⊕	⊕	⊕	⊕	⊕	⊕

Judgement

⊕ Low risk

⊖ Moderate risk

⊗ High risk

D1	Bias due to confounding
D2	Bias due to selection of participants
D3	Bias due to classification of intervention
D4	Bias due to deviation from intended interventions
D5	Bias due to missing data
D6	Bias in measurement of outcomes
D7	Bias in selection of the reported result

Figure 10.3 Risk of bias (RoB) traffic light plot. Assessment of the risk of bias via the traffic light plot of the RoB of each included clinical trial on the left and the weighted plot for assessing the overall risk of bias via the Cochrane Robins-I tool ($n = 12$ studies). The yellow circle indicates some concerns about the risk of bias, and the green circle represents a low risk of bias.

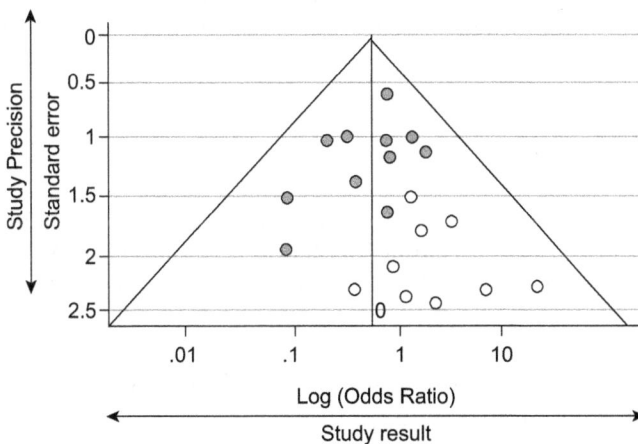

Figure 10.4 Funnel plot to assess the presence of publication bias.

Scatter of Studies: Individual studies are represented by dots or other markers scattered within the funnel. Ideally, they should form a mirror image on either side of the aggregate effect size.

Area of Potential Bias: If smaller studies are missing from the bottom corners of the plot (usually on one side of the effect size), this can indicate potential publication bias. It suggests that smaller studies with non-significant results might not have been published.

Other Tools

Software like RevMan (Review Manager) from the Cochrane Collaboration and online platforms, such as GRADEpro, can facilitate the creation of these visualizations.

Quality Control in Assessment

Having two independent reviewers assess the quality and risk of bias is a standard practice to reduce errors and improve reliability. Prior to starting the assessments, reviewers should undergo calibration exercises to ensure a consistent understanding of the assessment criteria. Disagreements between reviewers are typically resolved through discussion or by involving a third reviewer.

Data Synthesis

Synthesizing data from included studies can involve qualitative summaries for heterogeneous studies or quantitative methods like meta-analysis for studies with sufficient similarities. The choice of synthesis method depends on the nature of the research question and the consistency of the data available.

Qualitative Synthesis

Qualitative data synthesis in systematic reviews involves aggregating or interpreting non-numerical data from primary qualitative studies. The synthesis can reveal overarching themes, concepts, and constructs across multiple studies. It is a critical process for understanding complex phenomena, exploring heterogeneity, and providing context for quantitative findings.

Software Tools for Qualitative Synthesis
Covidence

Covidence is primarily designed to streamline the processes of systematic reviews in health and medical research, including qualitative study synthesis. While Covidence is more known for quantitative data handling, it can also support qualitative synthesis in the following ways:

Reference Management: Covidence can help manage references for qualitative studies and streamline the selection process.

Study Selection: It facilitates screening titles, abstracts, and full-text articles based on inclusion and exclusion criteria relevant to qualitative research.

Data Extraction: Although Covidence does not specifically analyze qualitative data, it can be used to extract relevant information, themes, or quotes from qualitative studies that can be further analyzed.

NVivo

NVivo is a powerful tool for qualitative data analysis and is especially useful for qualitative data synthesis in systematic reviews. It supports a range of functions that are beneficial for synthesizing qualitative data:

Data Importation: NVivo allows users to import data from various sources, including text documents, PDFs, and transcripts.

Coding: Researchers can code their data by tagging text segments (such as paragraphs, sentences, or words) with labels that summarize their content or theme.

Node Creation: Codes or "nodes" can be created to represent themes or concepts across different studies.

Queries: NVivo can run queries to find and explore coded data, helping to identify patterns or relationships within the data.

Models and Frameworks: NVivo supports the creation of models to visually represent the relationships between themes and structure the synthesis process.

Memoing: Researchers can write memos in NVivo to document their thoughts, interpretations, and analytical processes, essential in synthesizing qualitative evidence.

Qualitative Synthesis Approaches

Thematic Synthesis

This involves coding text "line-by-line" and then developing "descriptive themes". Eventually, "analytical themes" are generated, which can be interpreted and integrated into the systematic review's findings (Thomas and Harden 2008).

Framework Synthesis

This approach involves using a framework, either pre-existing or developed inductively from the data, to organize and synthesize findings (Brunton, Oliver, and Thomas 2020).

Meta-Ethnography

Developed by Noblit and Hare, meta-ethnography synthesizes interpretive qualitative research by translating studies into one another (Noblit and Hare 1999).

Grounded Theory Synthesis

This method involves developing a theory based on the data from the included qualitative studies, typically using coding and constant comparative analysis (Glaser and Strauss 2017).

Narrative Synthesis

It involves storytelling to synthesize findings, which is often useful when dealing with diverse studies. Software can help by organizing narratives and tracking themes (Popay et al. 2006).

Visualization Tools

Mind Maps: NVivo allows for the creation of mind maps to organize and connect ideas visually.

Models: Researchers can build models in NVivo to visualize the relationships between themes.

Charts: Both Covidence and NVivo can produce charts, such as coding frequency charts, to visualize data at a glance.

Best Practices for Qualitative Synthesis

Transparency: Documenting every step of the synthesis process is crucial for ensuring the reproducibility and credibility of the review.

Teamwork: Multiple coders should work on the data extraction and coding process to enhance reliability.

Audit Trail: Maintaining a comprehensive audit trail of decisions and interpretations made during the synthesis process.

Qualitative data synthesis, aided by software tools, offers a structured and systematic approach to understanding complex bodies of qualitative evidence. These tools help manage and analyze large volumes of text data, enabling researchers to identify key themes and patterns that emerge from the literature.

Section 3: Introduction to Meta-Analysis

Meta-analysis is a statistical technique that combines the results of multiple scientific studies. It is a critical component of systematic reviews, as it allows for a more objective appraisal of evidence by consolidating findings and identifying patterns across research studies.

Definition and Purpose of Meta-Analysis

Meta-analysis is a methodological approach that employs statistical techniques to aggregate and synthesize the findings from numerous studies. The primary objective of a meta-analysis is to determine an overarching effect size that reflects the strength of a treatment's impact or association across a range of research. This process enhances the sample size, increasing statistical strength and accurate estimates. Additionally, meta-analysis helps to clarify inconsistencies among study results, offering a clearer conclusion regarding the efficacy of a treatment or the robustness of an association.

Types of Data in Meta-Analysis

Meta-analysis can handle various types of data, including the following:

Continuous Data: Outcomes measured continuously, such as blood pressure or weight. The effect size can be expressed as a mean difference or standardized mean difference.

Binary Data: Dichotomous outcomes, such as the presence or absence of a disease. The effect size is often presented as an odds ratio, risk ratio, or risk difference.

Statistical Models in Meta-Analysis
There are two primary statistical models used to combine data in meta-analysis:

Fixed Effects Model:
Assume that all studies estimate the same underlying effect.
The observed variance between study results is due only to chance.
Appropriate when studies are functionally identical, and the between-study variance is insignificant.

Random Effects Model:
Recognize that studies estimate different yet related effects.
Assumes that the observed variance reflects real differences in study outcomes and chance. It is used when heterogeneity is present, which is often the case in medical research.

Understanding Heterogeneity
Heterogeneity refers to the variability in study outcomes. It is a key concept in meta-analysis for several reasons:

Source of Variation: Heterogeneity can arise from clinical differences (e.g., population characteristics), methodological differences (e.g., study design), or random variation.
Assessment Tools: The I^2 statistic quantifies the proportion of total variation in study estimates due to heterogeneity rather than chance. The Q Test is a statistical test that assesses whether observed differences in results are likely to have occurred by chance.
Implications: Significant heterogeneity can impact the validity of the meta-analysis and may suggest the need for subgroup analyses or a more refined approach to combining studies.

Section 4: Performing Meta-Analysis and Presenting the Result
Conducting a meta-analysis requires meticulous planning, a clear understanding of statistical methods, and careful interpretation of results. Each step is vital to ensure the reliability and validity of the conclusions drawn from the meta-analysis.

Statistical Methods

Choice of Effect Measure
The first step in the statistical analysis of a meta-analysis is to choose the appropriate effect measure, which is dependent on the nature of the outcome data:

For Dichotomous Outcomes: Odds ratios (OR), risk ratios (RR), and risk differences (RD) are commonly used.

For Continuous Outcomes: Mean differences (MD) if outcomes are measured in the same way across studies or standardized mean differences (SMD) if different scales are used.

Selection of Statistical Model

The next step is to decide on the statistical model:

Fixed Effects Model: Assumes that the true effect size is the same in all studies. It is typically used when studies are sufficiently similar, and the aim is to estimate the common effect size.

Random Effects Model: This model assumes that the true effect size varies from study to study. It is more appropriate when there is heterogeneity among the study results.

Pooling the Data

After choosing the effect measure and statistical model, data from the included studies are mathematically combined using appropriate tests. The Mantel-Haenszel and Peto odds ratio methods are generally used as statistical methods to get the pooled effect.

The Mantel-Haenszel method is a statistical approach used to estimate the pooled effect size in meta-analyses of studies that report categorical outcomes. It is particularly useful when studies have small sample sizes or when events are rare. The method provides a weighted average of the effect estimates from the individual studies, taking into account the size of each study, which ensures that larger studies have more influence on the overall estimate.

The Peto odds ratio method is a specialized tool in the meta-analyst's toolkit. It is useful for specific data types and under certain conditions, particularly rare events and situations where other methods may be less reliable or more cumbersome. However, it is crucial to understand its assumptions and limitations, apply them appropriately, and interpret the results correctly.

Weighting Studies: Each study's effect estimate is weighted by the inverse of its variance. This gives more weight to larger studies, which are assumed to provide more precise estimates.

Calculating the Pooled Estimate: The weighted effect sizes are summed across all studies to produce a pooled estimate and its confidence interval (CI).

Assessing Heterogeneity

Evaluating heterogeneity is crucial for understanding the variability in effect estimates across studies:

I^2 Statistic: This statistic describes the percentage of variation across studies that is due to heterogeneity rather than chance. 25%, 50%, and 75% values are considered low, moderate, and high heterogeneity, respectively.

Chi-Squared Test (Q Test): Tests whether the observed differences in results are compatible with chance alone. A low p-value (< 0.10) indicates significant heterogeneity.

Tau^2 (Tau-Squared): An estimate of the between-study variance in random effects models.

Forest Plot

Forest plots are graphical representations of the data from a series of studies pooled in a meta-analysis, with a graphical representation of the meta-analysis's result (Figure 10.5). They provide an easy-to-read visual summary of the estimated results from each study and how they contribute to the overall meta-analysis result. To understand it better, let us go through a forest plot adapted from a study by Goel et al. (2019). They conducted a systematic review and meta-analysis of the papers assessing the frequency of urethrocutaneous fistula formation (orange rectangles) following hypospadias repair surgeries, comparing patients who received caudal block pain relief (green rectangle next to the list of studies) to those who did not (navy blue rectangle).

Understanding and Interpreting a Forest Plot

Interpreting a forest plot involves analyzing a graphical representation of the results from multiple studies on a specific research question (orange rectangle on the left in the earlier example). The plot displays each study's effect sizes, confidence intervals, and an overall estimate of the combined effect. To interpret it, let us go through the earlier image (Figure 10.5) to understand the following:

1. Effect Sizes: Look at the central estimate of each study's effect size, typically represented by squares. The size of the square reflects the weight or size of the study (squares of varying sizes in blue colouring the center of the horizontal lines within the green rectangle in the extreme right of the image).
2. Confidence Intervals: Horizontal lines extending from each square indicate the confidence intervals. A wider interval suggests more uncertainty in the estimate (see within the green rectangle).
3. Overall Effect: The diamond at the bottom synthesizes all study results (red oval), showing the combined effect size and confidence interval. If the diamond crosses the line of no effect (magenta arrow), it indicates no significant overall effect.
4. Heterogeneity: Assess the variation between study results. Significant variability might necessitate a random effects model and cautious interpretation of the combined effect (blue rectangle).
5. Significance: Determine if the confidence intervals of individual studies or the overall effect exclude the line of no effect, indicating statistical significance.

By examining these elements, researchers can gain insights into the magnitude and reliability of the effect being studied, as well as the consistency of evidence across studies.

Advanced Techniques

For more sophisticated analyses, additional techniques may be used:

Subgroup Analysis: To explore whether the effect differs across subgroups defined by study or participant characteristics.

Meta-Regression: To investigate the relationship between study-level covariates (e.g., baseline risk, study quality) and the effect size.

Study or Subgroup	Caudal Analgesia		No Caudal Analgesia		Weught	Odds Ratio
	Events	Total	Events	Total	Weught	M-H, Random, 95% CI
Braga et al	32	357	5	151	15.5%	2.88 [1.10, 7.53]
Kim 2 et al	53	216	19	126	21.1%	1.83 [1.03, 3.26]
Kim et al	26	216	15	126	19.6%	1.01 [0.51, 1.99]
Kreysing et al	3	33	2	37	7.3%	1.75 [0.27, 11.18]
Kundra et al	5	27	0	27	3.4%	13.44 [0.70, 256.43]
Saavendra et al	9	91	2	101	9.2%	5.43 [1.14, 25.85]
Taicher et al	21	230	1	165	6.4%	16.48 [2.19, 123.76]
Zaidi et al	32	101	12	34	17.5%	0.85 [0.37, 1.93]
Total (95% CI)		1271		767	100.0%	2.08 [1.16, 3.74]
Total events	181		56			
Heterogeneity: Tau² = 0.34; Chi² = 15.86, df = 7 (P = 0.03); I² = 56%						
Text for overall effect: Z = 2.44 (P = 0.01)						

Heterogeneity: $Tau^2 = 0.34$; $Chi^2 = 15.86$, $df = 7$ ($P = 0.03$); $I^2 = 56\%$

Text for overall effect: $Z = 2.44$ ($P = 0.01$)

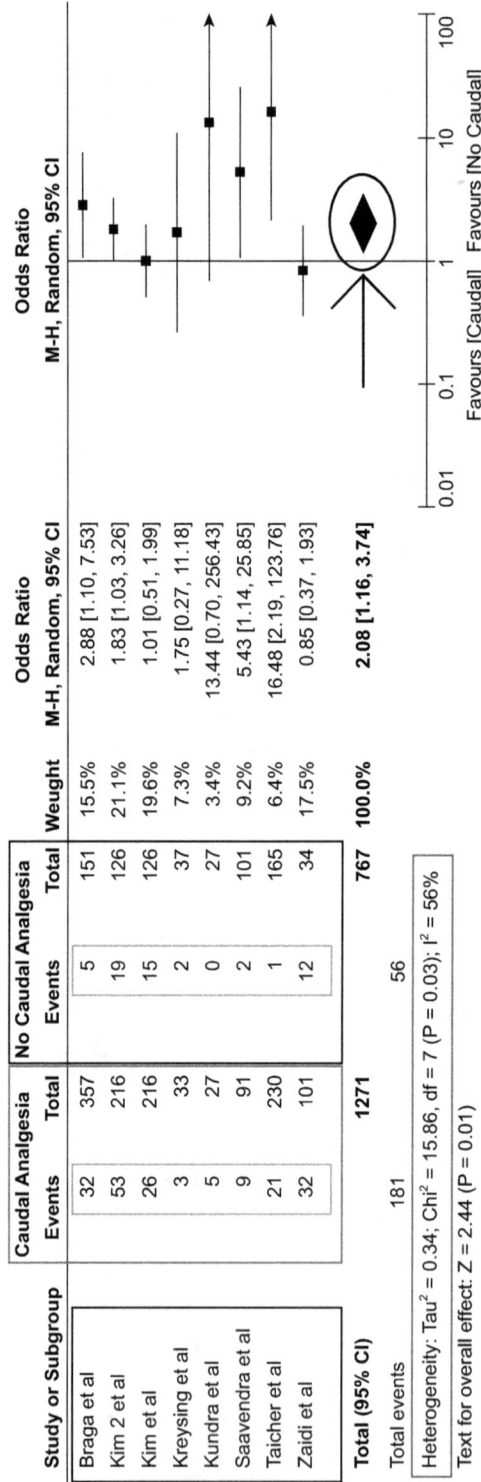

Figure 10.5 A representative forest plot used to visualize the summary of results of a meta-analysis. Note that the coloured annotations are not part of the forest plot but are added here to help understand the concepts.

Sensitivity Analysis

To test the robustness of the meta-analysis findings:

Leave-One-Out Analysis: Repeating the meta-analysis multiple times, each time leaving out a different study, to see if the results depend on a single study.

Influence Analysis: Identifying studies that have a large influence on the overall meta-analysis estimate.

Software for Conducting Meta-analysis

Here are some popular tools for conducting the statistical analysis in meta-analysis:

a. RevMan: Review Manager (RevMan), developed by Cochrane, is the designated software for crafting and updating Cochrane systematic reviews. RevMan supports creating protocols and systematic reviews encompassing text, study details, comparative tables, and research data. The software is capable of conducting meta-analyses on the inputted data and visually displaying the outcomes.

b. R (with meta and metafor packages): Offers extensive and flexible statistical programming capabilities for meta-analysis, including advanced graphics. The metafor package offers extensive tools for performing meta-analyses within the R programming environment. This package provides capabilities to compute different effect sizes or outcomes, apply a range of models, including equal-, fixed-, random-, and mixed-effects to the data, conduct analyses involving moderators and meta-regression, and generate a variety of charts for meta-analysis, such as forest and funnel plots, among others.

c. Stata: Commercial software with powerful commands for meta-analysis (metan, metareg, metafunnel, metabias).

d. Comprehensive Meta-Analysis (CMA): User-friendly paid software focused solely on meta-analysis.

Section 5: Reporting and Interpreting Results

Reporting and interpreting results is about presenting the data and providing insights and translating the findings into actionable knowledge. It is where the review speaks to the audience, conveying the nuances and intricacies of the evidence synthesized.

The reporting of systematic reviews and meta-analyses should adhere to established guidelines to ensure transparency and completeness. The most widely endorsed guidelines are as follows:

PRISMA (Preferred Reporting Items for Systematic Reviews and Meta-Analyses): A checklist of items that should be included in a report, such as the rationale, objectives, databases searched, total number of studies screened/included, risk of bias assessment, and synthesis of results. The PRISMA statement also includes a flow diagram to track the number of records identified, included, and excluded, as well as the reasons for exclusions. This diagram is an essential part of the PRISMA report as it provides a visual and clear method for readers to assess the reviewers' systematic search and selection processes (Page et al. 2021).

The checklist ensures that readers can assess the validity and applicability of a systematic review, which is crucial in the context of evidence-based practice. Authors are encouraged to adhere to this checklist to improve the quality of their systematic reviews and meta-analyses.

MOOSE (Meta-analysis Of Observational Studies in Epidemiology): Similar to PRISMA but tailored explicitly for observational studies.

(Brooke, Schwartz, and Pawlik 2021)

Conclusion

Conclusively, the chapter serves as an educational voyage through the structured landscape of systematic reviews and meta-analyses and as an affirmation of their role as cornerstones of evidence-based medicine. Through the meticulous application of these methodologies, healthcare professionals and researchers can navigate the complexities of medical research, ensuring that clinical decisions and policy directives are grounded in the most reliable, comprehensive, and up-to-date evidence available. As we advance, the continual refinement of these processes and the embrace of innovative analytical techniques will undoubtedly further solidify the foundation upon which evidence-based healthcare stands, promising a future where medical interventions are ever more effective, efficient, and aligned with patients' best interests worldwide.

Discussion Questions

- How do systematic reviews differ from narrative reviews in terms of methodology and reliability?
- What is the importance of using the PICO framework and protocol registration in conducting a systematic review?
- How can bias be identified and minimized during literature selection and data extraction?
- What role does heterogeneity play in choosing between fixed and random effects models in meta-analysis?
- How do forest and funnel plots help interpret results?
- Finally, how do advanced techniques like meta-regression and sensitivity analysis contribute to the credibility and applicability of systematic reviews in guiding clinical decision-making?

References

Akobeng, A. K. 2005. "Principles of evidence based medicine." *Arch Dis Child* 90 (8): 837–840. https://doi.org/10.1136/adc.2005.071761.

Beverley, J. Shea, C. Reeves Barnaby, Wells George, Thuku Micere, Hamel Candyce, Moran Julian, Moher David, Tugwell Peter, Welch Vivian, Kristjansson Elizabeth, and A. Henry David. 2017. "AMSTAR 2: A critical appraisal tool for systematic reviews that include randomised or non-randomised studies of healthcare interventions, or both." *BMJ* 358: j4008. https://doi.org/10.1136/bmj.j4008. http://www.bmj.com/content/358/bmj.j4008.abstract.

Brooke, Benjamin S., Todd A. Schwartz, and Timothy M. Pawlik. 2021. "MOOSE reporting guidelines for meta-analyses of observational studies." *JAMA Surgery* 156 (8): 787–788. https://doi.org/10.1001/jamasurg.2021.0522. https://doi.org/10.1001/jamasurg.2021.0522.

Brunton, G., S. Oliver, and J. Thomas. 2020. "Innovations in framework synthesis as a systematic review method." *Res Synth Methods* 11 (3): 316–330. https://doi.org/10.1002/jrsm.1399.

Glaser, Barney, and Anselm Strauss. 2017. *Discovery of grounded theory: Strategies for qualitative research.* Routledge.

Goel, P., S. Jain, M. Bajpai, P. Khanna, V. Jain, and D. K. Yadav. 2019. "Does caudal analgesia increase the rates of urethrocutaneous fistula formation after hypospadias repair? Systematic review and meta-analysis." *Indian J Urol* 35 (3): 222–229. https://doi.org/10.4103/iju.IJU_252_18.

Hartley, J. L., M. Davenport, and D. A. Kelly. 2009. "Biliary atresia." *Lancet* 374 (9702): 1704–1713. https://doi.org/10.1016/s0140-6736(09)60946-6.

Noblit, George W., and R. Dwight Hare. 1999. "Chapter 5: Meta-ethnography: Synthesizing qualitative studies." *Counterpoints* 44: 93–123. http://www.jstor.org/stable/42975557.

Page, Matthew J., David Moher, Patrick M. Bossuyt, Isabelle Boutron, Tammy C. Hoffmann, Cynthia D. Mulrow, Larissa Shamseer, Jennifer M. Tetzlaff, Elie A. Akl, Sue E. Brennan, Roger Chou, Julie Glanville, Jeremy M. Grimshaw, Asbjørn Hróbjartsson, Manoj M. Lalu, Tianjing Li, Elizabeth W. Loder, Evan Mayo-Wilson, Steve McDonald, Luke A. McGuinness, Lesley A. Stewart, James Thomas, Andrea C. Tricco, Vivian A. Welch, Penny Whiting, and Joanne E. McKenzie. 2021. "PRISMA 2020 explanation and elaboration: Updated guidance and exemplars for reporting systematic reviews." *BMJ* 372: n160. https://doi.org/10.1136/bmj.n160. https://www.bmj.com/content/bmj/372/bmj.n160.full.pdf.

Popay, Jennie, Helen Roberts, Amanda Sowden, Mark Petticrew, Lisa Arai, Mark Rodgers, Nicky Britten, Katrina Roen, and Steven Duffy. 2006. "Guidance on the conduct of narrative synthesis in systematic reviews." *A Product from the ESRC Methods Programme Version* 1 (1): b92.

Thomas, James, and Angela Harden. 2008. "Methods for the thematic synthesis of qualitative research in systematic reviews." *BMC Med Res Methodol* 8 (1): 45. https://doi.org/10.1186/1471-2288-8-45.

## CHAPTER 11

A Step-By-Step Guide on Writing a Systematic Literature Review for Prevalence Study

Abdulsalam Ahmed , Hafiz T.A. Khan and Nuha Ibrahim

Learning Outcomes

Learners will gain a clear understanding of how to conduct a systematic literature review (SLR) for prevalence studies, following a structured, step-by-step approach. They will learn how to form a research team, formulate a research question, and develop a protocol with defined inclusion and exclusion criteria. The chapter emphasizes practical application through the example of a published SLR on multimorbidity in older adults in Nigeria. Learners will acquire skills in literature searching, study selection, quality assessment, data extraction, and synthesis, enhancing their ability to produce rigorous, evidence-based reviews relevant to public health and social sciences.

Introduction

Academic writing can be challenging, especially when there is a deadline for its completion. This is especially the case for students trying to complete this task when they are up against competing schedules. One of the biggest challenges for some students is the review of literature, knowing which of the different types they should choose and which one to use at a particular time. For example, researchers can often show a level of inconsistency and confusion when choosing between a scoping review and a systematic review (Munn *et al.*, 2018). A scoping review can help identify research gaps, clarify research concepts, and be a precursor to a systematic review (Peterson *et al.*, 2017). The SLR may be linked to a research question or objective and be conducted to uncover evidence, confirm current practice, identify, and inform areas for future research, identify, and investigate conflicting results and produce statements to guide decision-making (Munn *et al.*, 2018; Lame, 2019). While scoping reviews answer larger, more complex, exploratory research questions, systematic reviews typically focus on research questions with a narrow parameter that usually fits into the PICO question format (Munn *et al.*, 2018).

DOI: 10.4324/9781032701004-14

A systematic review of the literature provides a way of synthesizing scientific evidence to answer a particular research question in a way that is transparent and reproducible, while also seeking to include all published evidence on the topic and appraising the quality of this evidence (Lame, 2019; Pati and Lorusso, 2018). It follows well-structured and predetermined guidelines that require a detailed approach to ensure results are robust, meaningful, reproducible, and transparent (Higgins, Altman and Sterne, 2011).

SLRs have been used in diverse disciplines, such as clinical research, social sciences advertising, education, international development, public policy, ecology, environmental sciences, engineering, and basic science research (Peričić and Tanveer, 2019; O'Hagan, Matalon and Riesenberg, 2018; Gilbody, Wilson and Watt, 2005; Pullin and Stewart, 2006). The focus of this article is the application of SLRs in prevalence/incidence studies. Postgraduate students do not always appreciate the need to keep SLRs up to date, and the aim of this article is to provide a step-by-step guide on writing them as an aid to this process. A detailed methodology of the chapter is linked with an earlier publication written by the authors (Ahmed, Khan and Lawal, 2023).

Step-by-Step Guide on Writing a Systematic Literature Review

Writing a systematic literature review can sometimes feel overwhelming, and the following steps are, therefore, recommended to help ease the path.

Formation of the Research Team

The first step is to discuss the SLR with your co-researchers because using multiple reviewers is essential to reduce bias and strengthen the analysis. A minimum of two is recommended. The research supervisor/lead will act as a tiebreaker to resolve conflicts around decisions in case of disagreement between the reviewers. Another expert on a relevant subject can be incorporated, but clear roles need to be assigned to each member of the team. This reduces ambiguity about roles and responsibilities, which improve team efficiency and reduce conflicts within the team. As an example from Ahmed, Khan and Lawal (2023), the research team was assigned different roles such as the following: conception of research idea (HK), literature review (AA), research protocol design (AA), study appraisal (HK, ML, and AA), data extraction (ML and AA), data analysis and interpretation of results (HK, ML, and AA), manuscript drafting (AA), and review of the initial and final drafts of the manuscript (HK and ML). Data was independently extracted, and study characteristics were assessed (AA and ML). The risks of bias were dealt with using the Joanna Briggs Institute, and areas of disparities were resolved by the third researcher (HK).

Formulate the Review Question

The review question should be defined with supporting evidence explaining why the research is necessary and to establish whether the same study has been carried out already recently. Many tools are used, for example, PITOS, PICOS, AND SPIDER, to aid the formulation of a well-defined review question: one tool is PICOTS (population, intervention, comparison, outcome, timing and setting) (Santos, Pimenta and Nobre,

Table 11.1 Illustrating PICOTS tool use in our previous study to formulate research questions

		Description	*Example in the previous publication*
P	Patient or Population or Problem/Disease	Who or what is the question about?	60 years and above
I	Intervention	Which main intervention or treatment are you considering for assessment?	Multimorbidity
C	Comparison(s) or Control	Is there an alternative intervention or treatment you're considering? Your systematic literature review doesn't have to contain a comparison, but you'll want to stipulate at this stage, either way.	Not applicable
O	Outcome(s)	What are you trying to measure or achieve? What's the wider goal for the work you'll be doing?	Primary outcome: prevalence of multimorbidity Secondary outcome: disease clusters and determinants
T	Timing	The timeframe for articles to be included are specific.	No limitation placed on timeframe
S	Setting	Where the studies were conducted.	Studies conducted in Nigeria

2007), used for quantitative studies, and the other is SPIDER (sample, phenomenon of interest, design, evaluation, research type), used for qualitative studies (Methley *et al.*, 2014). In our previous article, PICOTS was used, as illustrated in Table 11.1.

Develop Your Research Protocols

Once a clear research question has been formulated, the next stage is to develop a detailed research plan explaining all steps and the process, including a detailed strategy for searching the literature and evaluating the studies related to the question. This is called a study protocol. The reporting of a systematic review protocol should follow the Preferred Reporting Items for Systematic Reviews and Meta-Analyses (PRISMA) checklist or guidelines (Moher, 2009) and the PRISMA Protocols statement (Shamseer *et al.*, 2015). Elements of the protocol include the research question and objectives, proposed methods and processes that will be used, the eligibility criteria of the individual studies, data extraction and analyses plan (including tools to be used for quality appraisal of the included studies), and the theories, models, or frameworks to be used to map the findings of the included articles. While registering the scoping review protocol is optional, the SLR protocol must be registered with PROSPERO (https://www.crd.york.ac.uk/prospero/), an international database of prospectively registered systematic reviews, or with Cochrane, an international prospective database for the registration of systematic reviews. The advantage of registering with these prospective databases is that (1) protocols provide a detailed outline of how the SLR will be conducted, (2) it reduces research bias and goes through a vigorous review process, thereby uplifting the study standards promoting greater transparency, and (3) it checks for duplication of effort and resource waste. Our previous article protocol (Ahmed, Khan and Lawal, 2023) was registered at PROSPERO, and a link to it can be viewed via the article.

Set Up Inclusion and Exclusion Criteria

All final articles included in the SR contain information that will help in answering the research question. In addition, the exclusion criteria relate to duplicate articles, the availability and accessibility of full-text articles, and the exclusion of abstract-only papers (Tawfik *et al.*, 2019). Examples of inclusion and exclusion criteria are contained next in Table 11.2.

Literature Search

The aim of this stage in the SLR is to identify studies that have the ability to answer the research question. This is a demanding but critical stage of SLR. At this stage, the researcher conducts three steps in identifying databases, searching the databases using the key terms and search strategy in the protocol, and finally, managing the identified articles.

Use of Databases

There are several databases that can be used in a search of the literature, but the identification of relevant sources is dependent on the research question (Atkinson and Cipriani,

Table 11.2 Summary of inclusion and exclusion criteria

		Inclusion criteria	*Exclusion criteria*
P	Defined population	Studies with well-defined population aged 60 years and above	Studies without a clear description of the population
I	Study design/ Intervention	Observational cross-sectional studies	Any other studies besides cross-sectional studies, like longitudinal, cohort studies, and experimental studies
C	Study comparison	Peer-reviewed articles	Non-peer-reviewed articles and grey literature
O	Desire outcomes	Articles about multimorbidity	Papers with single review morbidity
T	Timeframe	No limitations placed on the year of publication	
S	Study location/ context	Only studies conducted in Nigeria	Exclude studies conducted outside Nigeria
	Language of communication	Only studies conducted in English will be conducted	Studies not published in English

Source: Ahmed, Khan and Lawal (2023)

2018). The search algorithm should be utilized in at least five electronic databases relevant to the subject. According to the A Measurement Tool to Assess Systematic Reviews (AMSTAR) guidelines, a minimum of two databases should be searched in the systematic literature review and meta-analysis (Shea *et al.*, 2017), but searching more databases will yield more robust results. Overall, the recommendation is to choose at least two generics (e.g., Web of Science), two specific (PubMed, PsycINFO, and CINHAL), and one regional database (e.g., Africa Index Medicus or Global Index Medicus). A previous study (Ahmed, Khan and Lawal, 2023) used the Web of Science (generic), PubMed (specific), CINAHL (specific), PsycINFO (specific), and Africa Index Medicus or Global Index Medicus (regional) databases. To ensure that relevant articles are not missed, a corresponding internet search should be done in Google Scholar and Google, and reference lists of those selected should be screened for other relevant articles.

The search strategy needs to be modified slightly, where necessary, according to the database or search engine being used, to suit the variation in truncation and wildcard techniques among different databases.

Identifying Search Terms

Having selected the databases for the search, the next step in the SLR process is to identify search terms or keywords. Searching the literature can be challenging especially with an enormous volume of published articles. Effective search strategy is critical to identify all relevant studies (Atkinson and Cipriani, 2018).

The search terms should consist of the words that are included in your research question plus the synonyms and other linguistic variations. An example of this approach is in the previous study (Ahmed, Khan and Lawal, 2023), where the search terms used included 'multimorbidity', 'multi-morbidity', 'multimorbidities', 'multi-morbidities', 'multi morbidity', 'multi morbidities', 'multiple morbidities', and 'multiple-morbidities'. Once keywords and phrases have been selected, they can then be combined with Boolean operators – words like AND, OR and NOT, where appropriate – to form a search string to widen or limit the search results. An example of search terms from our previous article include 'multimorbidity' and linguistic variations such as 'multi-multimorbidity', 'multi-morbidities', 'multi morbidity', 'multi morbidities', multiple morbidities', and 'multiple-morbidities'. Also included in the list are terms such as ' multiple conditions', 'multiple diseases', 'multiple chronic diseases', 'multiple chronic conditions', 'multiple illnesses', 'multiple diagnoses', 'multipathology', 'chronic condition', and 'chronic diseases'. These terms will be further restricted by location, for example, 'Nigeria' (Abia OR Adamawa

Table 11.3 Recommendation for databases used from the previous article

	Databases	Type of databases
1	Web of Science	Generic
2	CINAHL	Specific
3	PubMed	Specific
4	PsycINFO database	Specific
5	Africa Index Medicus or Global Index Medicus	Regional

Source: Ahmed, Khan and Lawal (2023)

OR Akwa Ibom OR Anambra OR Bauchi OR Bayelsa OR Benue OR Borno OR Cross River OR Delta OR Ebonyi OR Edo State OR Ekiti OR Enugu OR Gombe OR Imo OR Jigawa OR Kaduna OR Kano OR Katsina OR Kebbi OR Kogi OR Kwara OR Lagos OR Nasarawa OR Niger OR Ogun OR Ondo OR Osun OR Oyo OR Plateau OR Rivers OR Sokoto OR Taraba OR Yobe OR Zamfara OR ABUJA OR FCT), and also by method and study design, 'prevalence, epidemiology, pattern'.

Data Management

The literature search conducted by the two reviewers should be harmonized, and once the search is completed, citations should be transferred to a referencing tool such as RefWorks or Endnote, where duplicates will be removed. Afterwards, the publications can be exported from the reference manager into software tools like Covidence, Rayyan, EPPI-Reviewer, and CADIMA. That software will facilitate the rest of the systematic review processes. For our study, the citations were exported into Rayyan (Ouzzani *et al.*, 2016) for selection.

Study Selection and Extraction

The study selection should be conducted by two independent reviewers, and a third reviewer will decide about uncertainties in line with the documented criteria in the research protocol. The screening is done in two phases: (1) screening of all titles and abstracts and (2) selecting those appropriate and screening of the full-text articles of the selected studies. In essence, the full text of potentially relevant articles will be retrieved and independently reviewed by two review authors for eligibility. Documenting the reasons for excluding articles is recommended to ensure transparency and reliability of the screening process. A PRISMA flow diagram will detail the study selection decisions made as illustrated next in Figure 11.1. Detail of how to use Rayyan for study selection is attached in S1 supporting documentation.

Data Extraction

Data extraction is an essential step and includes the process of selecting key attributes uncovered in the search and organizing the information found in final articles included in the study to answer the review question in a structured and consistent format. In our previous study, the extraction of data was conducted simultaneously with full-text searching. The relevant information was extracted from each included article and recorded in the data extraction file (MS Excel). This was carried out by two independent reviewers, and one other checked the information to validate the extraction process. In the example review, the extracted information included were as follows: citation details (authors, title, journal, and year); details of the study (study setting [community or health facility]), study design, period of data collection, location of the study, sample size; case definition (how multimorbidity was defined and how disease conditions were measured); characteristics of the participants (age, sex, urban/rural, socio-economic characteristics); description of main results (percentage prevalence of multimorbidity [n/N] and 95% CIs).

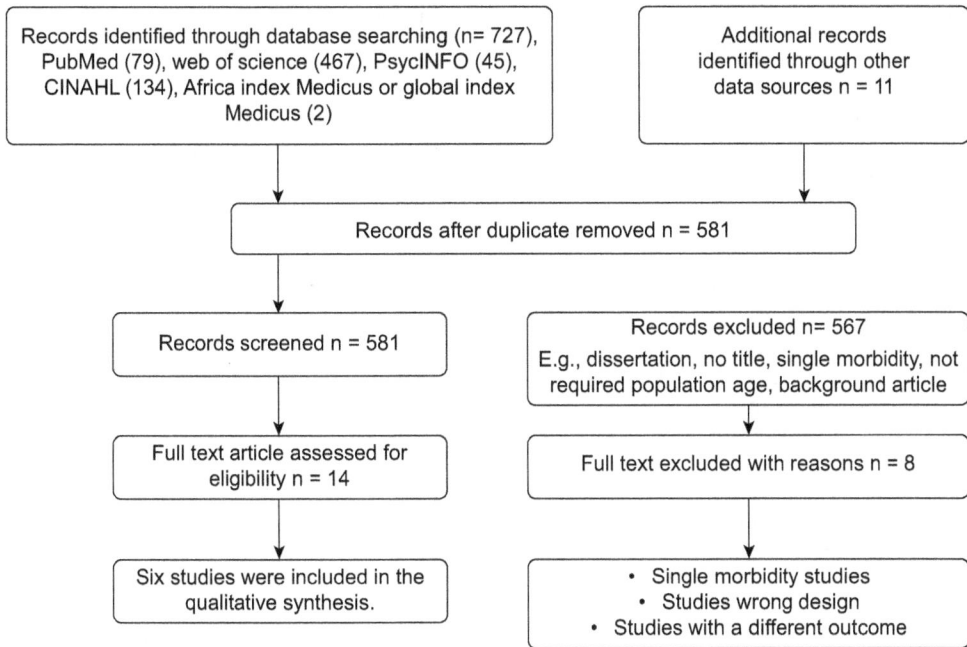

Figure 11.1 The PRISMA flow chart.

Assess the Quality of the Studies

After study selection, the quality of the articles needs to be assessed. Different types of quality assessment tools (QATs) have been developed to assess the quality of published articles, and finding the most suitable, non-cumbersome, and valid approach can be challenging. There is a lack of consensus among researchers as to which tools are best suited for different studies. Examples of QATs and their area of recommended applicability is shown next in Table 11.4.

Once a decision has been made on which QAT to use, an assessment of the risk of bias can be carried out that is usually conducted by two reviewers. The Joanna Briggs Institute (JBI) critical appraisal tool for prevalence studies was used to assess the quality of the included articles (see previous article, Ahmed, Khan and Lawal, 2023). The JBI uses nine items, and there are four possible answers to each of these items, which are 'yes', 'no', 'not clear', and 'not applicable'. The threshold for the conversion of the JBI means that any item with a 'yes' gets a score of 1, for 'no' and 'not clear', the score is zero, and those scoring 'not applicable' are not included in the percentage calculation. In our study, a score of 60% and above was regarded as good quality, and based on the JBI system, all six studies were rated good quality with four studies having a 100% score, one study having 88%, and another study with 62.5%. The results from the two reviewers were compared and differences discussed between them, and a consensus of the quality of the selected studies was reached as presented next in Table 11.5.

Table 11.4 Examples of QATs and recommended applicability

Quality assessment tools	Study type
Joanna Briggs Institute	Prevalence study (Joanna Briggs Institute, 2017)
The Cochrane Collaboration's tool	For assessing risk of bias is the best available tool for assessing RCTs (Zeng et al., 2015)
Newcastle-Ottawa Scale	For cohort and case-control studies
The Methodological Index for Non-Randomized Studies (MINORS)	An excellent tool for assessing non-randomized interventional studies (Zeng et al., 2015)
Agency for Healthcare Research and Quality (ARHQ) methodology checklist	cross-sectional studies (Zeng et al., 2015)
Quality Assessment of Diagnostic Accuracy Studies-2 (QUADAS-2) tool is recommended	For diagnostic accuracy test studies (Zeng et al., 2015)
SYstematic Review Centre for Laboratory animal Experimentation (SYRCLE) risk of bias tool	Animal studies (Zeng et al., 2015)
Assessment of Multiple Systematic Reviews (AMSTAR)	Systematic reviews/meta-analyses (Zeng et al., 2015)
Appraisal of Guidelines, Research and Evaluation (AGREE)-II instrument is widely used to evaluate	Clinical practice guidelines (Zeng et al., 2015)

Source: Joanna Briggs Institute (2017); Zeng *et al.* (2015)

Data Analysis

Data analysis for SLR is the process of synthesizing and reporting the evidence from existing published research. The aim is to summarize the characteristics of the included studies and bring the data together to produce a greater value than the individual study (Okoli and Schabram, 2010). The results should be presented as pre-specified in the research protocol, but the analysis will depend on the type of data, the type of analysis used, and the applicable reporting guidelines. The synthesized findings from included articles should be summarized in tables, which should be guided by the inclusion and exclusion criteria as shown in the example from the study (Ahmed, Khan and Lawal, 2023). They include the year of data collection, the study type and setting (community or health facility-based), geographical location of the study, how the outcome was measured, how multimorbidity was defined in each study, the diseases and number of diseases included in the studies, and how they were ascertained (e.g., measured, or self-reported).

Writing the Review

Summarizing the results is the final stage of the SLR process, and it is recommended that the summary is detailed enough to enable reproduction in a scientific manner (Okoli and Schabram, 2010). The SLR should also highlight the knowledge gleaned from the study. The use of PRISMA checklist is essential to ensure the adequate reporting of the different steps and needed information at the end of the study.

Table 11.5 Calculating the quality assessment of selected research from our previous study (Ahmed, Khan and Lawal, 2023) using the JBI tool

	Study 1	Study 2	Study 3	Study 4	Study 5	Study 6
Was the sample frame appropriate to address the target population?	YES	YES	YES	YES	YES	YES
Were study participants sampled in an appropriate way?	UNCLEAR	NOT APPLICABLE	YES	YES	YES	YES
Was the sample size adequate?	NOT APPLICABLE	NOT APPLICABLE	YES	YES	YES	YES
Were the study subjects and the setting described in detail?	NO	YES	YES	NO	YES	YES
Was the data analysis conducted with sufficient coverage of the identified sample?	UNCLEAR	YES	YES	YES	YES	YES
Were valid methods used for the identification of the condition?	YES	YES	YES	YES	YES	YES
Was the condition measured in a standard, reliable way for all participants?	YES	YES	YES	YES	YES	YES
Was there appropriate statistical analysis?	YES	YES	YES	YES	YES	YES
Was the response rate adequate, and if not, was the low response rate managed appropriately?	YES	YES	YES	YES	YES	YES
Overall appraisal:	62.5	100%	100%	88%	100%	100%

Conclusion

A systematic literature review (SLR) can be challenging, but the importance of doing it well and thoroughly cannot be over emphasized. The results will be beneficial for providing a comprehensive and robust overview of the available evidence on a given topic. It is of paramount importance to bear in mind that the whole process of SLR is tailored to answer research question. With the continuous need to generate evidence-based practice through SLRs, learners or students need to understand the steps required when preparing such reviews. This article highlights the necessary steps needed to perform a systematic review for prevalence study with a clear example from the Ahmed, Khan and Lawal (2023) study, which, it is hoped, will assist students, and early researchers, to understand the steps needed to conduct a robust SLR for prevalence studies.

Discussion Questions

- What distinguishes a systematic literature review from other types of literature reviews, particularly in the context of prevalence studies?
- Why is team collaboration critical in conducting an SLR, and how does the role of a third reviewer improve reliability?
- How do structured steps, such as defining criteria and assessing study quality, enhance the transparency and credibility of an SLR?
- What challenges might students face when conducting an SLR, and how can they be addressed?
- Lastly, how do real-world examples, like the SLR on multimorbidity in Nigeria, help in understanding the practical application of each review stage?

References

Ahmed, A., Khan, H.T.A. and Lawal, M. (2023) 'Systematic literature review of the prevalence, pattern, and determinant of multimorbidity among older adults in Nigeria', *Health Services Research & Managerial Epidemiology*, https://doi.org/10.1177/23333928231178774.

Atkinson, L.Z. and Cipriani, A. (2018) 'How to carry out a literature search for a systematic review: A practical guide', *BJPsych Advances*, 24(2), pp. 74–82.

Gilbody, S., Wilson, P. and Watt, I. (2005) 'Benefits and harms of direct to consumer advertising: A systematic review', *BMJ Quality & Safety*, 14(4), pp. 246–250.

Higgins, J., Altman, D.G. and Sterne, J. (2011) 'Assessing risk of bias in included studies', In: Higgins J.P.T., Green S. (editors). *Cochrane handbook for systematic reviews of interventions version 5.1. 0* (updated March 2011). The Cochrane Collaboration, 2011', Available from handbook.cochrane.org, pp. 243–296.

Joanna Briggs Institute (2017) 'Critical appraisal tools for use in JBI systematic reviews: Checklist for prevalence studies', *The Joanna Briggs Institute: Adelaide, Australia*.

Lame, G. (2019) *Systematic literature reviews: An introduction.* Cambridge University Press, pp. 1633.

Methley, A.M., Campbell, S., Chew-Graham, C., McNally, R. and Cheraghi-Sohi, S. (2014) 'PICO, PICOS and SPIDER: A comparison study of specificity and sensitivity in three search tools for qualitative systematic reviews', *BMC Health Services Research*, 14(1), pp. 1–10.

Moher, D. (2009) 'Liberati A, Tetzlaff J, Altman DG, Group TP, Preferred reporting items for systematic reviews and meta-analyses: The PRISMA statement.' *PLoS Med*, 6(7), pp. 1000097.

Munn, Z., Peters, M.D., Stern, C., Tufanaru, C., McArthur, A. and Aromataris, E. (2018) 'Systematic review or scoping review? Guidance for authors when choosing between a systematic or scoping review approach', *BMC Medical Research Methodology*, 18, pp. 1–7.

O'Hagan, E.C., Matalon, S. and Riesenberg, L.A. (2018) 'Systematic reviews of the literature: A better way of addressing basic science controversies', *American Journal of Physiology-Lung Cellular and Molecular Physiology*, 314(3), pp. L439–L442.

Okoli, C. and Schabram, K. (2010) 'A guide to conducting a systematic literature review of information systems research', *Working Papers Information Systems*, https://doi.org/10.2139/ssrn.1954824.

Ouzzani, M., Hammady, H., Fedorowicz, Z. and Elmagarmid, A. (2016) 'Rayyan – A web and mobile app for systematic reviews', *Systematic Reviews*, 5, pp. 1–10.

Pati, D. and Lorusso, L.N. (2018) 'How to write a systematic review of the literature', *HERD: Health Environments Research & Design Journal*, 11(1), pp. 15–30.

Peričić, T.P. and Tanveer, S. (2019) 'Why systematic reviews matter: A brief history, overview and practical guide for authors', *Cochrane International Mobility Programme*, https://www.cochrane.org/about-us/news/cochrane-international-mobility.

Peterson, J., Pearce, P.F., Ferguson, L.A. and Langford, C.A. (2017) 'Understanding scoping reviews: Definition, purpose, and process', *Journal of the American Association of Nurse Practitioners*, 29(1), pp. 12–16.

Pullin, A.S. and Stewart, G.B. (2006) 'Guidelines for systematic review in conservation and environmental management', *Conservation Biology*, 20(6), pp. 1647–1656.

Santos, C.M.d.C., Pimenta, C.A.d.M. and Nobre, M.R.C. (2007) 'The PICO strategy for the research question construction and evidence search', *Revista latino-americana de enfermagem*, 15, pp. 508–511.

Shamseer, L., Moher, D., Clarke, M., Ghersi, D. and Liberati, A. (2015) 'Research methods & reporting', *BMJ*, pp. 1–25.

Shea, B.J., Reeves, B.C., Wells, G., Thuku, M., Hamel, C., Moran, J., Moher, D., Tugwell, P., Welch, V. and Kristjansson, E. (2017) 'AMSTAR 2: A critical appraisal tool for systematic reviews that include randomised or non-randomised studies of healthcare interventions, or both', *BMJ*, 358.

Tawfik, G.M., Dila, K.A.S., Mohamed, M.Y.F., Tam, D.N.H., Kien, N.D., Ahmed, A.M. and Huy, N.T. (2019) 'A step by step guide for conducting a systematic review and meta-analysis with simulation data', *Tropical Medicine and Health*, 47(1), pp. 1–9.

Zeng, X., Zhang, Y., Kwong, J.S., Zhang, C., Li, S., Sun, F., Niu, Y. and Du, L. (2015) 'The methodological quality assessment tools for preclinical and clinical studies, systematic review and meta-analysis, and clinical practice guideline: A systematic review', *Journal of Evidence-Based Medicine*, 8(1), pp. 2–10.

## CHAPTER 12

Meta-Analysis

A Primer

Anoop Kumar and Denny John

Learning Outcomes

Learners will understand the diverse types of meta-analyses aligned with different systematic review questions. They will explore the distinction between random effects meta-analysis for intervention effectiveness, proportional meta-analysis for prevalence, and meta-analyses of correlation coefficients for identifying barriers and facilitators. The chapter also covers advanced forms, including diagnostic, prognostic, rare events, and individual patient data (IPD) meta-analyses. Students will gain familiarity with appropriate statistical techniques, use of ROC curves, and predictive modeling. Practical skills will be enhanced through examples and R code, equipping learners to select, perform, and present the right meta-analytic method for their research objectives.

Introduction

Meta-analysis is analysis of data from the already published studies having similar outcomes (Kumar, 2023a; Borenstein et al.,2021). Numerous meta-analyses have been published so far in different areas, which indicates its popularity. These analyses are helpful to draw a valid clinical decision to resolve conflicting findings across individual studies (Patel, 1989). Systematic literature review (SLR) is a must before conducting any kind of meta-analysis (Kumar, 2023b). The Preferred Reporting Items for Systematic Reviews and Meta-Analyses (PRISMA) guideline is the most well-known to be followed while conducting meta-analysis using PRISMA flow chart and checklist (Page et al., 2021). The quality assessment of individual studies is also required using available checklists for different types of studies, such as QUOROM, which is used to assess the quality reports of meta-analyses of randomized controlled trials (Moher et al., 2000); the MOOSE (Meta-AnalysesOf Observational Studies in Epidemiology) Checklist (Brooke et al., 2021); study quality assessment tools like the NIH quality assessment tools for case-control studies and controlled intervention studies (Zeng et al., 2015); cohort studies; the Newcastle-Ottawa Scale (NOS) (Lo et al., 2014); and so on (Kumar, 2023c).

DOI: 10.4324/9781032701004-15

Types of Meta-Analysis

Meta-analyses are broadly categorized into the following types: Interventional meta-analysis (Corona et al., 2018), diagnostic test accuracy meta-analysis (Campbell et al., 2015a), proportional meta-analysis (Barker et al., 2021), meta-analysis of correlational coefficients (Field, 2001), meta-analyses of prognostic studies (calculate a summary outcome or summary effects of predictive accuracy) (Sousa and Ribeiro, 2009), individual patient data (IPD) meta-analyses (Tudur et al., 2016), and meta-analyses of rare events (Efthimiou, 2018).

Interventional Meta-Analysis

Interventional meta-analysis is used to draw a valid clinical decision regarding the use of a particular intervention in a particular disease.

Study Designs

The research questions should be framed into PICO format, where P represents patient, I represents intervention, C represents comparator, and O represents outcome (Efthimiou, 2018).

Statistical Analysis

The analysis of data is done using various available software, such as RevMan, R package, etc. The weightage is given to the individual studies depending on the sample size of the trial. The results from studies with a small sample size are provided less weightage as compared to studies with a large sample size (Brockwell and Gordon, 2001).

Choose an Effect Size

The effect size should be comparable (i.e., measure same outcome) among multiple studies and should be relevant to the researchers or clinical practice. Broadly, if data is presented as mean and standard deviation in two groups in interventional studies, the appropriate effect size would be mean difference or standard mean difference. If data is dichotomous in individual interventional studies, the most appropriate effect sizes would be risk ratio, odds ratio, or risk difference.

Mean Difference (MD) vs. Standardized Mean Difference (SMD)

Mean difference (MD) is preferred if the outcome is measured using the same scale across the studies. The mean of the differences is equal to the difference in means and can be calculated by using the following mentioned formula:

$$MD = ME - MC$$

ME is mean of measurements of intervention E, whereas MC is mean of measurements of intervention C.

However, if the same outcome is measured using a different scale, in that case, SMD is preferred over MD. SMD actually divides the MD in each study by standard deviation, which will somewhat generate a similar index (Bakbergenuly et al., 2020; Takeshima et al., 2014; Sedgwick and Marston, 2013).

The SMD expresses the size of the intervention effect in each study relative to the variability observed in that study.

SMD = Difference in mean outcome between groups/standard deviation of outcome among participants

Response Ratios

When the outcome is unlikely to be zero and assessed on a physical scale, such as length, area, etc., the ratio of the means in two groups could be used as an impact size. These types of outcomes are usually observed in experimental ecology (Sánchez-Meca and Marín-Martínez, 2000; Bakbergenuly et al.,2020; Nakagawa et al., 2023).

Effects Sizes for Binary Data

The risk ratio, odds ratio, and risk difference are the most commonly used effect sizes for binary data (Fleiss and Berlin, 2009). Risk ratio is the ratio of two risks. We normally calculate the log risk ratio and, finally, convert back into risk ratio (O'Connor, 2013; Viera, 2008). Odds ratio is the ratio of two odds (Chinn, 2000; Haddock et al., 1998). For better understanding, let us start with a simple example.

Suppose the risk of death in a treated group out of 100 patients is 5, and the risk of death in a control group is 1/100. Then the risk ratio –5/1 = 5, and in case of odds ratio, the odds of death in the treated group would be 5/95 = 0.0526, and the odds of death in the control group would be 1/99 = 0.010

So odds ratio –0.0526/0.010 = 5.26

In most of cases, we calculate log odds ratio along with the standard error and finally convert it into the original measure (Chinn, 2000; Haddock et al., 1998).

Risk difference is the difference between two risks (Sánchez-Meca and Marín-Martínez, 2000). In this example, the risk in the treatment group is 0.05, whereas the risk in the control group is 0.01. The difference between these two = 0.04 risk difference. The risk difference is usually calculated in raw units, whereas risk ratios and odds ratios are calculated in log units.

The risk ratio and odds ratio are not affected by the variations in baseline occurrences, as these both are relative measures, whereas risk difference is sensitive to baseline risk, as it is an absolute measure.

Meta-analysis includes all the studies into one analysis. Therefore, researchers should use common effect six or convert the results into common effect size. However, sometimes conversion is not possible or feasible and should be examined on a case-by-case basis.

Models

The fixed effects and random effects models are the most used models in meta-analysis. The assessment of the fixed effects model is that all included studies share the common effect size as well as all factors are similar across the included studies that could influence the effect sizes. However, this assumption is implausible in most of the cases. Therefore, random effects model is frequently used in meta-analysis as compared to the fixed effects model. In both models, each study is weighted the inverse of its variance. Fixed effects model is preferred if the variation is low; otherwise, random effects model is preferred. The variation among included studies could be within and between the studies (Borenstein et al., 2010; Kelley and Kelley, 2012; Borenstein et al., 2010; Schmidt et al., 2009; Nikolakopoulou et al., 2014; Kumar, 2023d). The fixed effects model considered variations within the study only whereas random effects model considered the sources of variations within as well as between the studies. Therefore, if you are both models for the same data, you will find the range of confidence interval for random effects model will be wider as compared to the confidence interval for the fixed effects model.

In a fixed effects model, a single true effect size θ, the intercept-only fixed effects model can be denoted as follws: $yi = \theta + \varepsilon i$

where εi represents the sampling error for yi

In random effects model, θi differs between studies under the assumption of a normal distribution around θ.

Therefore, it can be denoted as follows: $yi = \theta + \varepsilon i + \mu i$, where μi represents the between-study variance τ^2.

Selection of Model

The selection of model should be done before the analysis of the data. It has been observed that many researches are choosing the model based on the results of heterogeneity. The model should be selected during the design of the meta-analysis by keeping all things in mind regarding variations among included studies.

Heterogeneity

Heterogeneity is one of the important aspects in any kind of meta-analysis (Higgins and Thompson, 2002; Higgins et al., 2003; Fletcher, 2007; Deeks et al., 2009; Lin et al., 2017; Von Hippel, 2015; Cohen et al., 2015; Kulinskaya and Dollinger, 2015). There are various tests for the identification and quantification of heterogeneity among included studies. The simpler test is the eyeball test in which, by just observing the forest plots, one can get an idea about the heterogeneity. The more overlapping confidence intervals of different studies indicate more homogeneity and vice-versa. The most used statistical methods to measure heterogeneity among studies are chi-squared (X^2) and I^2 tests.

The chi-squared test provides the p-value, based on which researchers can interpret the involvement of significant or non-significant heterogeneity. A p-value less than 0.05 indicates significant heterogeneity among included studies and vice-versa. In most of published meta-analysis, a cut-off value of 0.1 is often used instead of 0.05; this might be due to the low sensitivity of the chi-squared test. I^2 statistics tells us about the extent of heterogeneity among studies and does not depend on one factor. The most commonly used ranges in published papers are as follows: 0–40% (low heterogeneity), 30–60% (moderate), 60–90% (substantial), and 90–100% (considerable).

The formula for calculating heterogeneity is mentioned next:

$$I^2 = \tau^2/(\sigma^2 + \tau^2)$$

where τ^2 denotes the between-trial heterogeneity, σ^2 denotes some common sampling error across trials, and $\sigma^2 + \tau 2$ is the total variation in the meta-analysis

I^2 is usually calculated in percentage using the following mentioned formula:

$$I^2 = (Q - df)/Q \times 100$$

where Q is the Cochran's homogeneity test statistic and df is the degrees of freedom (the number of trials minus 1)

Cochrane Q Test

As another test to measure heterogeneity, this test estimates the weighted sum of squared differences between individual study effect and pooled effect across trials. If heterogeneity is too high even after subgroup analysis, my personal advice is researchers should restrict themselves to SLR.

Publication Bias

Publication bias is another important parameter in meta-analysis. Funnel plot is the most commonly used plot to assess the publication bias qualitatively. Whereas the Begg and Egger's test is widely used for the quantitative analysis of publication bias (Sedgwick, 2015; Duval and Tweedie, 2000; Lin and Chu, 2018; Ayorinde et al., 2020).

Meta-Analysis of Diagnostic Studies

Diagnostic tests are widely used in the diagnosis of various diseases, and there are so many queries regarding these tests by healthcare professionals, clinicians, policymakers, and patients. Therefore, the main objective of the diagnostic test accuracy review (DTA) is to analyze the diagnostic accuracy data from suitable studies and guidelines (Campbell et al., 2015b). As we have to follow PRISMA for the international meta-analyses, as mentioned in the earlier sections, in the case of diagnostics, we have to follow the Preferred Repurposing Items for Systematic Reviews and Meta-Analyses extension for Diagnostic Test Accuracy (PRISMA-DTA) statement (McInnes et al., 2018; Salameh et al., 2020).

Study Design

The research questions related to DTA renew should be framed into SPIRIT format, where S stands for study design, P stands for population, I stands for index test, R stands for reference standard, and T stands for target condition. Population is a single group which should be a representative of the target population or intended use population. The study is preferably performed in the setting in which the test is used or will be used.

Target condition is a particular disease:

Index test: test to be evaluated;
Reference standard: best available method. It can be single test or a combination of tests.

The QUADAS-2 contains three phases: Phase I (define the review questions), Phase II (draw a flow diagram), and Phase III (assessment of risk of bias and applicability). Applicability contains four domains, i.e., patient selection, index test, reference standard, flow, and timing. To perform DTA renews, one should follow a standard guideline like STARD, which refers to a standard (Rivera et al., 2020).

Quality Assessment Tools

QUADAS-2 (Quality Assessment of Diagnostic Accuracy Studies-2) is a well-known tool to access the quality of included studies. QUADAS-2 is a three-phased tool: Phase 1 (define the review question), Phase 2 (draw a flow diagram), and Phase 3 (assessment of risk of bias and applicability of four domains: patient selection, index test, reference standard, and flow and timing).

Cochrane Risk of Bias Tools for Diagnostic Test Accuracy (ROB 2) is another well-known tool to access the quality of included studies (Ge et al., 2021).

Guidelines

One should follow a STARD guidelines, which refers to Standards for Reporting of Diagnostic Accuracy Studies. It's not a quality assessment tool. It provides guidelines for reporting diagnostic accuracy studies. The objective is to improve the accuracy and completeness of the reporting of studies of diagnostic accuracy to allow readers to assess the potential for bias in the study (internal validity) and to evaluate the generalizability (external validity). The STARD statement consists of a checklist of 25 items and recommends the use of a flow diagram, which describes the design of the study and the flow of patients (Vali et al., 2021; Simel et al., 2008; Cohen et al., 2016).

Heterogeneity

The assessment of heterogeneity among studies is required to find out how test accuracy varies with the characteristics, which depends upon the availability of data and number of studies in each subgroup. The most used software to calculate heterogeneity is "R" package.

Statistical Models for Meta-Analysis of Diagnostic Studies

Two hierarchical models are recommended for the meta-analysis of studies of diagnostic accuracy, which are mentioned in the following:

a) Hierarchical summary ROC model (HSROC) (Macaskill, 2004).
b) Bivariate regression of sensitivity and specificity (Reitsma et al., 2005).

The models are "hierarchical" because they involve statistical distributions at two levels. At the lower level, they model the cell counts in the 2 × 2 tables extracted from each study using binomial distributions and logistic (log-odds) transformations of proportions. At the second (higher) level, the models assume random study effects to account for heterogeneity in diagnostic test accuracy between studies beyond that accounted for by sampling variability at the lower level

Bivariate vs. HSROC Model

The primary objective of HSROC model is to fit a summary ROC curve, whereas the primary objective of the bivariate model is to fit a summary point (summary estimates of sensitivity and specificity). The bivariate model is preferred where studies report a common threshold (or cut-off) for a positive result, whereas if studies report several different thresholds, use the HSROC model (Bauz-Olvera et al., 2018).

A properly conducted diagnostic test study should adhere with the following mentioned points:

- Patients must be selected using a consecutive or random sample of a target patient population.
- Index test should be interpreted without the knowledge of the results of the reference standard.
- The reference standard used in such studies must correctly classify the target condition and be interpreted without the knowledge of the results of the index test.
- The time intervals between each test should be as short as possible to avoid the clinical condition of the study subject to change.
- All patients must be analyzed and using the same reference standard.

Proportional Meta-Analysis

A transformation of data is required in a proportional meta-analysis as incidence and prevalence are reported in terms of their proportions. The prevalence/incidence always falls between the values of 0 and 1. The sum of the prevalence/incidence over different categories should always equal to 1. However, if the confidence interval falls outside of the established 0-to-1 range, then it will impact the readability and presentation of the pooled data. The variance from studies contributing proportional data at the extreme ends of the 0-to-1 range tends towards 0, therefore affecting the weightage of studies. The two most common methods which are being used for the transformation of data are as follows:

a) Double arcsine transformation
b) Logit transformation

These both methods calculate the pooled prevalence estimate with 95% confidence interval.

The double arcsine transformation is most commonly used, as it solves both the issue (mentioned earlier), obviously. After the completion of the meta-analysis, the back transformation should be done.

Meta-Analysis of Correlational Coefficients

If the linear association/relationship between two continuous/quantitative outcome variables is of interest, then the correlation coefficient is the appropriate effect size measure.

Methods

The most used methods for the meta-analysis of correlational coefficients are mentioned next:

a) The Hedges-Olkin method
b) The Hunter-Schmidt method

The Hedges-Olkin method is based on a conventional summary meta-analysis with a Fisher Z transformation of the correlation coefficient. The Hunter-Schmidt method is effectively a weighted mean of the raw correlation coefficient (Biggerstaff and Tweedie, 1997; Higgins and Thompson, 2002).

Neither of these methods is completely suitable for either a small number of studies (less than 30) or a heterogeneous set of studies. The Hedges-Olkin method tends to overestimate the pooled effect, whereas the Schmidt-Hunter method underestimates it a little when the correlation is greater than 0.5. The least biased estimate of the true population correlation is provided by the Schmidt-Hunter method. The Hedges-Olkin method reduces the risk of Type I error when compared with the Schmidt-Hunter method but only when the studies are homogeneous. For heterogeneous studies, you should consider consulting with a statistician about an alternative multilevel modeling approach.

The heterogeneity among studies is calculated by using the I-squared (I^2), H statistic, τ (tau), and τ^2 (tau-squared) statistics. The I^2 statistic quantified the proportion of total variation in effect sizes that was due to heterogeneity rather than chance. We considered I^2 values of 25%, 50%, and 75% to represent low, moderate, and high heterogeneity, respectively. The H statistic measured the influence of a single study on the overall results of a meta-analysis. The τ statistic measured the between-study variance in effect sizes and was used to estimate the degree of heterogeneity. A larger τ value indicated greater heterogeneity between studies. The τ^2 statistic was the estimated variance of true effects across studies after accounting for sampling error.

Meta-Analysis of Prognostic Studies

Prognostic studies are done to estimate the risk of an individual to develop a particular health outcome. These studies play a significant role in decision-making. Systematic renews of prognostic studies are helpful in drawing valid conclusions after analyzing data from individual studies (Sousa and Ribeiro, 2009; Damen et al., 2023).

Design of Study

The renew questions of SLR of prognostic studies should be framed into PICOTS format, where P is for population, I is for index model, C is for comparator model, O is for outcome(s), T is for timing, and S is for setting. The most commonly used checklist to perform SLR of prognostic studies is the Critical Appraisal and Data Extraction for Systematic Renews of Prediction Modeling Studies (CHARMS) checklist. The quality and risk of bias of included studies is usually done using the Prediction Model Risk OF Bias Assessment (PROBAST) tool (Wolff et al., 2019; Moons et al., 2019).

Statistical Analysis

The weighted average of a prediction model's performance is calculated where weights are considered as the standard error of the study. The heterogeneity between studies is usually found high due to the differences in population characteristics, measurement of predictors and outcomes, study designs, data sources, etc. Therefore, most of the meta-analysis of prognostic studies prefer the random effects model over the fixed effects model. The most commonly used software packages are the R-packages MetaMIS and metafor, which is freely available. The pooled discrimination and calibration estimates are also calculated in meta-analysis of prognostic studies if sufficient studies are available. The pooled prediction interval tells us about the uncertainty around the pooled estimate as well as the heterogeneity between studies. If heterogeneity is found high, then researchers should explore it further by performing subgroup analysis and meta-regression (Riley et al., 2019).

Individual Patient Data (IPD) Meta-Analysis

Individual patient data (IPD) meta-analysis includes data of each participant from the individual study. The IPD meta-analysis might be considered as an ideal approach; however, it's a time-consuming and expensive process. Further, since the main interest in any kind of meta-analysis is overall result, therefore, both IPD and aggregate data meta-analysis should yield similar findings. Therefore, most of published meta-analysis are aggregate data meta-analysis instead of IPO (Simmonds et al., 2005; Thomas et al., 2014; Riley et al., 2008).

Meta-Analysis of Rare Events

Most of the individual studies have less power to detect differences in rare outcomes. Therefore, meta-analysis, which includes data from multiple studies, may have better power to detect the difference in rare outcomes. The Peto method is the most suitable method for the meta-analysis of rare events. The choice of overall estimate measure depends upon the comparator group risk, size of the treatment effects, and so on. The odds and risk estimates are similar when events are rare. Therefore, results of both can be interpreted as ratios of probabilities. However, biases are more when events are rare in most commonly used methods, such as the inverse variance, DerSimonian, and Mantel-Haenszel methods in meta-analysis (Cai et al., 2010; Efthimiou, 2018).

Meta-Regression Approaches

Fixed effects and random effects approaches are used. Fixed effects method is based on logistic regression. Whereas, random effects refer to the inclusion of random study effect in the regression model. Control rate meta-analysis where outcome rate in the control group is the only covariate (Morton et al., 2004).

Network Meta-Analysis

The direct comparison among two interventions is not always feasible; however, indirect comparison can be done. For example, various classes of drugs are tested in randomized clinical trials with the same control group, but the efficacy of these drugs were not compared directly. So in that case, it is possible to compare interventions with each other's through a network meta-analysis (White, 2015; Rouse et al., 2017).

Limitations

The most common limitations of meta-analysis are dependence on the quality of included studies. The poor-quality studies can directly impact the meta-analysis results. Another important issue is heterogeneity among included studies, which depends upon various factors, such as study locations, sample size, methodology employed, and so on. Most of studies with negative findings are not published and create involvement of publication bias.

Conclusion

Meta-analyses are one of the important analyses which play a role not only in the medical field but also in other fields. It is a powerful tool to combine the results of individual studies to derive valid conclusions, particularly when individual studies are inconclusive. However, these studies should be planned and executed carefully, as the number of factors could affect the results of these studies. It's always recommended to involve a group of experts to conduct this analysis in a proper way.

Discussion Questions

- Why is a systematic review a prerequisite for conducting any type of meta-analysis?
- How does the review question determine the choice of meta-analytic method – for example, when should proportional or correlation meta-analyses be used?
- What are the methodological challenges in conducting diagnostic or rare event meta-analyses, and how can these be addressed?
- How does IPD meta-analysis enhance the quality and depth of research findings?
- Lastly, how can the inclusion of statistical tools like R improve the transparency, reproducibility, and accuracy of meta-analysis reporting in academic and clinical research?

References

Ayorinde AA, Williams I, Mannion R, Song F, Skrybant M, Lilford RJ, Chen YF. Assessment of publication bias and outcome reporting bias in systematic reviews of health services and delivery research: A meta-epidemiological study. PLoS One. 2020 Jan 30;15(1):e0227580. https://doi.org/10.1371/journal.pone.0227580.

Bakbergenuly I, Hoaglin DC, Kulinskaya E. Estimation in meta-analyses of mean difference and standardized mean difference. Stat Med. 2020 Jan 30;39(2):171–191. https://doi.org/10.1002/sim.8422.

Barker TH, Migliavaca CB, Stein C, Colpani V, Falavigna M, Aromataris E, Munn Z. Conducting proportional meta-analysis in different types of systematic reviews: A guide for synthesisers of evidence. BMC Med Res Methodol. 2021 Sep 20;21(1):189. https://doi.org/10.1186/s12874-021-01381-z.

Bauz-Olvera SA, Pambabay-Calero JJ, Nieto-Librero AB, Galindo-Villardón MP. Meta-analysis in DTA with hierarchical models bivariate and HSROC: Simulation study. In: Selected contributions on statistics and data science in Latin America: 33 FNE and 13 CLATSE, 2018, Guadalajara, Mexico, Octr 2019 1–5 (pp. 33–42). Springer International Publishing.

Biggerstaff BJ, Tweedie RL. Incorporating variability in estimates of heterogeneity in the random effects model in meta-analysis. Stat. Med. 1997;16:753–768.

Borenstein M, Hedges LV, Higgins JP, Rothstein HR. A basic introduction to fixed-effect and random-effects models for meta-analysis. Res Synth Methods. 2010 Apr;1(2):97–111. https://doi.org/10.1002/jrsm.12.

Borenstein, M, Hedges, LV, Higgins, JP, Rothstein, HR. Introduction to meta-analysis. John Wiley & Sons, New York. 2021.

Brockwell SE, Gordon IR. A comparison of statistical methods for meta-analysis. Stat Med. 2001 Mar 30;20(6):825–840. https://doi.org/10.1002/sim.650.

Brooke BS, Schwartz TA, Pawlik TM. MOOSE reporting guidelines for meta-analyses of observational studies. JAMA Surg. 2021 Aug 1;156(8):787–788. https://doi.org/10.1001/jamasurg.2021.0522.

Cai T, Parast L, Ryan L. Meta-analysis for rare events. Statistics in Medicine. 2010 Sep 10;29(20):2078–2089.

Campbell JM, Klugar M, Ding S, Carmody DP, Hakonsen SJ, Jadotte YT, White S, Munn Z. Diagnostic test accuracy: Mthods for systematic review and meta-analysis. Int J Evid Based Healthc. 2015a Sep;13(3):154–162. https://doi.org/10.1097/XEB.0000000000000061.

Campbell JM, Klugar M, Ding S, Carmody DP, Hakonsen SJ, Jadotte YT, White S, Munn Z. Diagnostic test accuracy: Methods for systematic review and meta-analysis. JBI Evidence Implementation. 2015b Sep 1;13(3):154–162.

Chinn SA. Simple method for converting an odds ratio to effect size for use in meta-analysis. Statistics in Medicine. 2000 Nov 30;19(22):3127–3131.

Cohen JF, Chalumeau M, Cohen R, Korevaar DA, Khoshnood B, Bossuyt PM. Cochran's Q test was useful to assess heterogeneity in likelihood ratios in studies of diagnostic accuracy. J Clin Epidemiol. 2015 Mar;68(3):299–306. https://doi.org/10.1016/j.jclinepi.2014.09.005.

Cohen JF, Korevaar DA, Altman DG, Bruns DE, Gatsonis CA, Hooft L, Irwig L, Levine D, Reitsma JB, De Vet HC, Bossuyt PM. STARD 2015 guidelines for reporting diagnostic accuracy studies: Explanation and elaboration. BMJ Open. 2016 Nov 1;6(11):e012799.

Corona G, Rastrelli G, Di Pasquale G, Sforza A, Mannucci E, Maggi M. Testosterone and cardiovascular risk: Meta-analysis of interventional studies. J Sex Med. 2018 Jun;15(6):820–838. https://doi.org/10.1016/j.jsxm.2018.04.641.

Damen JA, Moons KG, van Smeden M, Hooft L. How to conduct a systematic review and meta-analysis of prognostic model studies. Clin Microbiol Infect. 2023 Apr 1;29(4):434–440.

Deeks, JJ Higgins, JPT Altman, DG. Analysing data and undertaking meta-analyses. Cochrane Handbook for Systematic Reviews of Interventions Version 5.1.0. The Cochrane Collaboration. 2009.

Duval S, Tweedie R. Trim and fill: A simple funnel-plot-based method of testing and adjusting for publication bias in meta-analysis. Biometrics. 2000 Jun;56(2):455–463. https://doi.org/10.1111/j.0006-341x.2000.00455.x.

Efthimiou O. Practical guide to the meta-analysis of rare events. Evid Based Ment Health. 2018 May;21(2):72–76. https://doi.org/10.1136/eb-2018-102911.

Field AP. Meta-analysis of correlation coefficients: A Monte Carlo comparison of fixed- and random-effects methods. Psychol Methods. 2001 Jun;6(2):161–180. https://doi.org/10.1037/1082-989x.6.2.161.

Fleiss JL, Berlin JA. Effect sizes for dichotomous data. The Handbook of Research Synthesis and Meta-Analysis. 2009; 2:237–253.

Fletcher J. What is heterogeneity and is it important? BMJ. 2007 Jan 13;334(7584):94–96. https://doi.org/10.1136/bmj.39057.406644.68.

Ge MW, Ni HT, Huang JW, Fan ZH, Shen WQ, Chen HL. Diagnostic value of autofluorescence laryngoscope in early laryngeal carcinoma and precancerous lesions: A systematic review and meta-analysis. Photodiagnosis and Photodynamic Therapy. 2021 Sep 1;35:102460.

Haddock CK, Rindskopf D, Shadish WR. Using odds ratios as effect sizes for meta-analysis of dichotomous data: A primer on methods and issues. Psychol Methods. 1998 Sep;3(3):339.

Higgins JP, Thompson SG. Quantifying heterogeneity in a meta-analysis. Stat Med. 2002 Jun 15;21(11):1539–1558. https://doi.org/10.1002/sim.1186.

Higgins JP, Thompson SG, Deeks JJ, Altman DG. Measuring inconsistency in meta-analyses. BMJ. 2003 Sep 6;327(7414):557–560. https://doi.org/10.1136/bmj.327.7414.557.

Kelley GA, Kelley KS. Statistical models for meta-analysis: A brief tutorial. World J Methodol. 2012 Aug 26;2(4):27–32. https://doi.org/10.5662/wjm.v2.i4.27.

Kulinskaya E, Dollinger MB. An accurate test for homogeneity of odds ratios based on Cochran's Q-statistic. BMC Med Res Methodol. 2015 Jun 10;15:49. https://doi.org/10.1186/s12874-015-0034-x.

Kumar A. Introduction. In: Meta-analysis in clinical research: Principles and procedures. Springer, Singapore. 2023a. https://doi.org/10.1007/978-981-99-2370-0_1.

Kumar A. Models. In: Meta-analysis in clinical research: Principles and procedures. Springer, Singapore. 2023b. https://doi.org/10.1007/978-981-99-2370-0_5.

Kumar A. Quality assessment of studies. In: Meta-analysis in clinical research: Principles and procedures. 2023c. Springer, Singapore. https://doi.org/10.1007/978-981-99-2370-0_3.

Kumar A. Systematic Literature Review (SLR). In: Meta-analysis in clinical research: Principles and procedures. 2023d. Springer, Singapore. https://doi.org/10.1007/978-981-99-2370-0_2.

Lin L, Chu H. Quantifying publication bias in meta-analysis. Biometrics. 2018 Sep;74(3):785–794. https://doi.org/10.1111/biom.12817.

Lin L, Chu H, Hodges JS. Alternative measures of between-study heterogeneity in meta-analysis: Reducing the impact of outlying studies. Biometrics. 2017 Mar;73(1):156–166. https://doi.org/10.1111/biom.12543.

Lo CK, Mertz D, Loeb M. Newcastle-Ottawa scale: Comparing reviewers' to authors' assessments. BMC Med Res Methodol. 2014 Apr 1;14:45. https://doi.org/10.1186/1471-2288-14-45.

Macaskill P. Empirical Bayes estimates generated in a hierarchical summary ROC analysis agreed closely with those of a full Bayesian analysis. J Clin Epidemiol. 2004 Sep 1;57(9):925–932.

McInnes MD, Moher D, Thombs BD, McGrath TA, Bossuyt PM, Clifford T, Cohen JF, Deeks JJ, Gatsonis C, Hooft L, Hunt HA. Preferred reporting items for a systematic review and meta-analysis of diagnostic test accuracy studies: The PRISMA-DTA statement. Jama. 2018 Jan 23;319(4):388–396.

Moher D, Cook DJ, Eastwood S, Olkin I, Rennie D, Stroup DF. Improving the quality of reports of meta-analyses of randomised controlled trials: The QUOROM statement. Onkologie. 2000 Dec;23(6):597–602. https://doi.org/10.1159/000055014.

Moons KG, Wolff RF, Riley RD, Whiting PF, Westwood M, Collins GS, Reitsma JB, Kleijnen J, Mallett S. PROBAST: A tool to assess risk of bias and applicability of prediction model studies: Explanation and elaboration. Ann Intern Med. 2019 Jan 1;170(1):W1–W33.

Morton SC, Adams JL, Suttorp MJ, Shekelle PG. Meta-regression approaches: What, why, when, and how? Rockville (MD): Agency for Healthcare Research and Quality (US); 2004 Mar. Report No.: 04–0033.

Nakagawa S, Noble DWA, Lagisz M, Spake R, Viechtbauer W, Senior AM. A robust and readily implementable method for the meta-analysis of response ratios with and without missing standard deviations. Ecol Lett. 2023 Feb;26(2):232–244. https://doi.org/10.1111/ele.14144.

Nikolakopoulou A, Mavridis D, Salanti G. How to interpret meta-analysis models: Fixed effect and random effects meta-analyses. Evid Based Ment Health. 2014 May;17(2):64. https://doi.org/10.1136/eb-2014-101794.

O'Connor AM. Interpretation of odds and risk ratios. J Vet Inter Med. 2013 May;27(3):600–603.

Page MJ, McKenzie JE, Bossuyt PM, Boutron I, Hoffmann TC, Mulrow CD, Shamseer L, Tetzlaff JM, Akl EA, Brennan SE, Chou R, Glanville J, Grimshaw JM, Hróbjartsson A, Lalu MM, Li T, Loder EW, Mayo-Wilson E, McDonald S, McGuinness LA, Stewart LA, Thomas J, Tricco AC, Welch VA, Whiting P, Moher D. The PRISMA 2020 statement: An updated guideline for reporting systematic reviews. BMJ. 2021 Mar 29;372:n71. https://doi.org/10.1136/bmj.n71.

Patel MS. An introduction to meta-analysis. Health Policy. 1989;11:79–85.

Reitsma JB, Glas AS, Rutjes AW, Scholten RJ, Bossuyt PM, Zwinderman AH. Bivariate analysis of sensitivity and specificity produces informative summary measures in diagnostic reviews. J Clin Epidemiol. 2005 Oct 1;58(10):982–990.

Riley RD, Lambert PC, Staessen JA, Wang J, Gueyffier F, Thijs L, Boutitie F. Meta-analysis of continuous outcomes combining individual patient data and aggregate data. Stat Med. 2008 May 20;27(11):1870–1893.

Riley RD, Moons KG, Snell KI, Ensor J, Hooft L, Altman DG, Hayden J, Collins GS, Debray TP. A guide to systematic review and meta-analysis of prognostic factor studies. bmj. 2019 Jan 30;364.

Rivera SC, Liu X, Chan AW, Denniston AK, Calvert MJ, Ashrafian H, Beam AL, Collins GS, Darzi A, Deeks JJ, ElZarrad MK. Guidelines for clinical trial protocols for interventions involving artificial intelligence: The SPIRIT-AI extension. Lancet Digit Health. 2020 Oct 1;2(10):e549–e560.

Rouse B, Chaimani A, Li T. Network meta-analysis: An introduction for clinicians. Internal and Emergency Medicine. 2017 Feb;12:103–111.

Salameh JP, Bossuyt PM, McGrath TA, Thombs BD, Hyde CJ, Macaskill P, Deeks JJ, Leeflang M, Korevaar DA, Whiting P, Takwoingi Y, Reitsma JB, Cohen JF, Frank RA, Hunt HA, Hooft L, Rutjes AWS, Willis BH, Gatsonis C, Levis B, Moher D, McInnes MDF. Preferred reporting items for systematic review and meta-analysis of diagnostic test accuracy studies (PRISMA-DTA): Explanation, elaboration, and checklist. BMJ. 2020 Aug 14;370:m2632. https://doi.org/10.1136/bmj.m2632.

Sánchez-Meca J, Marín-Martínez F. Testing the significance of a common risk difference in meta-analysis. Computational Statistics & Data Analysis. 2000 May 28;33(3):299–313.

Schmidt FL, Oh IS, Hayes TL. Fixed- versus random-effects models in meta-analysis: Model properties and an empirical comparison of differences in results. Br J Math Stat Psychol. 2009 Feb;62(Pt 1):97–128. https://doi.org/10.1348/000711007X255327.

Sedgwick P. What is publication bias in a meta-analysis? BMJ. 2015 Aug 14;351:h4419. https://doi.org/10.1136/bmj.h4419.

Sedgwick P, Marston L. Meta-analyses: Standardised mean differences. BMJ. 2013; 347:f7257 https://doi.org/10.1136/bmj.f7257

Simel DL, Rennie D, Bossuyt PM. The STARD statement for reporting diagnostic accuracy studies: Application to the history and physical examination. J Gen Intern Med. 2008 Jun;23:768–774.

Simmonds MC, Higginsa JP, Stewartb LA, Tierneyb JF, Clarke MJ, Thompson SG. Meta-analysis of individual patient data from randomized trials: A review of methods used in practice. Clinical Trials. 2005 Jun;2(3):209–217.

Sousa MR, Ribeiro AL. Systematic review and meta-analysis of diagnostic and prognostic studies: A tutorial. Arq Bras Cardiol. 2009 Mar;92(3):229–238, 235–245. English, Spanish. https://doi.org/10.1590/s0066-782x2009000300013.

Takeshima N, Sozu T, Tajika A, Ogawa Y, Hayasaka Y, Furukawa TA. Which is more generalizable, powerful and interpretable in meta-analyses, mean difference or standardized mean difference? BMC Med Res Methodol. 2014 Feb 21;14:30. https://doi.org/10.1186/1471-2288-14-30.

Thomas D, Radji S, Benedetti A. Systematic review of methods for individual patient data meta-analysis with binary outcomes. BMC Med Res Methodol. 2014 Dec;14:1–9.

Tudur Smith C, Marcucci M, Nolan SJ, Iorio A, Sudell M, Riley R, Rovers MM, Williamson PR. Individual participant data meta-analyses compared with meta-analyses based on aggregate data. Cochrane Database Syst Rev. 2016 Sep 6;9(9):MR000007. https://doi.org/10.1002/14651858.MR000007.pub3.

Vali Y, Leeflang MM, Bossuyt PM. Application of weighting methods for presenting risk-of-bias assessments in systematic reviews of diagnostic test accuracy studies. Syst Rev. 2021 Dec;10:1–8.

Viera AJ. Odds ratios and risk ratios: What's the difference and why does it matter? South Med J.2008; 101(7):730–734.

von Hippel PT. The heterogeneity statistic I(2) can be biased in small meta-analyses. BMC Med Res Methodol. 2015 Apr 14;15:35. https://doi.org/10.1186/s12874-015-0024-z.

White IR. Network meta-analysis. The Stata Journal. 2015 Dec;15(4):951–985.

Wolff RF, Moons KG, Riley RD, Whiting PF, Westwood M, Collins GS, Reitsma JB, Kleijnen J, Mallett S, PROBAST Group†. PROBAST: A tool to assess the risk of bias and applicability of prediction model studies. Ann Intern Med. 2019 Jan 1;170(1):51–58.

Zeng X, Zhang Y, Kwong JS, Zhang C, Li S, Sun F, Niu Y, Du L. The methodological quality assessment tools for preclinical and clinical studies, systematic review and meta-analysis, and clinical practice guideline: A systematic review. J Evid Based Med. 2015 Feb;8(1):2–10. https://doi.org/10.1111/jebm.12141.

##R Codes for Meta

```
thr<- escalc(measure="OR", ai=T, bi=(Num-T), ci=T.1,
di=(Num.1-T.1), add=1/2, to="all", slab=paste(Studies),data=hep)
```

##Model

```
thr_ana<-rma(yi, vi,data=thr)
predict(thr_ana, transf=exp, digits=2)
```

##Forest plot

```
forest(thr_ana)
thr_ana<-rma(yi, vi, mods = ~Treatment, data=thr)
```

##sub group analysis

```
forest(thr_ana, xlim=c(-16, 6.5), at=log(c(0.05, 0.25, 1,
4)), ylim=c(-1.5,25), addpred=TRUE, header=TRUE, atransf =
exp, ilab=cbind(hep$T, hep$Num, hep$T.1, hep$Num.1), ilab.
xpos=c(-9.5,-8,-6,-4.5), cex=0.90, order=thr$Treatment,
rows=c(3,8:9,14:20), mlab = thr_fun("RE Model Overall", thr_ana),
psize=1)
```

##Label

```
text(c(-9.5,-8,-6,-4.5), 24,font=2, c("VTE+", "Total", "VTE+", "To-
tal")) text(c(-8.75,-5.25), 25, font=2, c("High Dose", "Low Dose"))
text(-16, c(21.5,10.5,4.5), font=4, pos=4, c("Therapeutic Dose
vs Prophylactic Dose", "Intermediate Dose vs Prophylactic Dose",
"Therapeutic Dose Vs Placebo"))
```

```
Thr.a<- rma(yi, vi, subset=(Treatment=="A"),data=thr)
Thr.b<- rma(yi, vi, subset=(Treatment=="B"),data=thr)
Thr.c<- rma(yi, vi, subset=(Treatment=="C"),data=thr)
Thr_fun<- function (text, thr_ana) {list(bquote(paste(.(text),"
(Q = ",.(formatC(thr_ana$QE, digits=2, format="f")),", df =
",.(thr_ana$k - ble_ana$p), ", p ",.(metafor:::.pval(thr_ana$QEp,
digits=2, showeq=TRUE, sep=" ")), "; ", I2, " = ",.(formatC(thr_
ana$I2, digits=1, format="f")), "%)")))}
```

##Sub group-overall effect size

```
addpoly(Thr.a, addpred=TRUE, row=1.5, cex=0.90, atransf=exp,
mlab=thr_fun("RE Model for Subgroup", Thr.a))
addpoly(Thr.b, addpred=TRUE, row=6.5, cex=0.90, atransf=exp,
mlab=thr_fun("RE Model for Subgroup", Thr.b))
addpoly(Thr.c, addpred=TRUE, row=12.5, cex=0.90, atransf=exp,
mlab=thr_fun("RE Model for Subgroup", Thr.c))
```

##Funnel

```
Funnel(thr_ana)
```

PART IV

Clinical Trials Design and Analysis

## CHAPTER 13

Conceptualization of Clinical Study Design

Insights and Utilities

Pratibha Prasad and Masuma Khanam

Learning Outcomes

Readers will understand the critical role of clinical research designs in generating reliable medical evidence, especially in stroke research. They will explore various study designs, including observational (cohort and case-control) and interventional (randomized controlled trials), learning when and how each is applied. Key statistical concepts, such as prevalence, incidence, risk ratios, and sample size calculations will be introduced. Learners will also gain insights into advanced trial designs, like crossover, superiority, noninferiority, and equivalence trials. By the end, students will be able to select appropriate study designs and apply statistical tools to improve the quality and interpretation of clinical research.

Introduction

Clinical research requires a systematic approach with proper planning, execution, and sampling in order to obtain reliable and validated results, as well as an understanding of each research methodology. This is because by selecting an inappropriate study type, any error that cannot be corrected after the beginning of a study will result in flawed methodology. The successful implementation of clinical research methodology depends upon several factors, which include the type of study, the objectives, the population, study design, methodology/techniques, and the sampling and statistical procedures. According to Campbell and Machin (2005), a well-designed study is more critical than the analysis of its results, as poor study planning can never yield correct results, while poorly analyzed data can often be re-examined and corrected. In clinical research, designs can broadly be classified into observational and interventional studies. Observational studies involve monitoring subjects without interference from the researcher, often used to identify risk factors and disease associations. Common types of observational studies include cohort studies, where groups of individuals are

DOI: 10.4324/9781032701004-17

followed over time to observe the development of diseases, and case-control studies, where patients with a specific condition are compared to a control group to identify potential risk factors (Lu, 2009; Noordzij et al., 2009). For example, cohort studies have been used to explore the association between risk factors, such as hypertension and stroke incidence (Yu et al., 2023).

Interventional studies, on the other hand, involve the active introduction of a treatment or intervention to study its effects on outcomes. Among these, randomized controlled trials (RCTs) are considered the gold standard for testing the efficacy of new treatments, ensuring that groups are similar at baseline to avoid bias. Different RCT designs include superiority trials, which test if a new treatment is better than an existing one, and noninferiority trials, which assess whether a new treatment is not worse than the standard by a preset margin (Senn, 2002; Chen et al., 2023). Advanced methodologies, such as crossover designs, where each participant receives multiple treatments in random order, are often used in stroke rehabilitation research to measure the effect of different interventions on patient outcomes (Nindorera et al., 2023). These designs, along with proper statistical tools, like risk ratios, prevalence, and incidence calculations, contribute to the robustness of clinical study findings, making it possible to draw reliable conclusions about treatment efficacy and risk factors (Altman, 1990).

In clinical studies, basically, the research is broadly divided into two types, viz., observational and experimental studies. Here, we discuss the different designs used in a clinical setup (Lu, 2009; Noordzij et al., 2009).

Taxonomy of research study designs is shown in the earlier **Figure 13.1**. Analytical studies are a primary category into which research can be classified. These studies explore the relationships between variables and test hypotheses to evaluate causal and associative theories (Lu, 2009). Analytical investigations can be observational or interventional in nature. Observational studies, such as cohort, case-control, and cross-sectional designs, involve the passive observation of subjects without intervention and are typically used to identify correlations and causal links between exposures and outcomes (Noordzij et al., 2009). In contrast, interventional research actively modifies or implements interventions, including but not limited to randomized controlled trials (RCTs), which use superiority, noninferiority, equivalence, and crossover designs to assess the effects of specific treatments or interventions (Senn, 2002; Altman, 1990).

Objective

To provide a comprehensive review of various clinical research study designs, including observational and interventional methods, with a particular focus on their application in stroke-related research. This paper aims to explore how different study designs – such as cohort, case-control, and randomized controlled trials – contribute to understanding risk factors, treatment efficacy, and patient outcomes in stroke care. Furthermore, the paper will assess the utility of advanced trial methodologies, statistical tools, and the impact of well-structured designs on enhancing the validity and reliability of clinical research findings.

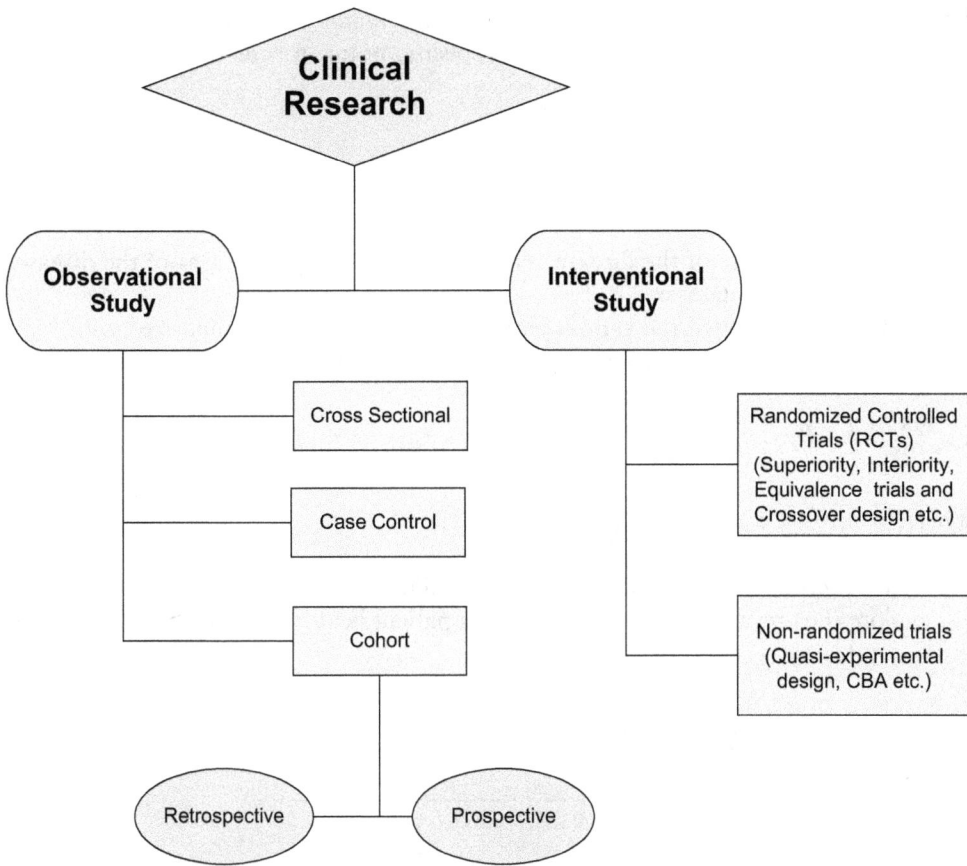

Figure 13.1 Classification of clinical research study designs.

Study Design
Observational Study
Cross-Sectional Study
A cross-sectional study is an observational research design that involves collecting data from a population, or a representative subset, at a single point in time or over a short period. This type of study aims to assess the prevalence of outcomes, conditions, or characteristics within the population. Cross-sectional studies are particularly useful for describing the current status of a disease or health condition in a population and can help identify potential associations between risk factors and outcomes (Lu, 2009; Noordzij et al., 2009). However, since data are collected at one time point, cross-sectional studies cannot determine causality or the temporal relationship between exposure and outcome.

Measure
Measure includes simple proportion or average with the respect to different characteristics of the population.

Prevalence – Prevalence is the proportion of individuals in a population who have a particular disease or condition at a specific point in time or over a specified period.

$$P_A = \frac{N_d}{N_t} \times 100 \tag{1}$$

where P_A = prevalence of the disease, N_d = number of existing cases of the disease, N_t = total populationat risk.

The difference between the various exposure strata could be summarized with 95% CI (confidence interval) and also tested for statistical significance for appropriate statistic.

$$95\%CI = \hat{p} \pm 1.96 \times SE(\hat{p}) \tag{2}$$

Where, $\hat{p} = \dfrac{a}{a+c}$ and $SE(\hat{p}) = \sqrt{\dfrac{\hat{p}(1-\hat{p})}{n}}$

Example – A cross-sectional study was conducted in 151 patients of stroke survivors to explore the prevalence of depression using patient health questionnaire-9 (PHQ-9) (see Table 13.1).

Table 13.1 Study of 151 stroke survivors

Depression	Stroke survivors
Yes	50
No	101
Total	151

$N_d = 50$, $N_t = 151$

$$P_A \, (\text{Prevalence of the disease}) = \frac{50}{151} \times 100 = 33.11\%$$

$$\hat{p} = \frac{50}{151} = 0.33$$

$$SE(\hat{p}) = \sqrt{\frac{0.33 \times 0.67}{151}} = 0.39$$

$$95\%CI = 0.33 \pm 1.96 \times 0.39$$

It was found that 50 participants (33.1%) had a score of ≥ 10, indicating the presence of clinical diagnosis of depression. 101 (66.9 %) patients had minimal to mild depression. The conclusion was that almost one-third of stroke survivors experience post-stroke depression (Sadanandan et al., 2021).

Case-Control Study

A case-control study is an observational research design in which persons with a specific condition or disease (cases) are compared to those who do not have the condition (controls) in order to discover and assess factors that may contribute to the development of the condition. This strategy is especially effective for researching uncommon diseases or ailments with a lengthy latency period since it allows researchers to look back at exposure factors (Grimes & Schulz, 2002). By comparing cases and controls, researchers can identify possible risk factors, such as lifestyle choices, environmental exposures, or genetic predispositions, offering vital insights into illness etiology (Schulz & Grimes, 2002a). Case-control studies are frequently used in epidemiological research because they are efficient, cost-effective, and produce rapid results. However, they are subject to certain limitations, including recall bias and difficulty in establishing causality (Mann, 2003).

Measure

Odds Ratio – The odds ratio (OR) is a measure of the relationship between exposure and outcome. It compares the chances of the result occurring in the exposed group to the non-exposed (or control) group.

$$OR = \frac{Odds_{exposed}}{Odds_{non-exposed}} = \frac{a \times d}{b \times c} \tag{3}$$

Such as,

$$Odds_{exposed} == \frac{a}{b} \text{ (odds of event in exposed group)}$$

$$dds_{non-exposed} == \frac{c}{d} \text{ (odds of event in exposed group)},$$

Where,

    a = number of exposed individuals who experienced the event
    b = number of exposed individuals who did not experience the event
    c = number of non-exposed individuals who experienced the event
    d = number of non-exposed individuals who did not experience the event

Statistical Tests

Chi-Square Test: For categorical outcomes

$$\chi^2 = \sum \frac{(0_i - E_i)^2}{E_i} \tag{4}$$

Example

For example, in a study by Coutinho et al. (2017), the objective was to determine whether there is an association between carotid artery web and ischemic stroke. Cases were the patients with ischemic stroke in anterior circulation of undetermined etiology. While the controls were consecutive patients diagnosed with cerebral aneurysms, arteriovenous malformations, or primary intracerebral haemorrhages. The exposure was the development of the carotid web. Hence, the conclusion of the study was that there is an association between carotid artery web and ischemic stroke in patients who lack an alternative cause of stroke (see Table 13.2).

Table 13.2 Carotid artery web and ischemic stroke association

Ischemic stroke	Carotid web		Total
	Yes	No	
Yes	11 (a)	69 (b)	80
No	1 (c)	79 (d)	80
Total	12	148	160

Here,

Cases (Ischemic Stroke) with Carotid Web (a): 11
Cases (Ischemic Stroke) without Carotid Web (b): 69
Controls (No Stroke) with Carotid Web (c): 1
Controls (No Stroke) without Carotid Web (d): 79

From the previous equation (2),

$$\text{Odds ratio} = \frac{11 \times 79}{69 \times 1} = \frac{869}{69} \approx 12.6$$

The odds ratio (OR) of 12.6 indicates that individuals with a carotid artery web are approximately 12.6 times more likely to have an ischemic stroke compared to individuals without the web. This suggests a strong association between carotid artery web and the occurrence of ischemic stroke, implying that the web might be a significant risk factor for stroke in these patients.

Cohort Study

A cohort study is a form of observational research strategy that aims to investigate the causes of illness or other health consequences. In this strategy, researchers track a group of people (the cohort) throughout time to see how different exposures influence the incidence of a certain outcome. Cohort studies can be either prospective (following individuals from the present into the future) or retrospective (analyzing previous data). A cohort study's main strength is its capacity to demonstrate a temporal link between exposure and result, which is essential for demonstrating causation (Mann, 2003). This approach is widely used in epidemiology to investigate illness incidence, etiology, and prognosis (Rothman et al., 2008). A famous example is the Framingham Heart Study, which has tracked participants for almost 70 years, resulting in substantial findings about cardiovascular risk factors (Dawber et al., 1951). Despite their advantages, cohort studies are not without limits. They can be expensive, have extensive follow-up periods, and are prone to attrition bias (Schulz and Grimes, 2002b). Nonetheless, they are still an important tool in public health research, providing critical data for the creation of preventative interventions (Szklo & Nieto, 2014).

Cohort studies are classified into two types: retrospective and prospective. In a retrospective cohort study, researchers look back at data that has already been collected in the past, identify the cohort based on past records, and then track outcomes to the present. This type of study is useful when the outcomes are rare or have a long latency period between exposure and disease onset (Wang et al., 2019).

A prospective cohort study, on the other hand, starts with the identification of a cohort in the present and tracks them into the future to evaluate outcomes. This design gives researchers more control over the data collection process and guarantees that all pertinent exposures and outcomes are documented as they occur; it is particularly useful when researching newly discovered diseases or exposures and their potential effects in the future (Smith & Johnson, 2020).

E.g., in a prospective cohort study (Yu et al., 2023), the subject was middle-aged and elderly (main respondents ≥ 45 years) individuals without diabetes, and exposure was insulin resistance measured by the triglyceride-glucose (TyG) index. The follow-up was for seven years, and the outcome was the risk of stroke occurrence. Hence, the conclusion was that TyG index was significantly associated with a higher risk of stroke among the middle-aged and elderly non-diabetic population.

E.g., for a retrospective study (Addisu and Mega, 2023), the subjects are patients diagnosed with acute ischemic stroke (AIS), the exposure is atrial fibrillation, and the outcome was incidence in hospital mortality. Hence, the conclusion was that hospital mortality was greater in AIS associated with atrial fibrillation.

Measure

Risk Ratio: The risk ratio (also known as the relative risk) is a measure used to compare the risk of a certain event occurring in two different groups. Specifically, it compares the risk of the event in an exposed group to the risk of the event in a non-exposed (or control) group.

$$RR = \frac{P_{exposed}}{P_{non-exposed}} = \frac{a(c+d)}{c(a+b)} \tag{5}$$

Such as,

$$P_{exposed} = \frac{a}{a+b} \text{ (The probability of the event occurring in the exposed group)}$$

$$P_{non-exposed} = \frac{c}{c+d}$$ (The probability of the event occurring in the non-exposed group)

Where,

a = number of exposed individuals who experienced the event
b = number of exposed individuals who did not experience the event
c = number of non-exposed individuals who experienced the event
d = number of non-exposed individuals who did not experience the event

Example

To calculate the risk ratio (RR) from the data in the prospective cohort study, we have the event rates in two groups: those in care homes and those living in their own homes. The primary event of interest is mortality in stroke survivors (see Table 13.3).
From the study:

Table 13.3 Risk ratio (RR)

Home residents death	Care home residents death		Total
	Yes	No	
yes	364 (a)	63 (b)	427
No	1,377 (c)	1,744 (d)	3,121
Total	1,741	1,807	3,548

Using the table values in equation 3 earlier:

$$\text{Risk ratio}(RR) = \frac{364 \times 3121}{1377 \times 427} = \frac{1136044}{587979} = 1.93$$

The risk ratio of 1.93 indicates that stroke survivors discharged to care homes have nearly 1.93 times the risk of mortality compared to those discharged to their own homes, suggesting significantly worse survival outcomes for care home residents.

For Sample Size Calculation

Odds ratio: case-control – For case-control study, the sample size calculation is based on the odds ratio and the proportion of exposure among controls. The formula is as follows:

$$n_{cases} = n_{controls} = \frac{\left(Z_{\alpha/2} + Z_\beta\right)^2}{[\log(OR)]} \left[\frac{1}{r p_T (1 - p_T)} + \frac{1}{p_C (1 - p_C)} \right]$$ (6)

p_T: Proportion of cases (patients with ischemic stroke) who have the exposure (carotid artery web)

$$O_T \left(\frac{p_T}{1 - p_T} \right) - \text{odd due to the cases}$$

p_C: Proportion of controls (patients with cerebral aneurysms, arteriovenous malformations, or primary intracerebral haemorrhages) who have the exposure (carotid artery web)

$$O_C \left(\frac{p_C}{1 - p_C} \right) - \text{odd due to control}$$

$$OR = \frac{O_T}{O_C} = \text{odds ratio between the patients with ischemic stroke and carotid artery web}$$

For prospective cohort study,

$$n = n_{cases} = n_{controls} = \frac{(Z_\alpha + Z_\beta)^2 \left[\dfrac{p_1(1 - p_1)}{r} + p_2(1 - p_2) \right]}{\varepsilon^2} \tag{7}$$

p_1: Proportion of individuals with high TyG index who develop a stroke
p_2: Proportion of individuals with low TyG index who develop a stroke

$$\sigma = \left(\sqrt{\frac{p_1(1 - p_1)}{r} + p_2(1 - p_2)} \right) - pooled$$

$\varepsilon = (p_2 - p_1)$ – difference between the proportion of TyG index and stroke.

As per the retrospective cohort study example:

$$n = n_{cases} = n_{controls} = \frac{(Z_\alpha + Z_\beta)^2 \left[\dfrac{p_1(1 - p_1)}{r} + p_2(1 - p_2) \right]}{\varepsilon^2} \tag{8}$$

p_1: Proportion of AIS patients with atrial fibrillation who experience in-hospital mortality

p_2: Proportion of AIS patients without atrial fibrillation who experience in-hospital mortality

$$\sigma = \left(\sqrt{\frac{p_1(1 - p_1)}{r} + p_2(1 - p_2)} \right) - pooled$$

$\varepsilon = (p_2 - p_1)$ – difference between the proportion of patients with and without atrial fibrillation who experience in-hospital mortality (Verma et al., 2024).

Interventional Study

Randomized Control Trial

Randomized controlled trials (RCTs) are considered the gold standard for assessing the efficacy of interventions in clinical research. By randomly allocating participants to intervention or control groups, RCTs minimize selection bias and confounding variables, thereby ensuring that the observed effects are attributable to the intervention being tested (Schulz & Grimes, 2002a). The randomization process, when properly implemented, helps in achieving comparable groups at the baseline, making the conclusions more robust. Moreover, the use of blinding, where possible, reduces performance and detection biases, enhancing the reliability of the results (Higgins et al., 2011). RCTs have been widely utilized in various fields of medical research, including cardiology, oncology, and neurology, to evaluate new therapies and treatments (Peto et al., 1995). The rigorous design of RCTs not only allows for causal inference but also provides essential evidence for the development of clinical guidelines and public health policies (Guyatt et al., 2008).

In randomized controlled trials (RCTs), the design choice plays a crucial role in addressing specific research questions. The superiority design aims to demonstrate that one intervention is more effective than another, typically a standard treatment or placebo. Researchers use this design to prove that a new treatment is better than the existing standard (Pocock, 2013). On the other hand, a noninferiority design is employed to show that a new treatment is not significantly worse than the standard of care within a predefined margin. This is often used when the new treatment may have other advantages, such as fewer side effects or lower cost, even if it isn't more effective (Piaggio et al., 2006). Finally, the equivalence design is used to prove that two treatments have no meaningful differences in efficacy, within a specified range. This design is essential when the goal is to show that a new intervention is as effective as an established one (Schumi & Wittes, 2011). The choice between these designs is driven by the research objectives and the clinical implications of the findings.

Example 1

Superiority Trials

Based on the study of Ranjbar et al., 2021, which is a randomized controlled trial comparing methylprednisolone (intervention group) and dexamethasone (control group) in hospitalized COVID-19 patients, we can structure a 2 × 2 contingency table (see Table 13.4) for treatment and outcome (e.g., clinical improvement vs. no improvement).

Table 13.4 Methylprednisolone group and dexamethasone group

	Clinical improvement (day ten)	No improvement (day ten)
Methylprednisolone Group	a = 36	b = 8
Dexamethasone Group	c = 24	d = 18

STUDY DETAILS
- *Intervention group (methylprednisolone)*: 44 patients
- *Control group (dexamethasone)*: 42 patients
- Clinical outcomes at day ten, based on the study's primary results

Where:

- a = Number of patients in the methylprednisolone group who showed clinical improvement at day ten
- b = Number of patients in the methylprednisolone group who did not show clinical improvement at day ten
- c = Number of patients in the dexamethasone group who showed clinical improvement at day ten
- d = Number of patients in the dexamethasone group who did not show clinical improvement at day ten

Example 2

Inferior Trials

In the context of the ARAMIS trial described in Chen et al., 2023, the study compares dual antiplatelet therapy (DAPT) to alteplase (a thrombolytic agent) for patients with minor nondisabling acute ischemic stroke. The objective would be to assess whether dual antiplatelet therapy is non-inferior or possibly superior to alteplase in preventing future stroke or complications.

In a typical trial comparing two treatments, the 2×2 contingency table (see Table 13.5) will compare the outcome of interest (e.g., stroke recurrence or functional outcome) between the two groups:

Table 13.5 2×2 contingency table

Treatment	Favourable outcome (e.g., no stroke recurrence, mRS 0–1)	Unfavourable outcome (e.g., stroke recurrence, mRS > 1)
Dual Antiplatelet Therapy (DAPT)	a = 130	b = 20
Alteplase	c = 120	d = 30

Where,

- a = Number of patients on dual antiplatelet therapy with favourable outcomes (e.g., no stroke recurrence or mRS score 0–1)
- b = Number of patients on dual antiplatelet therapy with unfavourable outcomes (e.g., stroke recurrence or mRS score > 1)
- c = Number of patients on alteplase with favourable outcomes
- d = Number of patients on alteplase with unfavourable outcomes

Example 3
Equivalence Trials
In a study of which compares yoga in the rehabilitation of post-stroke sequelae, the trial would aim to demonstrate that yoga is equivalent to a standard rehabilitation therapy in improving recovery from post-stroke complications. In this scenario, Table 13.6 would assess the outcomes (e.g., improvement vs. no improvement) for patients undergoing yoga therapy compared to those receiving standard rehabilitation therapy.

Table 13.6 Yoga therapy vs. standard rehabilitation therapy

Treatment	Improvement (e.g., mRS 0–1 or functional recovery)	No improvement (e.g., mRS > 1 or no functional recovery)
Yoga Therapy	a = 45	b = 5
Standard Rehabilitation Therapy	c = 42	d = 8

Where,

a = Number of patients receiving yoga therapy with improvement in post-stroke recovery
b = Number of patients receiving yoga therapy with no improvement
c = Number of patients receiving standard rehabilitation therapy with improvement
d = Number of patients receiving standard rehabilitation therapy with no improvement

Other Measures
For analysis, descriptive measures and some test statistics for continuous outcomes, such as for the following:
Noninferiority: t-test, Z-test/Wald test, confidence interval approach
Superiority: t-test, ANOVA, Z-test/Wald test, mixed effects models
Equivalence: TOST, t-test, Z-test/Wald test, confidence interval approach are used (Altman, 1990)

For proportions of outcomes:
Noninferiority: Z-test for proportions, chi-square test, Fisher's exact test, confidence interval approach
Superiority: Z-test for proportions, chi-square test, Fisher's exact test, log-rank test
Equivalence: TOST, Z-test for proportions, chi-square test, Fisher's exact test, confidence interval approach

The other statistics that are used as a measure and sample size calculation formulae are presented in **Table 13.7, Table 13.8 and Table 13.9 of Appendix.**

Conclusion

This paper presents a thorough review of clinical research study designs, emphasizing the need of both observational and interventional approaches in producing accurate and useful results in medical research, especially studies pertaining to stroke. Cohort, case-control, and cross-sectional studies are examples of observational designs that are very useful for determining risk factors and proving links between exposures and outcomes. Although these designs are successful and economical, they have drawbacks, including the inability to determine causation and possible biases. However, they are extensively used in epidemiology to comprehend health outcomes and illness trends. When assessing the effectiveness of a treatment, interventional studies – particularly randomized controlled trials (RCTs) – remain the gold standard. They are crucial for determining causal conclusions because of their strict design, which reduces biases and confounding variables. Advanced trial designs, superiority, noninferiority, and equivalency trials – all of which provide sophisticated ways to address various research questions – are covered in the study. The formulation of clinical recommendations is facilitated by these designs, which guarantee precise measurement of therapy effects.

Furthermore, the robustness of clinical study results is increased by the statistical methods that are frequently used, such as risk ratios, prevalence, incidence estimates, odds ratios, and sample size determination. These resources are essential for analyzing study results, particularly for determining how effective certain interventions or therapies are. Researchers may measure the accuracy and dependability of their findings with the use of confidence intervals and hypothesis testing, which helps to make better evidence-based therapeutic judgments. To sum up, the choice of a suitable study design is essential to the accomplishment of clinical research. Robust statistical analysis, in conjunction with well-structured research, yields more accurate insights into patient outcomes, treatment efficacy, and disease prevention, and precise study designs facilitate the investigation of the intricate connections among risk factors, therapeutic treatments, and long-term patient health in stroke care and rehabilitation, therefore enhancing patient care. Subsequent investigations have to persist in honing these designs and statistical techniques to augment their suitability across various medical domains.

Discussion Questions

- How do different clinical research designs, such as cohort, case-control, and RCTs, help address questions about stroke risk and treatment?
- What are the strengths and limitations of observational vs. interventional designs in stroke studies?
- Why are statistical concepts, like incidence and risk ratios, essential in interpreting clinical outcomes?
- In what situations would a crossover or noninferiority trial design be preferable?
- Finally, how can selecting the right research design and statistical approach influence the accuracy and applicability of findings in stroke care and rehabilitation?

References

Addisu, Z.D. and Mega, T.A., 2023. Clinical characteristics and treatment outcomes of acute ischemic stroke with atrial fibrillation among patients admitted to tertiary care hospitals in Amhara Regional State: Retrospective-cohort study. *Vascular Health and Risk Management*, pp.837–853.

Altman, D.G., 1990. *Practical statistics for medical research.* Chapman and Hall/CRC.

Campbell, M.J. and Machin, D., 2005. Medical statistics: a commonsense approach (Vol. 2). Chichester: Wiley.

Chen, H.S., Cui, Y., Zhou, Z.H., Zhang, H., Wang, L.X., Wang, W.Z., Shen, L.Y., Guo, L.Y., Wang, E.Q., Wang, R.X. and Han, J., 2023. Dual antiplatelet therapy vs alteplase for patients with minor nondisabling acute ischemic stroke: The ARAMIS randomized clinical trial. *Journal of the American Medical Association*, 329(24), pp.2135–2144.

Coutinho, J.M., Derkatch, S., Potvin, A.R., Tomlinson, G., Casaubon, L.K., Silver, F.L. and Mandell, D.M., 2017. Carotid artery web and ischemic stroke: A case-control study. *Neurology*, 88(1), pp.65–69.

Dawber, T.R., Meadors, G.F. and Moore Jr, F.E., 1951. Epidemiological approaches to heart disease: The Framingham Study. *American Journal of Public Health and the Nations Health*, 41(3), pp.279–286.

Grimes, D.A. and Schulz, K.F., 2002. Bias and causal associations in observational research. *The Lancet*, 359(9302), pp.248–252.

Guyatt, G.H., Oxman, A.D., Vist, G.E., Kunz, R., Falck-Ytter, Y., Alonso-Coello, P. and Schünemann, H.J., 2008. GRADE: An emerging consensus on rating quality of evidence and strength of recommendations. *BMJ: British Medical Journal*, 336(7650), pp.924–926.

Higgins, J.P., Altman, D.G., Gøtzsche, P.C., Jüni, P., Moher, D., Oxman, A.D., Savović, J., Schulz, K.F., Weeks, L. and Sterne, J.A., 2011. The Cochrane Collaboration's tool for assessing risk of bias in randomised trials. *BMJ: British Medical Journal*, 343.

Lu, C.Y., 2009. Observational studies: A review of study designs, challenges and strategies to reduce confounding. *International Journal of Clinical Practice*, 63(5), pp.691–697.

Mann, C.J., 2003. Observational research methods. Research design II: Cohort, cross sectional, and case-control studies. *Emergency Medicine Journal*, 20(1), pp.54–60.

Nindorera, F., Nduwimana, I., Sinzakaraye, A., Havyarimana, E., Bleyenheuft, Y., Thonnard, J.L. and Kossi, O., 2023. Effect of mixed and collective physical activity in chronic stroke rehabilitation: A randomized cross-over trial in low-income settings. *Annals of Physical and Rehabilitation Medicine*, 66(4), p.101704.

Noordzij, M., Dekker, F.W., Zoccali, C. and Jager, K.J., 2009. Study designs in clinical research. *Nephron Clinical Practice*, 113(3), pp.c218–c221.

Peto, R., Collins, R. and Gray, R., 1995. Large-scale randomized evidence: Large, simple trials and overviews of trials. *Journal of Clinical Epidemiology*, 48(1), pp.23–40.

Piaggio, G., Elbourne, D.R., Altman, D.G., Pocock, S.J., Evans, S.J. and CONSORT Group, F.T., 2006. Reporting of noninferiority and equivalence randomized trials: An extension of the CONSORT statement. *Journal of the American Medical Association*, 295(10), pp.1152–1160.

Pocock, S.J., 2013. *Clinical trials: A practical approach.* John Wiley & Sons.

Ranjbar, K., Moghadami, M., Mirahmadizadeh, A., Fallahi, M.J., Khaloo, V., Shahriarirad, R., Erfani, A., Khodamoradi, Z. and Gholampoor Saadi, M.H., 2021. Methylprednisolone or dexamethasone, which one is superior corticosteroid in the treatment of hospitalized COVID-19 patients: A triple-blinded randomized controlled trial. *BMC Infectious Diseases*, 21, pp.1–8.

Rothman, K.J., Greenland, S. and Lash, T.L., 2008. *Modern epidemiology* (Vol. 3). Philadelphia: Wolters Kluwer Health/Lippincott Williams & Wilkins.

Sadanandan, S., Silva, F.D. and Renjith, V., 2021. Depression among rural stroke survivors: A cross-sectional study. *Indian Journal of Community Medicine*, 46(2), pp.309–312.

Schulz, K.F. and Grimes, D.A., 2002a. Case-control studies: Research in reverse. *The Lancet*, *359*(9304), pp.431–434.

Schulz, K.F. and Grimes, D.A., 2002b. Generation of allocation sequences in randomised trials: Chance, not choice. *The Lancet, 359*(9305), pp.515–519.

Schumi, J., and Wittes, J. T., 2011. Through the looking glass: Understanding non-inferiority. *Trials*, *12*(1), pp.1–12. https://doi.org/10.1186/1745-6215-12-114

Senn, S.S., 2002. *Cross-over trials in clinical research*. John Wiley & Sons.

Smith, A., and Johnson, B., 2020. Prospective cohort studies and their role in medical research. *American Journal of Medical Studies*, *45*(2), pp.156–164. https://doi.org/10.1016/j.ajms.2020.01.006

Szklo, M. and Nieto, F.J., 2014. *Epidemiology: Beyond the basics*. Jones & Bartlett Publishers.

Verma, V., Mishra, A.K. and Narang, R., 2024. Determination of sample size for different clinical study designs. *The Journal of the Association of Physicians of India*, *72*(7), pp.34–40.

Wang, Q., Li, J. and Zhao, X., 2019. Retrospective cohort studies: Applications and challenges. *Clinical Epidemiology and Global Health*, *7*(1), pp.10–15. https://doi.org/10.1016/j.cegh.2019.01.001

Yu, Y., Meng, Y. and Liu, J., 2023. Association between the triglyceride-glucose index and stroke in middle-aged and older non-diabetic population: A prospective cohort study. *Nutrition, Metabolism and Cardiovascular Diseases*, *33*(9), pp.1684–1692.

Appendix I

Table 13.7 For continuous outcomes of the statistical measures

Design	Test statistics and confidence interval approach	Decision rule
Superiority	For superiority trial to demonstrate that a new treatment is better than a standard treatment. Such as the following: $$t = \frac{\overline{X}_1 - \overline{X}_2}{\sqrt{\dfrac{s_1^2}{n_1} + \dfrac{s_2^2}{n_2}}}$$ Confidence interval calculation: $$\left(\overline{X}_1 - \overline{X}_2\right) \pm t_{\alpha/2}\sqrt{\frac{s_1^2}{n_1} + \frac{s_2^2}{n_2}} \ \text{[lower bound > 0]}$$ $\overline{X}_1$: Mean outcome in the treatment group $\overline{X}_2$: Mean outcome in the control group s_1^2 : Variance in the treatment group s_2^2 : Variance in the control group n_1 : Sample size in the treatment group n_2 : Sample size in the control group	If t is greater than a critical value from the normal distribution (usually $t_{\alpha/2}$ for a two-sided test at $\alpha = 0.05$, which is approximately 1.96), the new treatment is considered superior.

(Continued)

Table 13.7 (Continued)

Design	Test statistics and confidence interval approach	Decision rule
Equivalence	Effects of two treatments are sufficiently similar, within a predefined margin (Δ). Such as the Two One-Sided Tests (TOST) procedure is commonly used for equivalence testing. Test 1: $t = \dfrac{(\overline{X}_1 - \overline{X}_2) + \Delta}{\sqrt{\dfrac{s_1^2}{n_1} + \dfrac{s_2^2}{n_2}}}$ Test 2: $t = \dfrac{(\overline{X}_1 - \overline{X}_2) - \Delta}{\sqrt{\dfrac{s_1^2}{n_1} + \dfrac{s_2^2}{n_2}}}$ Confidence interval calculation: $(\overline{X}_1 - \overline{X}_2) \pm t_\alpha \sqrt{\dfrac{s_1^2}{n_1} + \dfrac{s_2^2}{n_2}}$ [Entire interval within $- \Delta$ and Δ] Where, $\overline{X}_1$: Mean outcome in the first treatment group $\overline{X}_2$: Mean outcome in the second treatment group s_1^2: Variance in the first treatment group s_2^2: Variance in the second treatment group n_1: Sample size in the first treatment group n_2: Sample size in the second treatment group Δ: Equivalence margin	Both t_1 and t_2 must be less than the critical value from the normal distribution (usually t_α, typically 1.645 for $\alpha = 0.05$). If both conditions are met, the treatments are considered equivalent.

Source: Verma et al. (2024)

Table 13.8 For proportion of outcomes of the statistical measures

Design	Test statistics and confidence interval approach	Decision rule
Noninferiority	To demonstrate that the proportion of a positive outcome with a new treatment is not worse than the proportion with a standard treatment by more than a specified margin (Δ). Test Statistic is $Z = \dfrac{(p_1 - p_2) - \Delta}{\sqrt{\dfrac{p_1(1 - p_1)}{n_1} + \dfrac{p_2(1 - p_2)}{n_2}}}$	If Z is greater than a critical value from the normal distribution (usually Z_α is the significance level, typically 1.645 for a one-sided test at $\alpha = 0.05$), the new treatment is considered noninferior.

(Continued)

Table 13.8 (Continued)

Design	Test statistics and confidence interval approach	Decision rule
	Confidence interval calculation:	

$$CI = (p_1 - p_2) \pm Z_\alpha \sqrt{\frac{p_1(1-p_1)}{n_1} + \frac{p_2(1-p_2)}{n_2}}$$

p_1 : Proportion of positive outcomes in the treatment group

p_2 : Proportion of positive outcomes in the control group

n_1 : Sample size in the treatment group

n_2 : Sample size in the control group

Δ: Noninferiority margin

Design	Test statistics and confidence interval approach	Decision rule
Superiority	Superiority trial to demonstrate that the proportion of a positive outcome with a new treatment is better than the proportion with a standard treatment. Test statistic is	If Z is greater than a critical value from the normal distribution (usually Z_α for a two-sided test at $\alpha = 0.05$, which is approximately 1.96), the new treatment is considered superior.

$$Z = \frac{p_1 - p_2}{\sqrt{\frac{p_1(1-p_1)}{n_1} + \frac{p_2(1-p_2)}{n_2}}}$$

p : Pooled proportion of positive outcomes, calculated as $p = \frac{n_1 p_1 + n_2 p_2}{n_1 + n_2}$

Confidence interval calculation:

$$CI = (p_1 - p_2) \pm Z_{\alpha/2} \sqrt{\frac{p_1(1-p_1)}{n_1} + \frac{p_2(1-p_2)}{n_2}}$$

Design	Test statistics and confidence interval approach	Decision rule
Equivalence	*Equivalence trial* to demonstrate that the proportions of positive outcomes between two treatments are sufficiently similar, within a predefined margin (Δ). *Test statistic is* the Two One-Sided Tests (TOST) procedure, which is commonly used for equivalence testing.	Both Z_1 and Z_2 must be less than the critical value from the normal distribution (usually Z_α, typically 1.645 for $\alpha = 0.05$). If both conditions are met, the treatments are considered equivalent.

Test 1: $$Z_1 = \frac{(p_1 - p_2) + \Delta}{\sqrt{\frac{p_1(1-p_1)}{n_1} + \frac{p_2(1-p_2)}{n_2}}}$$

Test 2: $$Z_2 = \frac{(p_1 - p_2) - \Delta}{\sqrt{\frac{p_1(1-p_1)}{n_1} + \frac{p_2(1-p_2)}{n_2}}}$$

(*Continued*)

Table 13.8 (Continued)

Design	Test statistics and confidence interval approach	Decision rule
	Confidence Interval calculation –	

$$CI = (p_1 - p_2) \pm Z_{\alpha/2} \sqrt{\frac{p_1(1-p_1)}{n_1} + \frac{p_2(1-p_2)}{n_2}}$$

Where,

p_1 : Mean outcome in the first treatment group
p_2 : Mean outcome in the second treatment group
n_1 : Sample size in the first treatment group
n_2 : Sample size in the second treatment group
Δ : Equivalence margin

Source: Verma et al. (2024)

Table 13.9 Sample size calculation for different RCT designs for continuous and proportion of outcomes

Design	Sample size calculation formula
Continuous outcome in RCT test for noninferiority/ superiority	$$n = n_{cases} = n_{controls} = \left(\frac{r+1}{r}\right)\frac{(Z_\alpha + Z_\beta)^2 \sigma^2}{(\varepsilon - \delta)^2}$$ Superiority trials ($\delta > 0$) Noninferiority trial ($\delta < 0$) μ_1: Mean of continuous outcome of the dual antiplatelet therapy (DAPT) treatment μ_2: Mean of continuous outcome of the intravenous thrombolysis σ: SD of the continuous outcome of the dual antiplatelet therapy (DAPT) treatment $\varepsilon = (\mu_2 - \mu_1)$: Difference between the means of dual antiplatelet therapy (DAPT) treatment and intravenous thrombolysis δ: Clinically meaningful difference (largest change from the reference value that is trivial) Assumption: σ is known
Proportions of outcome in RCT test for noninferiority/ superiority	$$n = n_{cases} = n_{controls} = \frac{(Z_\alpha + Z_\beta)^2 \left[\frac{p_1(1-p_1)}{r} + p_2(1-p_2)\right]}{(\varepsilon - \delta)^2}$$ p_1: Proportion of response due to the dual antiplatelet therapy (DAPT) treatment p_2: Proportion of response due to the intravenous thrombolysis

(Continued)

Table 13.9 (Continued)

Design	Sample size calculation formula
	$\varepsilon = (p_2 - p_1)$: Difference between the proportion of responses due to dual antiplatelet therapy (DAPT) treatment and intravenous thrombolysis $$\sigma = \left(\sqrt{\frac{p_1(1-p_1)}{r} + p_2(1-p_2)} \right) - pooled$$ δ: Clinically meaningful difference (largest change from the reference value that is trivial)
Continuous outcome in RCT test for equivalence design	$$n = n_{cases} = n_{controls} = \left(\frac{r+1}{r} \right) \frac{\left(Z_\alpha + Z_{\beta/2} \right)^2 \sigma^2}{\left(\delta - |\varepsilon| \right)^2}$$ μ_1: Mean of continuous outcome of the dual antiplatelet therapy (DAPT) treatment μ_2: Mean of continuous outcome of the intravenous thrombolysis σ: SD of the continuous outcome of the dual antiplatelet therapy (DAPT) treatment $\varepsilon = (\mu_2 - \mu_1)$: Difference between the means of dual antiplatelet therapy (DAPT) treatment and intravenous thrombolysis δ: Clinically meaningful difference (largest change from the reference value that is trivial) Assumption: σ^2 is known
Proportions of outcome in RCT test for equivalenc edesign	$$n = n_{cases} = n_{controls} = \frac{\left(Z_\alpha + Z_{\beta/2} \right)^2 \left[\frac{p_1(1-p_1)}{r} + p_2(1-p_2) \right]}{\left(\delta - |\varepsilon| \right)^2}$$ p_1: Proportion of response due to the dual antiplatelet therapy (DAPT) treatment p_2: Proportion of response due to the intravenous thrombolysis $$\sigma = \left(\sqrt{\frac{p_1(1-p_1)}{r} + p_2(1-p_2)} \right) - pooled$$ $\varepsilon = (p_2 - p_1)$: Difference between the proportion of responses due to dual antiplatelet therapy (DAPT) treatment and intravenous thrombolysis. δ: Clinically meaningful difference (largest change from the reference value that is trivial)

Source: Verma et al. (2024)

Sample Size

Basic Concepts

Prativa Choudhury, Anjan Kumar Dhua and Prabudh Goel

Learning Outcomes

Readers will understand the importance of accurate sample size determination in biomedical studies and its role in ensuring valid, reliable, and generalizable results. They will explore key statistical principles, such as statistical power, effect size, significance levels, and error types. The chapter introduces formula-based and software-assisted methods for calculating sample size across different study designs and objectives. Students will also recognize how factors like study design, outcome measures, population characteristics, and resource availability influence sample size decisions. By the end, learners will be equipped to appropriately plan powered studies that minimize sampling error and optimize research quality.

Introduction

The biomedical studies are conducted on a small cohort of subjects or individuals referred to as a 'sample', which is derived from a larger population. The sample is considered to be representative of the entire population in a manner that the inferences derived through experiments conducted upon this sample are applicable to the population at-large and are key factors differentiating a census study from the inferential analysis. The size of this sample population is crucial to the accuracy and reliability of the results. Logically, a larger sample size will lead to more precise estimates and greater statistical power. Besides, a precise estimation of the sample size is required to predict the quantum of manpower, time, and financial allocation for the study (**Figure 14.1**).

Sampling Error

While a census study gathers data from every member of the population, it provides a complete and accurate picture of the entire population and leaves no scope for questioning the accuracy of the results on this front. However, during inferential analysis,

DOI: 10.4324/9781032701004-18

Smaller Sample Size

- Cost-effectiveness of study (resources, time, and manpower)
- Feasibility of the study
- Congruence with capacity for data collection, analysis and interpretation (resource optimization)
- Setting the tone for later studies (pilot); identify the feasibility, practicality, challenges, and refinement
- Research into rare diseases and specific genetic conditions
- Ethical considerations

Sample Size

Larger Sample Size

- Representativeness of the parent population
- Statistical power (probability of detecting true effect when it exists)
- Larger precision and accuracy
- Reliability and reproducibility of research findings
- Permits subgroup analysis
- Capability of detecting rare events
- Scientific validity and ethical soundness of research

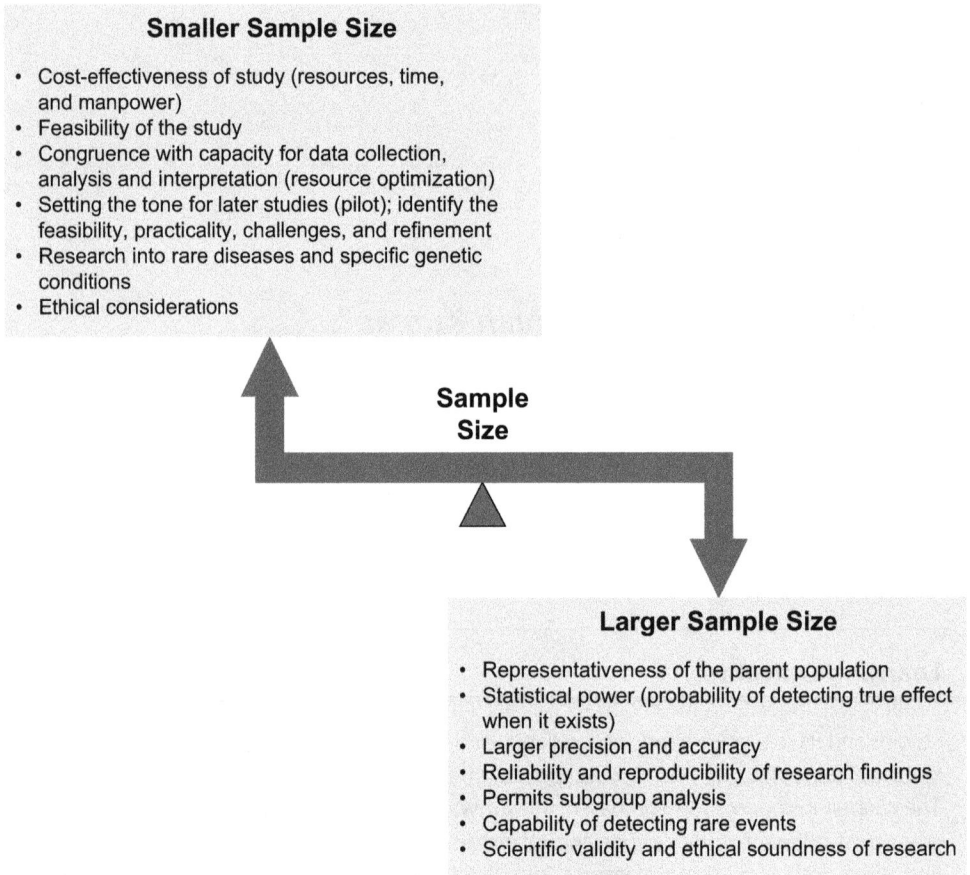

Figure 14.1 Sample size classification.

the study is conducted on a small subset considered representative of the entire population. The applicability of the results to the parent population is determined by the representativeness of the sample population. This introduces the possibility of sampling error, which represents the discrepancy between the sampling statistics and the population characteristics. The more the difference between the sample and the parent population, the more will be the sampling error. The quantum of the sampling error is dependent upon the sample size, methods used to sample the population, and the population characteristics, such as inherent variability.

Statistical Considerations While Estimating the Sample Size

Type I (α, alpha) and Type II error (β, beta): Type I error represents the probability of *incorrectly rejecting the null hypothesis (H$_0$)* (false positive result) or the probability of concluding that there is an intervention-driven significant difference between the outcomes of the study and control groups while there are actually none. The quantitative estimate (significance level) of the Type I error is provided by α, which is the maximum probability of making a Type I error. The usually acceptable values of α are 0.05 (5%) or 0.01 (1%).

An α of 0.05 or 5% implies that there is a 5% chance of rejecting the null hypothesis, while it is true (Suresh et al., 2012).

Type II error represents the probability of *failing to reject the null hypothesis (H$_0$)* (false negative result) or the probability of failing to detect an intervention-driven significant difference between the outcomes of the study and control groups. It is the probability of missing the real effect. The power of a study is quantitatively estimated by [1-β]; it is the probability of correctly rejecting the null hypothesis or the probability of detecting the real effect.

A high-power study has a lower probability of failing to detect a real effect and vice-versa.

While the sample size has little or no bearing on the probability of Type I error, the larger the sample size, the lesser is the probability of Type II error and the more is the statistical power.

Effect Size: Effect size signifies the difference between the study group and control group; a larger effect size would imply a substantial difference between the two groups which is observed with a smaller sample size and vice-versa. A sensitivity analysis may be deployed to explore the bearing of the effect size upon the sample size.

Standard Deviation or Variability: Standard deviation signifies the degree of dispersion of data or spread of observations around the mean; a larger standard deviation makes it more challenging to detect small effects or differences and requires larger sample sizes to achieve the same statistical power.

Confidence Interval Width and Confidence Level: Width of the confidence interval signifies the precision of the estimate of the population parameter. The relationship between the sample size and confidence interval is 'inverse'. A larger sample size will provide more information and reduce the uncertainty in the results. They cater to a narrower confidence interval. The probability that the confidence interval correctly captures the true population parameter is reflected by the confidence level; a 95% confidence level implies that if the same study was repeated upon 100 samples derived from the same population, the true population parameter estimate will be captured in the confidence interval in 95 results. Higher confidence levels require wider confidence intervals. The relationship between sample size, width of confidence interval, and confidence level is interconnected and complex; the researcher has to strike a trade-off to optimize the three parameters.

Other Prerequisites for Sample Size Estimation

Understanding the Research Question and Study Objectives: While the subsection is self-explanatory, studies with multiple objectives may require a unique sample size for each objective. In such situations, the researcher may calculate the minimum sample size for each objective and go ahead with the largest value. Alternatively, the minimum sample size for the primary objective may be considered relevant.

Study Design: Observational (cross-sectional, case-control, or cohort) or experimental (randomized controlled trial)

Outcome Measure of Interest: A small sample size is appropriate for outcome measures of interest which are more variable or have larger effect sizes and vice-versa.

Statistical Methods to Be Deployed for the Analysis: The approach to sample size calculation is different for different statistical tests or estimation techniques.

Estimated Dropout Rates: Relevant especially in the context of longitudinal or intervention studies.

Logistics: To work out parameters, such as the availability of budget, time allocation for participant enrolment, and manpower.

Ethical Considerations: Factors such as the participant burden, potential risks, and optimal trade-off between scientific gains and participant welfare should be factored into sample size calculation and ensure that the proposed sample size is ethically justified.

Statistical Formula-Based Approach to Sample Size Calculation

The formulae that best fit the study design and objectives must be selected. Various types of studies and analyses have different formulae related to parameters like effect size, variability, desired confidence level, and power (Charan et al., 2013).

■ **Means/Proportions:** Formulas like Z-test, t-test, or formulae for estimating proportions are used based on the desired confidence level, margin of error, variance, and effect size.

Sample Size for Estimating Population Mean with Predefined Precision

$$n = \left(Z_{\alpha/2}\right)^2 s^2 / d^2$$

- ■ n = minimum sample size
- ■ Z = Z-score (1.96 for a 95% CI or 2.576 for a 99% CI, etc.)
- ■ σ = standard deviation of the population
- ■ E = desired margin of error (precision)

Illustration 1: A researcher wishes to assess the effectiveness of a new medication in reducing blood pressure over six weeks among patients diagnosed with hypertension. He needs to calculate the sample size for a study to detect 5 mm reduction in systolic pressure with a SD of 10 mm of mercury and a 95% confidence interval.

Using the formula:

$$n = (1.96)^2 \times (10)^2/(5)2$$

$$n \approx 15.3664$$

The health officer would need a sample size of approximately 15 patients to achieve the desired precision in estimating the mean reduction in systolic blood pressure with a 95% confidence level.

Additionally, accounting for a 10% allowance for missing data, losses to follow-up, and withdrawals, the corrected sample size is adjusted to 27 subjects, obtained by dividing the initial sample size of 15 by (1.0–0.10), resulting in approximately 17 subjects. For a 20% allowance, the corrected sample size would be adjusted to 19 subjects.

Sample size for comparing means between two independent groups:

$$n = \frac{2\left(Z_{\frac{\alpha}{2}} + Z_{\beta}\right)^2 \sigma^2}{\delta^2}$$

- n = minimum sample size per group
- $Z_{\alpha/2}$ = Z-score corresponding to significance level (1.96 for a 5% significance level)
- Z_{β} = Z-score corresponding to the desired power (0.84 for 80% power)
- σ^2 = pooled variance of the two groups
- δ = minimum clinically or scientifically meaningful difference between the two groups

Illustration 2: An investigator is interested in comparing the efficacy of two diet programs for reducing obesity. With the aforementioned formula, the sample size can be calculated for each group:

- $Z_{1-\alpha/2} = 1.96$ (For a 5% significance level)
- Note: (Z_{α} is 1.96 for a 5% level of significance and 2.58 for a 1% level of significance)
- $Z_{1-\beta} = 0.84$ (For 80% power)
- Note: $Z_{1-\beta}$ is the normal deviate at 1-b% power with b% of Type II error (0.84 at 80% power and 1.28 for 90% power)
- $M_1 = 176$ (Mean of obesity of group 1)
- $M_2 = 166$ (Mean of obesity of group 2)
- $\sigma 1 = 15.2$ (Standard deviation of group 1)
- $\sigma 2 = 13.1$ (Standard deviation of group 2)

$n = [1.96 + 0.84]^2. [(15.2)^2 + (13.1)^2]/[176 - 166]^2$
$n = [2.8]^2. (231.04 + 171.61)/100$
$n = 7.84 \times 402.6/100$
$n = 3156.7/100$
$n = 31.56$
$n = 32$

A sample size of 32 for each group would be needed.

Sample size for estimating proportions: $n = \dfrac{Z^2 \cdot p \cdot (1-p)}{E^2}$

- n = required sample size
- Z = Z-score corresponding to the desired confidence level
- p = estimated proportion of the population with the characteristic of interest
- E = desired margin of error

Illustration 3: To calculate a sample size of a large population (infinite population) whose degree of variability is not known. Assuming the maximum variability, which is equal to 50% (p = 0.5), and taking a 95% confidence level with ± 5% precision, the calculation for the required sample size will be as follows:

$p = 0.5$ and hence $1 - \hat{p} = 1 - 0.5$; $e = 0.05$; $z = 1.96$

where:
$\hat{p}$= 50% or 0.50 (This value is often taken from previous research studies. If unsure, use 50%)
$z = 1.96$ (According to a 95% confidence interval, the z score table value is 1.96)
$e = 5\%$ or 0.05

$$n_0 = \dfrac{(1.96)^2 * (0.5)(1-0.5)}{(0.05)^2}$$

$$n = 384.16$$

Again, taking a 99% confidence level with ± 5% precision, the calculation for the required sample size will be as follows:

$p = 0.5$ and hence $1 - \hat{p} = 1 - 0.5$; $e = 0.05$; $z = 2.58$

$$n_0 = \dfrac{(2.58)^2 * (0.5)(1-0.5)}{(0.05)^2}$$

$$n = 665.64$$

Note: With the increase of CI, the sample size increases.

Regression Analysis: Factors relevant to sample size estimation in regression analysis include the number of predictors, effect sizes (of the predictors), statistical power, and level of significance.

Sample size $n = \dfrac{c.k}{R^2}$

- n = minimum sample size
- c = constant (usually 10–20, representing the desired events per predictor)
- k = number of predictor variables
- R^2 = expected coefficient of determination (proportion of variance explained by the model)

Sample Size Estimation Based Upon Statistical Power Analysis
The algorithm for sample size estimation based upon statistical power analysis has been given in **Figure 14.2**.

Statistical power analysis formula for estimating the sample size for predefined statistical power, effect size, and significance for a two-sample t-test:

$$n = \frac{2\left(Z_{\frac{\alpha}{2}} + Z_{\beta}\right)^2 \sigma^2}{\delta^2}$$

- n = minimum sample size
- $Z_{\alpha/2}$ = Z-score corresponding to the significance level
- Z_{β} = Z-score corresponding to the desired power
- σ^2 = estimated variance or standard variation
- δ = effect size

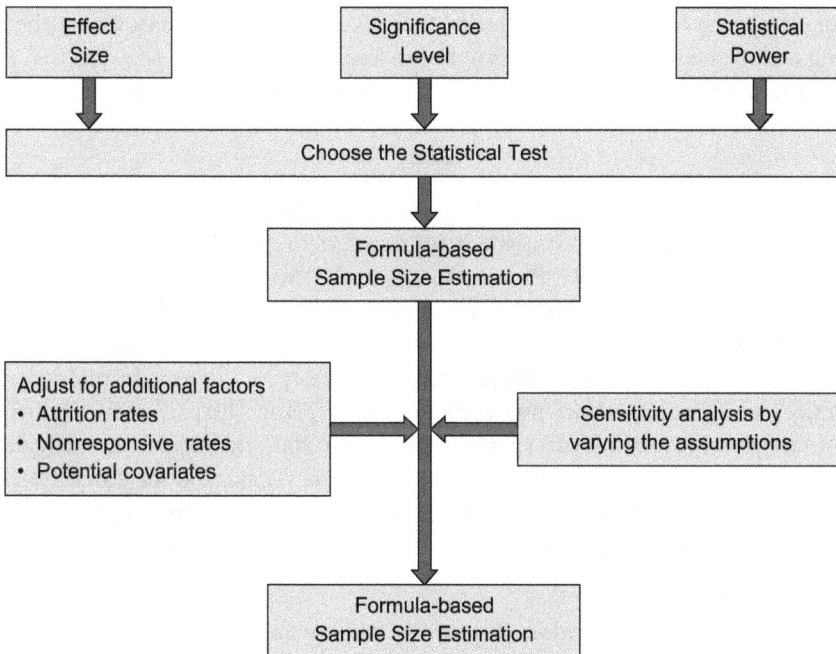

Figure 14.2 Components of sample size calculation.

The formula for regression analysis:

$$N = f^2 \left(Z_{\frac{\alpha}{2}} + Z_\beta \right)^2 + 2k(k-1)$$

where;
- N = sample size
- $Z_{\alpha/2}$ = critical value of the normal distribution at α/2 (for a two-tailed test)
- Z_β = critical value of the normal distribution at β (power of the test)
- f^2 = effect size
- k = number of predictors

Sample Size Estimation with Sample Size Tables

Sample tables are structured for sample size determination, and they provide pre-calculated values for sample sizes based on various combinations of parameters, such as statistical power, effect size, and significance level. These tables are available in textbooks, research method guides, and online resources. They are commonly used in research and experimental design to facilitate the process of sample size estimation.

Sample tables may include different columns or rows corresponding to different significance levels (alpha values), such as 0.05 (5%) or 0.01 (1%), or different rows or columns corresponding to different levels of statistical power (1-beta), such as 0.80 (80%) or 0.90 (90%) and effect size.

Researchers can use sample tables to interpolate or extrapolate sample sizes based on their specific study requirements. For example, if a researcher aims for a power of 0.90, an effect size of 0.50, and a significance level of 0.05, they can locate the corresponding cell in the sample table to find the recommended sample size.

While the sample size tables provide a convenient estimate of the sample size for different situations, they do not cover all possible combinations of parameters.

Sample Size Estimation with Online Calculators and Software

Several online calculators and statistical software are available that can assist in sample size estimation, such as G*Power (Kang, 2021; https://stats.oarc.ucla.edu/other/gpower/), ClinCalc (https://clincalc.com/stats/samplesize.aspx), Power Analysis and Sample Size (PASS) (https://www.ncss.com/software/pass/), and R packages like pwr (https://cran.r-project.org/web/packages/pwr/vignettes/pwr-vignette.html; https://cran.r-project.org/web/packages/pwr/pwr.pdf) and also pRoc (https://stats.oarc.ucla.edu/sas/seminars/proc-power/). It can vary in terms of the statistical tests and study designs, as well as their user interface and accessibility (online vs. standalone software). When compared to sample size tables, these tools offer greater convenience, flexibility, and precision in sample size estimation.

Data From Pilot Studies/Simulation Studies to Estimate Sample Size

Researchers use data from previous studies (pilot studies) to estimate sample sizes when there is limited prior information available or the study/experiment involves complex or novel methodologies. The estimates obtained from the pilot studies are subject to power analysis for estimation of sample size.

Similarly, simulation studies involve generating data based on assumed distributions or parameters and then performing the statistical analysis multiple times to evaluate the power and sample size requirements under different scenarios.

Rule of Thumb for Sample Size

In some cases, researchers use general guidelines or rules of thumb based on field-specific norms or practical constraints, viz., ten participants per variable (for observation studies, regression analysis), 30 participants per groups (comparative studies, such as t-test or ANOVA), 5–20% of the population (such as in surveys), or estimation of minimum detectable effect size for a given statistical power and level.

Such rules, however, may not always be appropriate for every situation.

Resource Constraints

The choice of sample size in research projects can be greatly impacted by resource limitations. Sample size determination is influenced by many factors, including financial resources (a larger sample size typically necessitates more funding for participant recruitment, compensation, data collection tools, salaries, and facilities), time constraints, human resources, and participant availability (the size and accessibility of the target population can affect sample size determination). If the population of interest is small or difficult to reach, researchers may need to settle for a smaller sample size, equipment and materials, and statistical power considerations (need to balance the desire for a larger sample size, which increases statistical power with the available resources).

Difference in Sample Size for One-Tailed and Two-Tailed Tests

A one-tailed test requires fewer subjects to reach a significance level of 0.05, as it allows the entire alpha to test the statistical significance in one direction of interest.

A two-tailed test splits the significance level since it applies in two directions. Thus, each direction is only half as strong as a one-tailed test. To overrule this, two-tailed tests require a larger sample size with greater resources.

Impact of Historical Data Upon Sample Size

Incorporating historical data into sample size determination can be valuable for several reasons: analyzing previous studies to estimate the effect size more accurately, reducing uncertainty in sample size estimation by providing empirical evidence of the variability and distribution of the outcome variable, increasing the statistical power of study without necessarily increasing the sample size by incorporating historical data, and revealing trends in the outcome variable over time. This can lead to more precise estimates of sample size requirements compared to relying solely on theoretical assumptions.

Bayesian Methods

It is applied to sample size determination in research studies, as it is flexible and offers an alternative approach to traditional frequentist methods, which focus on estimating sample size based on fixed parameters, such as effect size, significance level, and power. Bayesian methods incorporate prior knowledge from studies about the parameters of interest into the analysis and updating of beliefs (Bayes' theorem) on the observed data to obtain posterior distributions of parameters of interest.

The implications of and problems associated with inadequate sample size have been summarized in **Table 14.1**, while the effect of bias on the determination of sample size has been tabulated in **Table 14.2**.

Table 14.1 Implications of inadequate sample size

Reduced Generalizability	Studies with small sample sizes may lack external validity or generalizability to the broader population. Findings from underpowered studies may not be representative of the whole population, limiting the applicability of the results to the real world.
Low Statistical Power	Inadequate sample size decreases the statistical power of a study, which is the probability of detecting a true effect when it exists. Studies with low power are less likely to identify true effects, leading to an increased risk of Type II errors (false negatives).
Increased Risk of Type I Errors	Inadequate sample size can inflate the risk of Type I errors (false positives), where a significant result is detected when there is no true effect. This occurs when multiple statistical tests are conducted without appropriate adjustment for multiple comparisons, increasing the likelihood of spurious findings.
Wrong Conclusions	Wider confidence intervals around impact estimates are the outcome of smaller sample sizes, which lowers the precision (deviation towards incorrect estimates or conclusions) of study findings. As a result, the projected effect size may be less trustworthy and not a real representation of the population.
Sampling Bias	Sampling bias occurs when the sample selected for a study does not represent the whole population from which it is drawn. This can lead to systematic errors in research findings and affect the validity and generalizability of study results. The types of sampling bias are selection bias, response bias, survivorship bias, and others. The risk can be minimized by employing random sampling methods (simple random sampling, stratified sampling, or cluster sampling), by ensuring adequate sample size and representation across relevant demographic or subgroup categories, or by transparent reporting of documentation (including sampling methods and participant characteristics).
Shrinkage	A reduction in the number of participants in a study after data collection due to various reasons. It can occur during the data cleaning and preparation process or as a result of attrition, dropout, or exclusion of participants. Implications of shrinkage are reduced statistical power, decreased precision, and limited generalizability.

(Continued)

Table 14.1 (Continued)

Inefficient Resource Allocation	Researchers invest resources (time, money, and participants) in conducting studies that should not yield non-meaningful results.
Publication Bias and Reproducibility Issues	Studies with small sample sizes are more likely to suffer from publication bias, where statistically significant results are more likely to be published than non-significant results. This can lead to an overestimation of effect sizes. Additionally, underpowered studies are less likely to be reproducible and reliable.
Ethical Considerations and Feasibility	Sometimes the practicality or ethical constraints might limit the sample size that can be obtained. Participants contribute their time and effort to research studies with the expectation that meaningful knowledge will be gained. Failing to achieve meaningful results due to inadequate sample size may be considered a misuse of participant resources.

Table 14.2 Effect of bias on determination of sample size

Sl.	Type of bias	Description	Effect on sample size
1	Selection Bias	Certain groups or individuals are systematically included or excluded from the sample Non-representative sample	Larger sample sizes required
2	Measurement Bias	Measurement methods used to collect data systematically over- or underestimate the true values of variables	Larger sample sizes required to account for increased uncertainty introduced by biased measurements, ensuring that the study has sufficient power to detect true effects
3	Response Bias	Participants provide inaccurate or misleading responses: social desirability bias, non-response bias, interviewer bias, or cognitive bias	Larger sample sizes required to offset the impact of biased responses
4	Publication Bias	Selective publication of studies based on the direction or significance of their findings Overrepresentation of statistically significant results or conclusions	Larger sample sizes required to ensure that the study has sufficient power

Conclusions

Sample size estimation is a fundamental aspect of research design, ensuring that studies produce robust and reliable results. One of the prevalent issues found in clinical trial reports is the absence of adequate justification for the chosen sample size. This concern underscores the possibility that significant therapeutic effects or the actual outcome might be overlooked due to the inclusion of insufficiently sized studies.

This chapter is expected to serve as valuable guidance for researchers to plan and execute high-quality research endeavours. Well-sized samples are crucial for confidently inferring that the estimated sample values accurately represent the underlying population parameters. Inadequately sized studies can lead to unrealistic assumptions about treatment efficacy, misjudgments of parameter variability, and failure to predict noncompliance or high dropout rates. Ethically and scientifically, it's crucial to understand minimum sample size requirements and employ appropriate sampling methods for robust results and resource conservation.

Discussion Questions

- Why is sample size determination crucial in biomedical research, and how does it impact study outcomes?
- How do factors like effect size, power, and significance level contribute to sample size calculations?
- What are the implications of underpowered or overpowered studies in clinical and public health research?
- In what ways can Type I and Type II errors affect the interpretation of research results?
- How can researchers balance ideal sample size requirements with practical limitations such as funding, time, and participant availability?

References

Charan, J. and Biswas, T., 2013. How to calculate sample size for different study designs in medical research?. *Indian Journal of Psychological Medicine*, 35(2), pp.121–126.

Kang, H., 2021. Sample size determination and power analysis using the G* Power software. *Journal of Educational Evaluation for Health Professions*, 18.

Suresh, K.P. and Chandrashekara, S., 2012. Sample size estimation and power analysis for clinical research studies. *Journal of Human Reproductive Sciences*, 5(1), pp.7–13.

PART V

Diagnostic Tests

## CHAPTER 15

Inter-Observer and Intra-Observer Reliability

Prativa Choudhury, Anjan Kumar Dhua and Prabudh Goel

Learning Outcomes

Learners will gain a comprehensive understanding of inter-observer and intra-observer reliability, crucial for ensuring measurement consistency in both research and clinical settings. They will learn how to assess reliability using statistical tools such as the intraclass correlation coefficient, Cohen's kappa, and Bland-Altman plots. The chapter also emphasizes the influence of observer expertise, measurement methods, and contextual factors on reliability. Students will explore strategies like protocol standardization, training, and calibration to reduce variability. By the end, learners will understand the distinction between variability and reliability and apply best practices to enhance data quality and study validity.

Background

Accuracy and reliability of the observations are paramount in research. The discrepancies and inconsistencies in observations of different observers (inter-observer variability) or multiple observations by the same observer at different times (intra-observer variability) may affect the study conclusions. Inter-observer and intra-observer reliability is a reflection of the quality of measurement data generated by the study and is indispensable for ensuring the integrity of results (see Table 15.1).

A good measurement possesses several key characteristics that ensure its reliability, validity, and usefulness.

Inter-observer and intra-observer variability are highly relevant in the context of all measurements: research, clinical, or otherwise. The relevance is exaggerated in the context of fields wherein the observations are vulnerable to human error or interpretation. The two measurements are related closely; together, they play a pivotal role all along the spectrum, extending from scientific research to clinical practice in enhancing the credibility of research findings, assessments, and decision-making processes.

DOI: 10.4324/9781032701004-20

Table 15.1 Essential characteristics of effective measurements

Sl.	Characteristic	Definition	Implications	Impact upon intra-observer variability	Impact upon inter-observer variability
1	Reliability	Consistency, dependability, and trustworthiness of the collected data to perform consistently over time or in different situations	1) Consistent measurements enhance reliability, validity, and generalizability. 2) Reduced observer variations improve confidence in research findings.	Yes High reliability, lower intra-observer variation	Yes High reliability, lower inter-observer variation
2	Reproducibility	Ability to obtain consistent and similar results when the same measurement procedure is repeated multiple times, by the same or different observers, under similar conditions	1) Supports reliable and trustworthy data. 2) Critical for scientific progress, decision-making, and improvement of knowledge.	Yes Lower reproducibility, higher intra-observer variation	Yes Lower reproducibility, higher inter-observer variation
3	Validity	The extent to which a measurement tool or instrument accurately assesses the construct or concept it intends to measure	Ensures meaningful and interpretable results that guide informed decision-making.	Yes Higher validity, low intra-observer variation	Yes Higher validity, low inter-observer variation
4	Accuracy	The degree of closeness between a measured value and the true or accepted value of the measured quantity	1) Ensures reliable data for decision-making. 2) Supports quality control and problem-solving.	Yes Higher accuracy, low intra-observer variation	Yes Higher accuracy, low inter-observer variation
5	Precision	Degree of consistency or agreement among various observers when taking measurements or making observations	Contributes to data reliability and validity. Indicates minimal fluctuation or disagreement.	Yes Higher precision, low intra-observer variation	Yes Higher precision, low inter-observer variation
6	Objectivity	Extent to which the measurement is free of subjective judgments, bias, or interpretation	Promotes reliability, validity, and integrity. Improves quality and trust in assessments.	Yes Higher objectivity, low intra-observer variation	Yes Higher objectivity, low inter-observer variation

Intra-Observer Reliability: Conceptual Framework

Intra-observer reliability (Miglior *et al.*, 2004) refers to the objective reflection of the consistency or repeatability of two or more measurements made by the same observer over time (**Figure 15.1**). The concept is grounded in the notion that reliable measurements should yield consistent or stable results when applied by the same observer under similar conditions.

When the same parameter is assessed repeatedly by the same observer, the degree of agreement between the readings is referred to as intra-observer reliability. It indicates the dependability and consistency of a single observer's judgments or ratings over time. The concept is a reflection of the robustness of the technique or the technology.

Closely linked to intra-observer reliability is intra-observer variability, which reflects the quantum of variation or fluctuation between two measurements recorded by the same observer.

Illustration: A paediatric urologist was trying to standardize the technique for measurement of stretched penile length in patients with a particular disease. He was concerned if the measurements taken by his technique were objective or subject to the variations in position of the examiner, fatigue, distractions, or other such factors. He took measurements in triplicate; one per day on three consecutive days. The mean difference between the three measurements is the intra-observer variability.

Intra-observer variation may arise due to some influencing factors, such as slight variations or fluctuations in the positioning of the ruler or measuring tape, differences in the

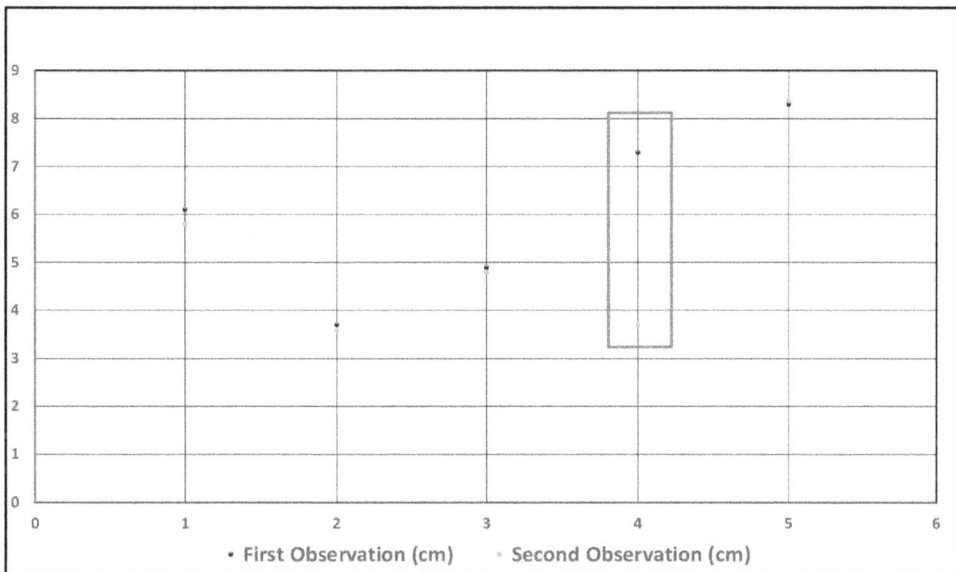

Figure 15.1 Graphical representation of intra-observer variation between two readings taken in five patients: the mathematical difference between the two readings (blue and orange dots, respectively) is minimum (0.1) in Patients 2, 3, and 5, and it is maximum (3.6) in Patient 4 (highlighted by the box).

level of penile arousal, patient comfort, environmental conditions (room temperature, setting of the room, or others), or maybe the variations in the level of tension applied during measurement.

Addressing intra-observer variability improves the reliability and accuracy of data in studies related to penile measurements.

Significance of Intra-Observer Reliability

- **Data Reliability:** Intra-observer variability influences the reliability of data collected in research studies. If the variability increases, the efficacy potentially influences the interpretation of outcomes. Consistency in measurements by the same observer is crucial for accurately assessing whether observed changes are due to treatment effects or variations in measurement techniques.
- **Clinical Applications:** Consistent measurements by healthcare professionals or clinicians are vital for accurate diagnosis, treatment planning, and monitoring of patients' conditions over time.
- **Longitudinal Studies:** For measuring the stability in longitudinal studies, tracking the changes over time and maintaining consistency in measurements by the same observer ensures accurate and reliable data for the analysis.
- **Data Reproducibility:** Minimizing the intra-observer variability is critical for ensuring the reproducibility, reliability, and accuracy.
- **Treatment Efficacy:** Intra-observer variations might affect the perceived effectiveness of treatment if measurements fluctuate due to inconsistencies in observation or measurement techniques.
- **Accuracy in Decision-Making:** Inaccurate or inconsistent data due to intra-observer variations can lead to flawed decision-making processes or guideline formulations.

Indices of Intra-Observer Reliability

The indices used to assess intra-observer variation are summarized in **Figure 15.1**.

- **Test-Retest Reliability:** The same test is administered to the same group of individuals more than once to assess the consistency and stability of the outcomes (Matheson, 2019).
- **Intraclass Correlation Coefficient (ICC):** This is a statistical reflection of the consistency of measurements (in this case: across repeated measurements by the same observer on the same patient). It is mostly applied to continuous data cases and the computation of quantitative measurements (Meesters *et al.,* 2020).
- **Coefficient of Variation (CV):** Calculates the ratio of the standard deviation to the mean of repeated measurements by the same observer. It reflects the relative variability of the dataset on either side of the mean (Reed *et al.,* 2002).
- **Pearson Correlation Coefficient:** Measures the strength and direction of the linear relationship between two continuous variables (Mukaka, 2012).
- **Bland-Altman Limits of Agreement (LOA):** Graphical and quantitative approach to estimate the level of agreement between two sets of continuous data. Often used with Bland-Altman plots (Gerke, 2020; Giavarina, 2015).

■ **Kendall's Coefficient of Concordance:** A statistical estimate of the degree of agreement between two sets of ordinal data (Gerylovová *et al.*, 1991).

Factors Can Influence Intra-Observer Reliability
That influences the reliability and agreement between the same observers when measuring or assessing the same phenomenon, such as the following:

■ **Observer characteristics:** Observer characteristics, such as experience, training, expertise, and cognitive biases, can impact the consistency of measurements.
■ **Measurement characteristics:** The characteristics for measurement (instruments or tools), such as complexity, ambiguity, and subjectivity, affect the reliability of measurement or interpretations.
■ **Contextual factors:** Factors such as environmental conditions and participant characteristics may also influence intra-observer reliability.
■ **Methodological factors:** To reduce variability and increase reliability, standardization of measuring protocols, blinding techniques, and quality control measures are essential fundamental components.

Inter-Observer Reliability: Conceptual Framework

Inter-observer or inter-rater reliability refers to the consistency or agreement between measurements pertaining to the same phenomenon or object taken by two or more observers under the same or similar conditions (see Table 15.2).

Inter-observer variability reflects the quantum of variation or fluctuation between two or more measurements recorded by multiple observers.

Illustration: In the illustration highlighted in the section earlier, the paediatric urologist assigned the task of measurement of stretched penile length to the four fellows in his team. The readings of the stretched penile length of the first patient visiting the clinic on a particular day were recorded as 5.7 cm, 5.2 cm, 5.2 cm, and 5.3 cm by the four fellows, respectively.

Despite following the same measurement protocol, variations in measurements are observed amongst multiple observers. Two fellows have made exactly the same measurement (5.2 cm); the observation of one fellow is close (5.3 cm) and that of the fourth one is distant (5.7 cm). This is an inter-observer variation.

Inter-observer variation may be ascribed to a multitude of factors, such as differences in technique, instrument calibration, and subjectivity in landmark identification.

Significance of Inter-Observer Reliability
■ **Quality Control and Assurance:** Recognizing the inter-observer variation is essential in maintaining consistent quality standards and ensuring product reliability.
■ **Research Validity and Reproducibility:** In scientific research, inter-observer reliability enhances and contributes to the validity and reproducibility of findings, ensuring that studies yield consistent results.

Table 15.2 Measure of indices for assessing the intra-observer and inter-observer reliability

Measure of indices	Description	Formula/Range	Interpretation	Methodology
Intra-observer reliability				
Test-Retest Reliability	Assesses the consistency of a measure when the same test is administered to the same participants on two occasions.	Depends on statistical method used (e.g., correlation coefficients: Pearson, ICC)	High values (closer to 1) indicate strong consistency between the repeated tests	Conduct identical tests on the same individuals twice
Intraclass Correlation Coefficient (ICC)	Measures how consistently different individuals or methods get the same results when measuring the same findings.	ICC = Variance between subjects/(Variance within subjects + Variance between subjects)	ICC < 0.5: Poor, 0.5–0.75: Moderate, 0.75–0.9: Good, > 0.9: Excellent	Collect measurements from same subjects by different observers or across different testing conditions
Coefficient of Variation (CV)	Measures spread/variability relative to the mean. Expressed as a percentage.	CV = (SD/Mean) × 100	Lower CV: less variability relative to mean; more consistent data	Calculate SD and mean, then express SD as a percentage of the mean
Pearson Correlation Coefficient	Measures the linear relationship between two continuous variables	Pearson formula	1: Perfect positive, –1: Perfect negative, 0: No linear relationship	Collect paired data points from continuous variables; compute Pearson correlation
Bland-Altman Limits of Agreement (LOA)	Statistical method to assess agreement between two measurement techniques	LOA = Mean Difference ± 1.96	A small mean difference and narrow limits suggest good agreement	Compare measurements from two methods for same subjects and plot difference against mean
Kendall's Coefficient of Concordance	Measures degree of agreement among raters using ranks	W = SS/(n(n²–1)/12)	0 to 1 (1 = perfect agreement)	Assemble rankings; assign ranks to items; compute W

Inter-observer reliability

	Description	Formula	Interpretation	Steps
Cohen's Kappa Coefficient	Measures agreement between two raters beyond chance (categorical data)	Kappa = (Observed Agreement – Expected Agreement)/(1 – Expected Agreement)	1: Perfect, 0: No agreement, < 0: Less than chance agreement	Compute observed (Po) and expected agreement (Pe), then calculate K
Fleiss' Kappa Coefficient	Extension of Cohen's Kappa to multiple raters	Same as earlier	Similar interpretation; higher values = better agreement	Determine rating proportions for each category and calculate agreement
Intraclass Correlation Coefficient (ICC)	Same formula and interpretation as for intra-observer reliability	ICC = Variance between subjects/(Variance within subjects + Variance between subjects)	Same: < 0.5: Poor, 0.5–0.75: Moderate, 0.75–0.9: Good, > 0.9: Excellent	Collect all ratings for all subjects and compute ICC (inter-observer version)
Percentage Agreement	% of times raters agree (simple but does not account for chance agreement)	% Agreement = (Number of Agreements/Total Ratings) × 100	80–100%: Strong, 60–79%: Moderate, < 60%: Poor	Count the number of times all observers agree; divide by total observations
Bland-Altman Plot	Graphical method to assess agreement between two continuous measurement methods	Mean Difference = Measurement 1 – Measurement 2	Mean difference should be close to 0 with narrow limits of agreement	Plot measurement differences vs. means; assess bias and limits

- **Diagnostic Consistency:** Understanding inter-observer variation is crucial for assessing the consistency of data collected by multiple observers. Consistent observations enhance data quality and trustworthiness in the measurement techniques.
- **Subjectivity:** Different observers may interpret the same event or data differently based on their subjective understanding, leading to variations in observations. Subjectivity introduced from individual biases, preconceptions, or prior experiences in inter-observer variation can impact the quality and reliability of data collected, and these differing subjective interpretations may lead to discrepancies in measurements.
- **Quality Improvement:** Improving inter-observer variation involves strategies to minimize differences among multiple observers when collecting data or making assessments. Enhancing consistency among observers is crucial for improving data quality.
- **Assessing Observer Agreement:** Inter-observer reliability helps to measure the level of agreement (LOA) among different observers. Understanding the extent of variation aids in evaluating the reliability of measurements.

Indices of Inter-Observer Reliability
The indices for assessing the inter-observer variations are represented in **Figure 15.2:**

- **Cohen's Kappa Coefficient:** Cohen's kappa is used to assess the inter-observer agreement for categorical (qualitative) items after correction for chance agreement (De Raadt *et al.*, 2019). The value of kappa ranges from –1 to +1; 0 represents an inter-observer agreement that is no greater than what would have been expected based on chance. A value of +1 represents perfect agreement between the observers (Al-Khawari *et al.*, 2010; Buntinx *et al.*, 1993).
- **Fleiss' Kappa:** It is an extension of the Fleiss kappa coefficient to accommodate more than two observers (Obuchowicz *et al.*, 2020).
- **Intraclass Correlation Coefficient (ICC):** Assesses the consistency and agreement between multiple observers for continuous data. It measures the proportion of total variance across observations that can be attributed to differences among observers (Koo *et al.*, 2016).
- **Percentage Agreement:** A straightforward technique that shows, for nominal or categorical data, the percentage of agreement or disagreement among multiple observers (Birkimer *et al.*, 1979).
- **Bland-Altman Plot:** Illustrates the agreement between two measures by plotting the difference between the measures against their mean. Aids in the visualization of disparities between observers.
- Inter-observer variability study results can be easier to grasp with graphical representation.

Factors Can Influence Inter-Observer Reliability
That influences the consistency and agreement between different observers when measuring or assessing the same phenomenon, such as the following:

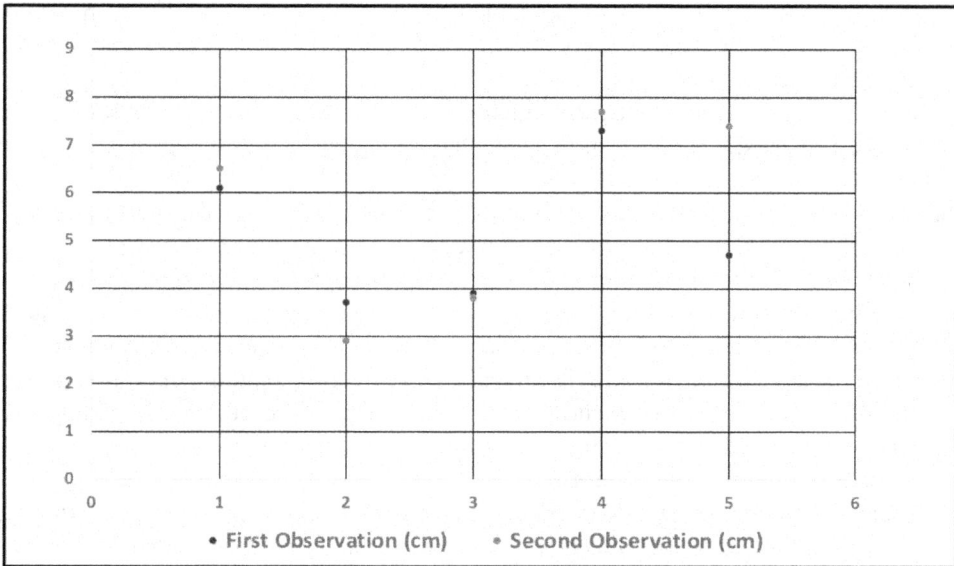

Figure 15.2 Graphical Illustration of Inter-observer variability varying from 0.1 cm (Patient 3) to 2.7 cm (Patient 5).

- **Observer Characteristics:** This component encompasses the characteristics or attributes of the observers involved, which may include factors such as the level of expertise, training, experience, cognitive biases, and personal interpretations.
- **Equipment and Technique:** Variability in design, functionality, and calibration of measurement devices or standardization of working protocol can affect the consistency and reliability of observations made by different observers.
- **Contextual Factors:** The environmental factors and characteristics of the subjects or stimuli being observed when the measurement is taken.
- **Communication and Consensus:** The extent to which observers communicate and collaborate to reach an agreement on their interpretations of measurements undertaken.

Addressing the Intra- and Inter-Observer Variability

These strategies play crucial roles in mitigating and managing the intra-observer and inter-observer variations:

- **Standardization of Protocols:** Clear and uniform protocols, measuring techniques, and evaluation standards ensure consistency and reduce ambiguity. The important aspects of the technique, such as key concepts, assessment criteria, and instructions for data recording, must be specified in detail.
- *Comprehensive training and education* of the observers to familiarize them with protocols, standards, and assessment methods.
- *Regular and periodic calibration sessions with* a reference standard to identify the discrepancies and to address them by optimizing their performance and ensuring accuracy or effectiveness.

- *Pilot studies before* full-scale implementation assist in the identifying potential issues, refining of study protocols, and enhancing observer consistency before actual data collection.
- **Blinding:** Information on concealment might cause bias among the observers. To reduce this bias, leading to more impartial and consistent observations, objective assessments need to be ensured.
- *Optimal utilization of measurement tools and technology* to reduce human-induced variations or errors and improve accuracy, employ standardized tools (digital instruments or software), and minimize subjective interpretation when appropriate.
- **Quality Control:** The quality control processes are implemented, and the measurement tools are calibrated regularly to ensure uniformity among the observers.
- **Continuous Monitoring and Feedback:** Implementing ongoing monitoring and feedback mechanisms to identify variations and provide necessary guidance to reinforce adherence to measurement protocols or correction to observers.
- **Statistical Analysis and Assessment:** Employ statistical methods, such as Cohen's kappa, intraclass correlation coefficient, or others, to assess, quantify, and analyze the variations. Observer agreement can also be measured independently to assess the reliability and validity of the observations.
- **Collaboration and Consensus-Building:** Encourage observers to work together to discuss observations, encourage candid dialogue, and come to an agreement on interpretations as a group to minimize variations and preserve consistency or uniformity
- **Ongoing Education, Training, and Improvement:** Encourage ongoing education and skill development among observers to stay updated with abreast of protocols, new developments, and best practices and to foster competency and consistency.
- **Documentation and Audit Trials:** Maintain comprehensive documentation of protocols, procedures, and observations, including the rationale behind the decisions. To optimize consistency, develop transparency, and evaluate and regularly review and refine these procedures.

Uncoupling of Reliability and Variability

It is easier to assume that efforts targeted towards reducing variability will lead to increased reliability. However, intra-observer reliability and intra-observer variability do not always go hand in hand. An understanding of the concept of 'uncoupling' is relevant to experimental design, data analysis, and interpretation of results.

For instance, an instrument designed to measure the stretched penile length may give consistent readings (minimal intra-observer and inter-observer variability). An erroneous calibration of the 'zero' point may introduce a systematic error across all measurements; despite low variability, reliability is jeopardized. Conversely, the study results may still be reliable despite high variability if appropriate statistical methods have been used to account for this inadequacy.

For instance, in a controlled experimental design, the researcher established a reliable association between the stretched penile length and serum level of testosterone during the formative years of life. However, this association may not be generalizable to the universal population due to variability introduced by the presence of additional underlying factors, such as genetic distancing, geography, and ethnicity.

Conclusion

Inter-observer and intra-observer reliability are critical considerations in research. The variations might have an impact on the reliability, validity, and accuracy of research findings.

It is possible to mitigate and manage such variations through systematic standardization of protocols, comprehensive training, utilization of technology, continuous monitoring, and performing statistical analyses. Strategies aimed at minimizing biases, fostering collaboration amongst observers, and promoting ongoing training and education contribute to enhancing the accuracy and reliability of data collected or assessments made by multiple observers.

Discussion Questions

- Why is it important to assess both inter- and intra-observer reliability in clinical and research measurements?
- How do statistical tools, like ICC, Cohen's kappa, and Bland-Altman plots, help quantify reliability?
- What are the common sources of measurement variability, and how can they be minimized?
- In what ways can training and protocol standardization improve measurement consistency?
- Finally, what does it mean to 'uncouple' reliability from variability, and why is this concept critical in interpreting study outcomes and maintaining data integrity?

References

Al-Khawari, H., Athyal, R.P., Al-Saeed, O., Sada, P.N., Al-Muthairi, S. and Al-Awadhi, A., 2010. Inter-and intraobserver variation between radiologists in the detection of abnormal parenchymal lung changes on high-resolution computed tomography. *Annals of Saudi Medicine, 30*(2), pp.129–133.

Birkimer, J.C. and Brown, J.H., 1979. Back to basics: Percentage agreement measures are adequate, but there are easier ways. *Journal of Applied Behavior Analysis, 12*(4), pp.535–543.

Buntinx, F., Schouten, H.J., AndréKnottnerus, J., Crebolder, H.F. and Essed, G.G., 1993. Interobserver variation in the assessment of the sampling quality of cervical smears. *Journal of Clinical Epidemiology, 46*(4), pp.367–370.

De Raadt, A., Warrens, M.J., Bosker, R.J. and Kiers, H.A., 2019. Kappa coefficients for missing data. *Educational and Psychological Measurement, 79*(3), pp.558–576.

Gerke, O., 2020. Reporting standards for a Bland–Altman agreement analysis: A review of methodological reviews. *Diagnostics, 10*(5), p.334.

Gerylovová, A. and Holčík, J., 1991. Use of nonparametric methods in medicine. VII. Kendall's coefficient of concordance in several sequences. *Vnitrni Lekarstvi, 37*(2), pp.186–191.

Giavarina, D., 2015. Understanding bland altman analysis. *Biochemia Medica, 25*(2), pp.141–151.

Koo, T.K. and Li, M.Y., 2016. A guideline of selecting and reporting intraclass correlation coefficients for reliability research. *Journal of Chiropractic Medicine, 15*(2), pp.155–163.

Matheson, G.J., 2019. We need to talk about reliability: Making better use of test-retest studies for study design and interpretation. *PeerJ, 7*, p.e6918.

Meesters, A.M., Ten Duis, K., Banierink, H., Stirler, V.M., Wouters, P.C., Kraeima, J., de Vries, J.P.P., Witjes, M.J. and IJpma, F.F., 2020. What are the interobserver and intraobserver variability of gap and stepoff measurements in acetabular fractures. *Clinical Orthopaedics and Related Research®*, 478(12), pp.2801–2808.

Miglior, S., Albe, E., Guareschi, M., Mandelli, G., Gomarasca, S. and Orzalesi, N., 2004. Intraobserver and interobserver reproducibility in the evaluation of ultrasonic pachymetry measurements of central corneal thickness. *British Journal of Ophthalmology*, 88(2), pp.174–177.

Mukaka, M.M., 2012. A guide to appropriate use of correlation coefficient in medical research. *Malawi Medical Journal*, 24(3), pp.69–71.

Obuchowicz, R., Oszust, M. and Piorkowski, A., 2020. Interobserver variability in quality assessment of magnetic resonance images. *BMC Medical Imaging*, 20, pp.1–10.

Reed, G.F., Lynn, F. and Meade, B.D., 2002. Use of coefficient of variation in assessing variability of quantitative assays. *Clinical and Vaccine Immunology*, 9(6), pp.1235–1239.

A Biostatistical Evaluation of Diabetes Medication Based on HbA1c and Glucose Levels Among US Adults

Vivek Verma, Masuma Khanam,
Gagan Gunjan and Divya Jain

Learning Outcomes

By the end of this chapter, readers will understand the relationship between HbA1c and glucose measurements in diagnosing and classifying diabetes and how these factors impact clinical decision-making. They will be able to apply biostatistical techniques, including descriptive statistics, correlation analysis, and classification methods (TP, FP, FN, TN), to interpret health data. The study will also help in understanding the importance of medication in diabetes diagnosis and classification, providing a deeper insight into potential misdiagnoses in both medicated and non-medicated groups.

Introduction

Diabetes is a metabolic condition with several root factors. Chronic and recurring hyperglycemia as well as abnormalities in the metabolism of carbohydrates, fats, and proteins brought on by deficiencies in insulin production, insulin action, or both are its defining characteristics (Holt *et al.* 2017). A few fatty and amino acids, in addition to glucose, also control the release of insulin. Because it is the main dietary replacement and may accumulate right away after diet administration, glucose is the main factor that stimulates the release of insulin (Chakrabarti *et al.* 2020).

According to World Health Organization (WHO), an estimated number of diabetes in the world in year 2014 was more than 400 million, which raised from 108 million in 1980. Since 1980, the global era standardization of diabetes has approximately doubled ascent from a percentage of 4.7 to 8.5 in the adult population. As diabetes can affect almost every organ system in the body leading to various serious complications, it therefore became a single cause for an additional 2.2 million deaths worldwide (WHO, 2016).

Diabetes mellitus is classified into two types, viz., Type 1 and Type 2, where Type 1 is caused by an autoimmune disorder and Type 2 is mainly due to lifestyle change. In a Type 1 diabetes situation, one has to mostly dependent on insulin (Centers for Disease Control and Prevention, 2019), and its occurrence is linked to environmental variables and exposure to certain viral infections or disorders (WHO, 2019). In the case of Type 2 diabetes, the body generates insulin resistance, where the body does not completely respond to insulin, and its occurrence is linked with family history and change in lifestyle conditions, such as ageing, overweight, eating poorly, not exercising, hypertension, impaired glucose tolerance (IGT), etc. Diabetic retinopathy is a well-known ocular complication of diabetes mellitus. The annual incidence of diabetic retinopathy ranges from 2.2% to 12.7% (Sabanayagam et al., 2018). It can present with signs of retinal ischemia and/or signs of increased retinal vascular permeability on evaluation (Eye disease prevalence research group, 2004).

Diabetes is the seventh (Centers for Disease Controland Prevention, 2019) most common cause of mortality in the United States of America (USA), with an average loss of 4.6 years of life among adults with diabetes. Out of the total diabetes cases in 2018, 34.2 million persons (diagnosed or undiagnosed) were from USA, which was 13% of the total USA adult population. Among them, 7.3 million had diabetes but were unaware.

The common test used to diagnose diabetes in an individual includes fasting plasma glucose (FPG), postprandial blood glucose, and hemoglobin A1c (HbA1C). According to American Diabetes Association, FPG < 100 mg/dl is considered normal, 100–125 mg/dl as prediabetes, and ≥ 126 mg/dl as diabetes (Engelgau et al. 1997). The HbA1c test yields the blood glucose average over the previous three months. HbA1C levels less than 5.7% are considered as normal, 5.7%–6.4% as prediabetes, and more than or equal to 6.5% as diabetes.

It has been assumed that the improvement in diabetes status either due to medication or non-medication among diabetic patients can be assessed by FPG and HbA1c levels. If the individual with diabetes is under medication (not in control), then it acts as a risk factor for a number of illnesses. As per the existing literature, patients with diabetes are more susceptible to death in some diseases, such as stroke (Shou et al. 2015), kidney disease (Molitch et al. 2015), vision disorder (Klein et al.1995), heart attack (Lundberg et al. 1997), dementia (Cheng et al. 2012), COVID-19 (Guo et al. 2020), etc., compared to non-diabetic patients. When assessing for and diagnosing diabetes, HbA1c should be used properly and in combination with standard glucose measurements (William et al. 2012). If diabetes is misdiagnosed then due to over-medication, the patient will develop other diseases, which will also lead to death. Overdose of insulin, metformin (Cusi et al. 1998), sulfonylureas (Harrigan et al. 2001), thiazolidinediones (Hussein et al. 2004), etc., medicines have different harmful impacts on the human body (Spiller, 1998).

Methodology
Prior to empirical model building, we applied descriptive statistics to summarize key features of the dataset and correlation analysis to explore the linear relationship between HbA1c and fasting blood sugar (FPG). Additionally, we utilized both categorical and continuous bivariate measures to assess the joint relation of HbA1c and glucose levels. These statistical tools serve practical purposes by providing insights into the

underlying data structure, ensuring the accuracy of the classification model for diabetes diagnosis and prediction.

Data: In the present study, the database of the Centre for Disease Control (CDC) conducted by the National Health and Nutrition Examination Survey (NHANES) has been used. NHANES database has been used for assessment as well as evaluation of the health and nutritional qualities of the non-institutionalized population in the United States. NHANES program was initiated to obtain information on various clinical and non-clinical health and nutritional related parameters in the United States. Here, NHANESs conducted from 2005 to 2018 have been considered, in which a total of 70,190 individuals participated, out of which 67,203 completed the interview (see Figure 16.1).

Study Population: Participants aged less than and equal to 35 ($n = 38,248$), and information on measurements of Hba1c or FPG levels were missing ($n = 28,153$), have been excluded. There were only 802 participants found eligible, and their complete information about Hba1c and glucose measurement is available.

Method: Let X_i and Y_i denote the measurement of FPG and HbA1C level, respectively, of ith individual, for all $i = 1, 2, \ldots, n$, where n denotes the total number of individuals surveyed. Here, both univariate and bivariate exploration have been made to characterize under both categorical and continuous measurements of HbA1C and FPG. Even though the methods of measuring glucose levels in the body using HbA1C and FPG are different, both are measuring the same parameters; therefore, we have assumed that they are linearly related and have a correlation denoted as 'r'. For the categorical analysis, sensitivity and specificity were used for measure of bivariate classification, where diagnostic result (FBG) vs. actual truth (HbA1C) can be assessed by the following:

i. When the diagnostic test result is positive:
    - If the actual condition is positive, the outcome is a true positive (TP_i).
    - If the actual condition is negative, the outcome is a false positive (FP_i).
ii. When the diagnostic test result is negative:
    - If the actual condition is positive, the outcome is a false negative (FN_i).
    - If the actual condition is negative, the outcome is a true negative (TN_i).
    The total number of test-positive individuals is denoted as a (i.e., $TP_i + FN_i$).
    The total number of test-negative individuals is denoted as b (i.e., $FP_i + TN_i$).

Results

The results presented in **Table 16.1** show that the prevalence of diabetes among males (51.7%) is comparatively higher than among females. As per the self-reported history of diabetes medication, no statistically significant differences have been observed based on gender and age. The mean age of the population is 62.6 ± 12 under both diabetes groups who were on medication or not. Most of the diabetes population (65.02%) belongs to the older age group (> 55 years). Out of them, 72.9% are on diabetes medication, which is close to those who are not on medication. According to race/ethnicity, most individuals (49.4%) taking diabetic medication belonged to the non-Hispanic

Table 16.1 Demographical and clinical distribution of participants based on diabetes medication status

Variable		Total (n = 802)	Diabetes		p-value
			Non-medicated (52.9%) n(%)	Medicated (47.1%) n(%)	
Gender	Male	412	220 (51.8%)	192 (50.8%)	0.76
	Female	390	204 (48.1%)	186 (49.2%)	
Age (Mean ± SD)		802	62.6 ± 11.7	62.8 ± 11.6	0.89
Age	36 to 55	220	115 (27.1%)	105 (27.7%)	0.84
	> 55	582	309 (72.9%)	273 (72.2%)	
Race	Mexican American	82	45 (10.6%)	37 (9.8%)	0.007
	Hispanic	71	33 (7.9%)	38 (10%)	
	non-Hispanic white	374	187 (44.1%)	187 (49.4%)	
	non-Hispanic black	168	85 (20%)	83 (21.1%)	
	non-Hispanic multiracial	107	74 (17.4%)	33 (8.7%)	
Education Level	< 9th grade	62	32 (7.5%)	30 (7.9%)	0.0002
	9th–12th grade (with no diploma)	88	33 (7.7%)	55 (14.5%)	
	High school grad	191	85 (20%)	106 (28%)	
	College degree	263	152 (35.8%)	111 (29.3%)	
	College graduate or above	198	122 (28.7%)	76 (20.1%)	
Marital Status	Married	502	266 (62.7%)	236 (62.4%)	0.74
	Widowed	91	42 (9.9%)	49 (12.9%)	
	Divorced	101	56 (13.2%)	45 (11.9%)	
	Separated	23	12 (2.8%)	11 (2.9%)	
	Ne'er married	58	34 (8%)	24 (6.3%)	
	Living with partner	27	14 (3.3%)	13 (3.4%)	
Taking	Insulin	297	0 (0.0%)	297 (78.5%)	<.0001

		n			p
Taking	Diabetic pills	109	0 (0.0%)	109 (80.1%)	< .0001
Consulted	Yes	676	344 (81.1%)	332 (87.8%)	0.0093
Diabetic Classification	Normal	108	78 (18.4%)	30 (7.9%)	< .0001
Based on	Glucose	137	80 (18.8%)	57 (15%)	
	HbA1C	137	61 (14.3%)	76 (20.1%)	
	Glucose-HbA1C	420	205 (48.3%)	215 (56.8%)	
Age of diabetes declared (Mean ± SD)		802	52.3 ± 12.7	45.9 ± 14.2	< .0001
Fasting glucose (mg/dL) (Mean ± SD)		802	156.1 ± 57.2	170.9 ± 73.1	0.0014
HbA1C (Mean ± SD)		802	7.02 ± 2.1	7.8 ± 2.08	< .0001

white group. Among non-medicated diabetes patients, 64.5% have a college degree and higher educational qualification, while 49.4% of those on diabetes medication have the same level of education. 62.7% of married individuals belong to the group of those who are not taking medicine for diabetes. Among the total population, 37% of individuals are taking insulin, and 13.6% of individuals are taking diabetic pills. Among those who were taking medicine, 78.5% are taking insulin and 80.1% are taking diabetic pills. As per the diabetic medication, 87.8% of those who are taking medicine have shown only a specific doctor. Based on the measurement, the diabetes status has been classified, which shows that out of the total population, only 13.4% found diabetes was under control (normal), 52.3% of individuals having both FPG and HbA1C measurements high, and in the remaining, either of FPG or HbA1C levels are elevated from the normal range. Among the medicated group, 7.9% are normal, whereas it is twice among the non-medicated group. And even after medication, 56.8% was having both glucose and HbA1C measurement high, whereas among the non-medicated group, it was 48.3%. The mean age of diabetes declared among the non-medicated group is 52.3 ± 12.7 and for those who are taking medicine is 45.9 ± 14.2. Statistically significant different and higher FPG (mg/dL) and HbA1c levels have been found among the medicated group (170.9 ± 73 and 7.8 ± 2.08, respectively) than non-medicated group (156.1 ± 57.2 and 7.02 ± 2.1, respectively).

Table 16.2 presented the descriptive measurements of FPG and HbA1C and their correlation and compared the differences among diabetes-medicated and non-medicated subgroups under different diabetes classification classes. Under the true negative class, clinically considered as normal or under control, the mean FPG and HbA1C levels across the medicated and non-medicated groups are statistically close, but their correlation is higher among the medicated group. Among the true positive class, where both glucose and HbA1C level are above the normal limits, they are significantly higher among and correlated in the medicated group [glucose 206.9 ± 69.5; HbA1c 8.53 ± 1.94] as compared to the non-medicated group [glucose 184.9 ± 59.96; HbA1c 7.83 ± 2.57].

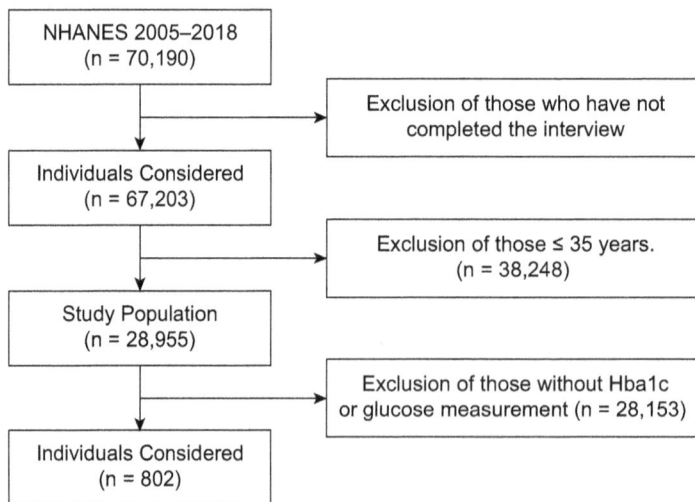

Figure 16.1 Procedure of sampling from the NHANES 2005–2018.

Table 16.2 Classical evaluation of diabetes medication differences in the association of glucose and HbA1c measurement among patients with diabetes

Diabetes classification			Diabetes medication					
			Medicated (n = 378; 47.1%)		*Non-medicated (n = 424; 52.9%)*			*p-value*
Classification	*Status*	*Measurement*	*Mean ± SD*	*Correlation*	*Mean ± SD*	*Correlation*		
True Negative	Normal (13.4%)	Glucose	102.7 ± 16.5	0.46	106.5 ± 13.5	0.08		0.26
		HbA1C	5.6 ± 0.9		5.7 ± 0.6			0.47
True Positive	Glucose and HbA1C (52.3%)	Glucose	206.9 ± 69.5	0.37	184.9 ± 59.96	0.18		0.0006
		HbA1C	8.53 ± 1.94		7.83 ± 2.57			0.002
False Negative	HbA1C (17.0%)	Glucose	99.76 ± 20.8	−0.109	111.4 ± 10.62	0.07		<.0001
		HbA1C	7.90 ± 1.67		7.42 ± 1.42			0.09
False Positive	Glucose (17.9%)	Glucose	165.9 ± 49.48	−0.507	164.9 ± 41.96	0.07		0.90
		HbA1C	5.58 ± 0.86		5.90 ± 0.39			0.008

In the false positive class (only glucose level is above the normal limit), statistically, no significant difference was observed among medicated [glucose 165.9 ± 49.48] and non-medicated [glucose 164.9 ± 41.96] groups, but a significant difference has been found in HbA1C levels. In the false negative class (only HbA1C level is above the normal limit), a statistically significant difference was observed among medicated [glucose 99.76 ± 20.8; HbA1c 7.90 ± 1.67] and non-medicated [glucose 111.4 ± 10.62; HbA1c 7.42 ± 1.42] groups, with a significant difference found in HbA1c levels. Furthermore, the normality has been checked by using the Kolmogorov-Smirnov test (P > 0.05), which says both FPG and HbA1C follow univariate normal distribution for different diabetes classifications. Here, the Statistical Analysis Software University Edition (SAS) and R version 4.1.2 have been used for data extraction and computational purposes.

Discussion

Literature on the impact of diabetes and its related diagnosis has been well explored. In the diagnosis plan and follow-up, the pathological tests FPG and HbA1c tests play a significant role. The daily change in glucose level is usually monitored by glucose measurement, which may be affected by various factors, like stress, anxiety, sleep, etc. Therefore, the HbA1c measurement has been considered comparatively more reliable for accessing the diabetes level as well as the impact of medication and/or daily life intervention (non-medicated). Medication and non-medication are two broader classes in diabetes diagnosis, but the purpose is to control the glucose level in two different ways. In the medicated group, any drug or insulin is prescribed to a diabetic patient along with their daily life routine changes, whereas in the non-medicated group, only daily life routine changes are recommended. In order to do so, proper and regular monitoring of FPG and HbA1c levels are very necessary. In the present study, we have considered the adults above 35, including the elderly population of the United States of America, and tried to measure the impact, association, and classification of diabetes patients based on Hba1c (normal < 6.5%) and FPG (normal < 126 mg/dL). In comparison to the diabetes-medicated (47.1%) group, non-medicated patients are more prevalent (52.9%) but are statistically similar in figure terms of their gender, age composition, and marital status. The majority of diabetes-medicated or non-medicated patients belong to either non-Hispanic white or non-Hispanic black and have a college degree and higher qualifications.

Among the diabetes-medicated group, patients who are taking pills or insulin are almost the same, and as compared to the non-medicated group, they preferred to consult a specialized doctor for treatment. The age of getting aware of their diabetes is earlier among the medicated group than non-medicated. It is interesting to note that the patients on medication have reported higher mean FPG and HbA1c levels than the non-medicated group. In classifying the diabetes patients based on their FPG and HbA1c levels, we have found that as compared to medicated patients, more than twice have normal FPG and HbA1c levels (TN) in non-medicated patients. Among those having FPG and HbA1c levels above the normal range (TP), the non-medicated group is comparatively less than the medicated group. Higher FPG level (FP), even with normal HbA1c level, is mostly reported in the non-medicated group than medicated. On the other hand, a higher HbA1c level (FN), even with normal FPG level, is mostly reported in the medicated group than non-medicated. In the situation of TP and FN, the medicated group needs more attention to their doses of medication, and non-medicated therapy should be started. For the FN situation, precaution is required, and a decision should be made based on the HbA1c level.

Conclusion

Demographically, no differences were observed among medicated and non-medicated groups based on their characteristics, like gender, age, race, and marital status. But in of terms clinical characteristics of diabetic patients – viz., medication types (pills or insulin), and diabetes classification based on measurements, FPG, and HbA1c levels – significant differences have been found between medicated and non-medicated groups. The study clearly suggests that even after medication, it is virtual to believe about the efficacy of drugs because in the non-medicated group, more people are normal (TN), fewer have diabetes levels above normal limit (TP), have only HbA1c above normal (FN), and augmentation has been observed in the diabetes-medicated group. A significant percentage of individuals having only high FPG levels (FP) is of serious concern in both ed and non-medicated groups, as they may be wrongly diagnosed as uncontrolled diabetic patients.

> ## Discussion Questions
>
> - How do HbA1c and glucose measurements complement each other in diagnosing diabetes?
> - What are the potential consequences of misclassifying diabetes patients as TP, FP, FN, or TN?
> - How does medication influence the accuracy of diabetes classification based on glucose and HbA1c levels?
> - Why is it important to consider both medicated and non-medicated groups in diabetes research?

References

Centers for Disease Controland Prevention. (2019). *Diabetes Report Card 2019*. Retrieved from Centers for Disease Control and Prevention: https://www.cdc.gov/diabetes/library/reports/reportcard.html.

Chakrabarti, S., & Ghosh, S. (2020). Physiology of insulin secretion. *RSSDI's Insulin Monograph: A Complete Guide to Insulin Therapy*, 11.

Cheng, G., Huang, C., Deng, H., & Wang, H. (2012). Diabetes as a risk factor for dementia and mild cognitive impairment: A meta-analysis of longitudinal studies. *Internal Medicine Journal*, 42(5), 484–491.

Cusi, K., & DeFronzo, R. A. (1998). Metformin: A review of its metabolic effects. *Diabetes Reviews*, 6(2), 89–131.

Engelgau, M. M., Thompson, T. J., Herman, W. H., Boyle, J. P., Aubert, R. E., Kenny, S. J., . . . & Ali, M. A. (1997). Comparison of fasting and 2-hour glucose and HbA1c levels for diagnosing diabetes: Diagnostic criteria and performance revisited. *Diabetes Care*, 20(5), 785–791.

The Eye Diseases Prevalence Research Group*. (2004). The prevalence of diabetic retinopathy among adults in the United States. *Archives of Ophthalmology*, 122(4), 552–563. https://10.1001/archopht.122.4.552.

Guo, W., Li, M., Dong, Y., Zhou, H., Zhang, Z., Tian, C., . . . & Hu, D. (2020). Diabetes is a risk factor for the progression and prognosis of COVID-19. *Diabetes/Metabolism Research and Reviews*, 36(7), e3319.

Harrigan, R. A., Nathan, M. S., & Beattie, P. (2001). Oral agents for the treatment of type-2 diabetes mellitus: Pharmacology, toxicity, and treatment. *Annals of Emergency Medicine*, 38(1), 68–78.

Herman, W. H., & Cohen, R. M. (2012, 1 April). Racial and ethnic differences in the relationship between HbA1c and blood glucose: Implications for the diagnosis of diabetes. *The Journal of Clinical Endocrinology & Metabolism*, 97(4), 1067–1072. https://doi.org/10.1210/jc.2011-1894.

Holt, R. I., Cockram, C., Flyvbjerg, A., & Goldstein, B. J. (Eds.). (2017). *Textbook of diabetes*. John Wiley & Sons.

Hussein, Z., Wentworth, J. M., Nankervis, A. J., Proietto, J., & Colman, P. G. (2004). Effectiveness and side effects of thiazolidinediones for type-2 diabetes: Real life experience from a tertiary hospital. *Medical Journal of Australia*, 181(10), 536–539.

Klein, R., & Klein, B. E. (1995). Vision disorders in diabetes. *Diabetes in America*, 1, 293.

Lundberg, V., Stegmayr, B., Asplund, K., Eliasson, M., & Huhtasaari, F. (1997). Diabetes as a risk factor for myocardial infarction: Population and gender perspectives. *Journal of Internal Medicine*, 241(6), 485–492.

Molitch, M. E., Adler, A. I., Flyvbjerg, A., Nelson, R. G., So, W. Y., Wanner, C., . . . & Mogensen, C. E. (2015). Diabetic kidney disease: A clinical update from Kidney Disease: Improving Global Outcomes. *Kidney International*, 87(1), 20–30.

Sabanayagam, C., Banu, R., Chee, M. L., Lee, R., Wang, Y. X., Tan, G., . . . & Wong, T. Y. (2018). Incidence and progression of diabetic retinopathy: A systematic review. *The Lancet Diabetes & Endocrinology*. https://doi.org/10.1016/s2213-8587(18)30128-1.

Shou, J., Zhou, L., Zhu, S., & Zhang, X. (2015). Diabetes is an independent risk factor for stroke recurrence in stroke patients: A meta-analysis. *Journal of Stroke and Cerebrovascular Diseases*, 24(9), 1961–1968.

Spiller, H. A. (1998). Management of antidiabetic medications in overdose. *Drug Safety*, 19(5), 411–424.

World Health Organization, (2016). *Global report on diabetes: executive summary*. In Global report on diabetes: executive summary.

World Health Organization. (2019). *Classification of Diabetes Mellitus*. WHO.

PART VI

Bayesian Methods and Machine Learning

Applying Bayesian Methods in Diagnostics Tests for Clinical Decision-Making

*Vivek Verma, Prabudh Goel,
Dilip C. Nath, and Hafiz T.A. Khan*

Learning Outcomes

Learners will understand the practical application of Bayes' rule in clinical diagnosis, particularly the transition from pre-test to post-test probability. They will grasp how diagnostic decisions are based on probability rather than certainty and how test sensitivity, specificity, and disease prevalence affect diagnostic accuracy. The chapter will help learners calculate and interpret predictive values, enhancing diagnostic reasoning. By mastering Bayes' rule, students will be equipped to make more informed clinical decisions, evaluate diagnostic test utility, and appreciate the probabilistic nature of medical diagnosis in everyday clinical practice.

Introduction

Clinical practice diagnostics are rife with uncertainty since they are reliant on probabilities (Matthews, 2020; Mengel et al, 2007). When a diagnosis is being made, the likelihood of the condition of interest is continuously changing, upward or downward, based on the particular data gathered. The information from the results is crucial for making a specific medical diagnosis one or more examinations for diagnosis (Sox et al, 2024). Diagnose or rule out the existence of a disease with a high enough degree of confidence is the primary goal of diagnostic testing (Swets, 1988).

In general, the more accurate the diagnostic test, the more certain the resultant diagnosis will be. Two common characteristics of high-quality diagnostic tests are their sensitivity and specificity. The likelihood of a profoundly good outcome in an individual with the condition is referred to as sensitivity, while the likelihood of a truly negative outcome in an individual without the disease is referred to as specificity. But in fact, it is evident that the disease is unknown at the time of testing; if it were known, there would be no reason to perform the test (Wilson and Jungner, 1968). Rather, the chance that the disease is present or missing should be estimated based on the predictive value of a positive or negative test result.

One of the main objectives of diagnostic testing is to determine the posterior probability, or probability of disease based on test results, as opposed to the prior probability, or chance of disease before the diagnostic test (Gelman and Carpenter, 2020; Bours, 2021). It is exceedingly challenging to objectify these changes in probability within the context of the diagnostic reasoning that physicians use to increase their level of confidence in a diagnosis. When they fail to sufficiently account for the previous probability of sickness, doctors frequently tend to overestimate the predictive value of a diagnostic test result (Morgan et al, 2021; Whiting et al, 2015). Here is when a well-known statistical theorem comes in handy: the Bayesian rule (Bours, 2021). Quantifying the diagnostic procedure of converting a priori probabilities into posterior probabilities is one application of Bayes' rule (Herrle et al, 2011; Joseph et al, 1995).

Applying Bayesian methods to diagnose decisions involves incorporating prior knowledge or beliefs about a situation, updating these beliefs with new evidence (data), and then making decisions based on the updated beliefs. In medical diagnosis, Bayesian methods can be particularly useful because they allow for the integration of prior knowledge, such as the prevalence of a disease in a population, with diagnostic test results to estimate the probability of a patient having the disease.

Bayes' Theorem of Conditional Probability

Reviewing marginal, joint, and conditional probability is necessary before delving into the Bayes' theorem.

Joint Probability: This refers to the probability of two or more events happening simultaneously. For example, the joint probability of event A and event B occurring together is denoted as $P(A\,and\,B)$.

Marginal Probability: This refers to the probability of a single event occurring irrespective of the occurrence of other events. It is obtained by summing (or integrating, in the case of continuous variables) the joint probabilities over all values of the other events. For instance, if we have events A and B, the marginal probability of A is denoted as $P(A)$ and is calculated as the sum of all joint probabilities where A occurs, regardless of the outcome of B.

Conditional probability: This refers to the probability of an event occurring given that another event has already occurred. It is denoted by $P(A\,|\,B)$, which reads as "the probability of event A given event B." The formula for conditional probability is as follows:

$$P(AB) = \frac{P(A\,and\,B)}{P(B)} \tag{1}$$

where:
- $P(A\,|\,B)$ is the conditional probability of A given B.

- $P(A \, and \, B)$ is the joint probability of A and B occurring together.
- $P(B)$ is the probability of event B occurring.

This formula says that the probability of A occurring given that B has occurred is equal to the probability of both A and B occurring together, divided by the probability of B occurring.

It is important to note that conditional probability can be interpreted as a new probability distribution that reflects the updated probabilities of events based on added information (i.e., the occurrence of event B).

Marginal probabilities are fundamental in probability theory and are often used in Bayesian statistics, hypothesis testing, and other statistical analyses. They provide insight into the likelihood of individual events occurring, regardless of the occurrence of other events. Conditional probability is particularly important in Bayesian statistics, where it forms the basis of updating prior beliefs with new evidence. Additionally, conditional probability is fundamental to understanding concepts like independence and dependence between random variables.

Bayes' Theorem in Diagnostic Tests

Bayes' rule, also known as Baye' theorem or Bayes' law, is indeed fundamental in understanding the probabilistic aspect of diagnostic reasoning. It provides a way to update the probability of a hypothesis considering new evidence. The theorem is mathematically expressed as follows:

$$P(AB) = P(BA) \times \frac{P(A)}{P(B)} \qquad (2)$$

where:

- $P(A \mid B)$ – probability of hypothesis A being true given the observed evidence B.
- $P(B \mid A)$ – probability of observing evidence B given that hypothesis A is true.
- $P(A)$ – prior probability of hypothesis A being true before considering the evidence.
- $P(B)$ – prior probability of observing evidence B before considering any hypotheses.

Bayes' rule tells us how to revise our beliefs about the probability of a hypothesis given new evidence. This is crucial in diagnostic reasoning, where we often need to update our beliefs about the likelihood of a disease or condition being present based on observed symptoms or test results.

For example, in medical diagnosis, Bayes' rule can help calculate the probability of a patient having a certain disease, diabetes, given their symptoms and test results, say fasting glucose reading, considering both the prior probability of the disease in the population and the accuracy of the tests. It allows for a more nuanced and probabilistic approach to diagnostic reasoning, incorporating both prior knowledge and new evidence.

The relationship between the probabilities that govern the diagnostic process is expressed by this equation (2), which demonstrates that the test's characteristics and the prior probability are the primary factors that determine the posterior probability of disease. The vocabulary used to describe Bayes' rule in diagnostic testing frequently includes posterior probabilities (predictive values), sensitivity (S_n), specificity (S_p), and prior probabilities (prev), which are frequently referred to as prevalence (*Prev*).

Absolutely, in the context of diagnostic testing, Bayes' rule is often used to calculate posterior probabilities, also known as predictive values, based on prior probabilities, sensitivity, and specificity of the test.

Here, we break down the terms for understanding:

- **Prior Probability (prev)**: This is the probability of the disease or condition being present in the population before any diagnostic test is performed. It represents our initial belief about the likelihood of the disease.
- **Sensitivity (S_n)**: This is the probability that the test correctly identifies individuals with the disease, i.e., the probability of a positive test result given that the individual has the disease.
- **Specificity (S_p)**: This is the probability that the test correctly identifies individuals without the disease, i.e., the probability of a negative test result given that the individual does not have the disease.

Given these terms, Bayes' rule of equation (2) can be expressed in the context of diagnostic testing as follows:

$$P(Disease\,Positive\,Test) = P(Positive\,Test\,Disease) \times \frac{P(Disease)}{P(Positive\,Test)}$$

where:
- $P(Disease \mid Positive\,Test)$ is the posterior probability of the disease given a positive test result (predictive value positive).
- $P(Positive\,Test \mid Disease)$ is the sensitivity of the test.
- $P(Disease)$ is the prior probability of the disease.
- $P(Positive\,Test)$ is the overall probability of obtaining a positive test result, calculated as follows:

$$P(Positive\,Test) = P(Positive\,Test\,Disease) \times P(Disease)$$

$$+ P(Positive\,Test\,No\,Disease) \times P(No\,Disease) \qquad (3)$$

where:
$$P(Positive\,Test\,No\,Disease) = 1 - Specificity \qquad (4)$$

$$P(No\,Disease) = 1 - P(Disease) \qquad (5)$$

Similarly, we can calculate the posterior probability of not having the disease given a negative and resulted to the following:

$$P(Positive\,Test\,Disease) = Sensitivity \qquad (6)$$

Bayes' as Statistical Metric for Classification

Positive Predictive Value (PPV): It is a statistical metric used in binary classification tasks, such as medical testing or machine learning models. It represents the proportion of true positive predictions (correctly predicted positive cases) out of all positive predictions made by the model. Mathematically, PPV is calculated as follows:

$$PPV = \frac{True\,Positives}{True\,Positives + False\,Positives}$$

In medical testing, for example, if a test for a disease is positive for 90 patients and 80 of those patients have the disease while 20 do not, the PPV would be 80/90 = 0.889 or 88.9%. This indicates that when the test predicts a positive result, there is an 88.9% chance that the patient has the disease.

Negative Predictive Value (NPV): It is another statistical metric used in binary classification tasks, like PPV, but focusing on the performance of negative predictions. NPV represents the proportion of true negative predictions (correctly predicted negative cases) out of all negative predictions made by the model. Mathematically, NPV is calculated as follows:

$$NPV = \frac{True\,Negatives}{True\,Positives + False\,Positives}$$

In medical testing, for instance, if a test for a disease is negative for 110 patients, and 100 of those patients truly do not have the disease while 10 do, the NPV would be 100/110 = 0.91 or 91%. This implies that when the test predicts a negative result, there is a 91% chance that the patient truly does not have the disease.

Like PPV, NPV is crucial in evaluating the performance of classifiers or diagnostic tests, especially in scenarios where accurate negative predictions are vital. However, like other metrics, NPV should be considered alongside sensitivity, specificity, and PPV for a comprehensive assessment of model performance.

Bayes' rule equations (2–6) are typically presented as follows (see Table 17.1):

Table 17.1 Diagnostic and disease classification table based on Bayes' rule

Test result	Disease status	
	Present (D+)	Absent (D–)
Positive (T+)	Probability of true positive (TP) $P(T+\mid D+) = S_n X Prev$	Probability of false positive (FP) $P(T+\mid D-) = (1-S_p) X (1-Prev)$
Negative (T–)	Probability of false negative (FN) $P(T-\mid D+) = (1-S_n) X Prev$	Probability of true negative (TN) $P(T-\mid D-) = S_p X (1-Prev)$
Prior Probability	$TP + FN = P(D+) = Prev$	$FP + TN = P(D-) = (1-Prev)$

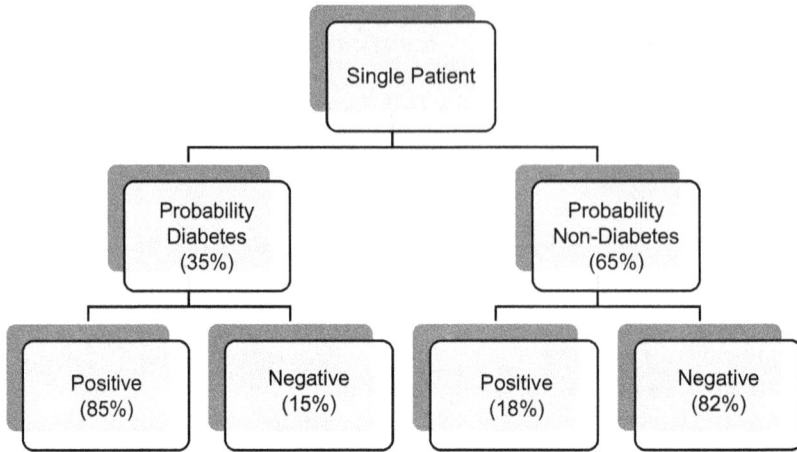

Figure 17.1 Probability of diabetes based on random glucose measurement.

$$Positive\ Predictive\ Value\,(PPV) = \frac{S_n \times Prev}{S_n \times Prev + (1 - S_p) \times (1 - Prev)}$$

$$Negative\ Predictive\ Value\,(NPV) = \frac{S_p \times (1 - Prev)}{(1 - S_n) \times (Prev) + S_p \times (1 - Prev)}$$

Illustrations

Example 1: In a community-based study, let us consider that there is a 35% a priori chance that a randomly selected patient seen by the general practitioner has diabetes. Also referred to as the "base rate" or pre-test probability, this represents the (previous) prevalence of diabetes in the general practitioner community. This 35% risk of diabetes is depicted in Figure 17.1. The likelihood that a patient who genuinely experiences diabetes will answer "yes" on the diabetes questionnaire is represented by the test's 85% sensitivity. The test's 82% specificity is represented by the right arm, which shows the likelihood that a patient without diabetes will have a negative result.

Here,

- Assume the prevalence of diabetes is 35% ($p = 0.35$).
- Sensitivity (true positive rate): Probability that the test correctly identifies a person with the diabetes is 90% ($S_n = 0.85$).
- Specificity (true negative rate): Probability that the test correctly identifies a person without diabetes is 95% ($S_p = 0.82$).

Bayesian inference:

$$P(Diabetes) = 0.35$$

$$P(No\,Diabetes) = 1 - P(Diabetes) = 0.65$$

$$P(Positive \mid Diabetes) = Sensitivity = 0.85$$

$$P(Positive \mid No\,Diabetes) = 1 - Specificity = 1 - 0.82 = 0.18$$

$$P(Positive) = P(Positive\,Diabetes) \times P(Diabetes) + P(Positive \mid No\,Diabetes)$$
$$\times P(No\,Diabetes) = (0.85 \times 0.35) + (0.18 \times 0.65) = 0.415$$

$$P(Diabetes\,Positive) = Sensitivity \times \frac{P(Diabetes)}{P(Positive)} = 0.85 \times \frac{0.35}{0.415} = 0.718$$

Now we can find the PPV and NPV:

$$Positive\,Predictive\,Value\,(PPV) = \frac{S_n \, X\,Prev}{S_n \, X\,Prev + (1 - S_p) X (1 - Prev)}$$

$$= \frac{0.85 \times 0.35}{(0.85 \times 0.35 + 0.18 \times 0.65)} = 0.718$$

$$Negative\,Predictive\,Value\,(NPV) = \frac{S_p \, X (1 - Prev)}{(1 - S_n) X (Prev) + S_p \, X (1 - Prev)}$$

$$= \frac{0.82 \times 0.65}{(0.15 \times 0.35 + 0.82 \times 0.65)} = 0.91$$

So the PPV is 71.8% and NPV is 91%. These values illustrate how the prevalence of diabetes affects the predictive values of the test results. Even with a sensitive and specific test, both PPV and NPV are found to be quite high.

Example 2: The concept may be best understood using the illustration derived from the study by Madžar et al (2016) on the diagnosis of acute appendicitis in women. Acute appendicitis is a clinical condition characterized by an acute inflammation of the appendix and warrants immediate appendicectomy to prevent further complications. However, till (to) date, there is (has been) no single test which may be considered absolute, and this leads to a significant number of patients undergoing anesthesia and surgery without there being a need for appendicectomy. Fenyö et al. (1997) and Teicher et al. (1983) are two scoring systems to assist the surgeon in pre-operative decision-making. These scores have been validated on a cohort of 130 patients by Madnar et al. Based upon the gold standard for final diagnosis of acute appendicitis (intraoperative findings and histological diagnosis), the authors concluded that 27 of 130 participants did not have acute appendicitis.

Fenyo et al. (1997) was evaluated at cut-offs of –17, –2, and –15. The teacher score was evaluated at a cut-off value of –3. The quoted sensitivity, specificity, positive predictive value, and negative predictive value have been summarized in Table 17.2. Let us consider the case of Fenyo-Lindberg score with a cut-off of –17.

Table 17.2 Positive predictive value and negative predictive value

Sl.	Cut-off	Sensitivity	Specificity	Positive predictive value	Negative predictive value
Fenyo-Lindberg score					
1.	−17	84.5%	55.6%	87.9%	48.4%
2.	−2	59.2%	77.8%	91.0%	33.3%
3.	−15	78.5%	70.4%	91.0%	46.3%
Teicher score					
4.	−3	89.3%	22.2%	81.4%	35.3%

a. **Size of cohort:** $n = 130$: of which acute appendicitis (AA): $n = 103$, non-specific pain (NS): $n = 27$ [referred to as Fact A]

b. **Sensitivity:** 84.5%
   Derivation: True Positive: $n = 87$

$$\left[\left(\frac{True\,Positive}{Total\,positive}\right) \times 100 = 84.5; \text{ wherein Total positive } n = 103 \text{ as per Fact A}\right]$$

   [referred to as Derivation A]

c. **Specificity:** 55.6%
   Derivation: True Negative: $n = 15$

$$\left[\left(\frac{True\,Negative}{Total\,negative}\right) \times 100 = 55.6; \text{ wherein Total negative } n = 27 \text{ as per Fact A}\right]$$

   [referred to as Derivation B]

Based upon the Derivations A and B, we can compute the contingency Table 17.3.

The authors have provided the positive and negative predictive values; however, the same could have been calculated by the reader from the contingency table also:

a. **Positive Predictive Value:** $\left(\frac{True Positive}{Total\,Positive}\right) \times 100 = (87 / 99) * 100 = 87.9\%$

b. **Negative Predictive Value:** $\left(\frac{True\,Negative}{Total\,Negative}\right) \times 100 = (15 / 31) * 100 = 48.4\%$

Similar calculations are possible for the other cut-off values used to validate the Fenyo-Lindberg score or the Teicher score.

Conclusion

Bayesian methods incorporate prior information (like patient history or prevalence of a condition) with new evidence (test results) to provide individualized probabilities of a disease. This personalized approach offers a clearer risk assessment for patients. Bayesian approaches help clinicians make more informed decisions by focusing on the posterior probability of disease after test results are known. This approach allows for better interpretation of diagnostic test outcomes, especially when dealing with

Table 17.3 Contingency table

	Fenyo-Lindberg positive	Fenyo-Lindberg negative	Total
Acute Appendicitis (Gold Standard)	87 (True Positive)	16 (False Negative)	AA $n = 103$
Non-Specific Pain (Gold Standard)	12 (False Positive)	15 (True Negative)	NS $n = 27$
Total	Positive on Fenyo-Lindberg: $n = 99$	Negative on Fenyo-Lindberg: $n = 31$	130

uncertain or ambiguous results. Bayesian methods are effective in managing diagnostic uncertainty. By using probability distributions, clinicians can update their beliefs about a patient's condition iteratively, as new data (such as follow-up tests) become available. These methods factor in test sensitivity and specificity and adjust the decision-making process based on the likelihood of false positives or false negatives, leading to a more nuanced interpretation of diagnostic accuracy. The present study demonstrated that Bayesian methods offer a powerful tool for enhancing the accuracy and reliability of diagnostic testing, ultimately leading to more tailored and effective patient care. They emphasize the dynamic updating of knowledge and integrate prior information with test outcomes to support better clinical decisions.

Discussion Questions

■ Why is understanding probability essential for accurate diagnosis in clinical settings?
■ How does Bayes' rule guide the transition from pre-test to post-test probability in diagnostic reasoning?
■ What roles do sensitivity, specificity, and disease prevalence play in determining post-test probability?
■ How can clinicians apply Bayes' rule to improve the selection and interpretation of diagnostic tests?
■ Finally, what are the challenges in applying probabilistic thinking in real-world clinical practice, and how can these be addressed through training or decision-support tools?

References

Bours, M.J., 2021. Bayes' rule in diagnosis. *Journal of Clinical Epidemiology*, 131, pp.158–160.
Fenyö, G., Lindberg, G., Blind, P., Enochsson, L. and Oberg, A., 1997. Diagnostic decision support in suspected acute appendicitis: Validation of a simplified scoring system. *The European Journal of Surgery= Acta Chirurgica*, 163(11), pp.831–838.
Gelman, A. and Carpenter, B., 2020. Bayesian analysis of tests with unknown specificity and sensitivity. *Journal of the Royal Statistical Society: Series C (Applied Statistics)*, 69(5), pp.1269–1283.
Joseph, L., Gyorkos, T.W. and Coupal, L., 1995. Bayesian estimation of disease prevalence and the parameters of diagnostic tests in the absence of a gold standard. *American Journal of Epidemiology*, 141(3), pp.263–272.

Herrle, S.R., Corbett Jr, E.C., Fagan, M.J., Moore, C.G. and Elnicki, D.M., 2011. Bayes' theorem and the physical examination: Probability assessment and diagnostic decision making. *Academic Medicine*, 86(5), pp.618–627.

Madžar, Z., Kopljar, M., Madžar, T., Mesić, M., Muina Mišić, D., Čiček, S. and Zovak, M., 2016. Sensitivity and specificity of Fenyö-Lindberg and Teicher scores in the diagnosis of acute appendicitis in women. *Acta Clinica Croatica*, 55(4), pp.593–599.

Matthews, R.A., 2020. The origins of the treatment of uncertainty in clinical medicine–Part 2: The emergence of probability theory and its limitations. *Journal of the Royal Society of Medicine*, 113(6), pp.225–229.

Mengel, M.B., Holleman, W.L. and Fields, S.A. eds., 2007. *Fundamentals of clinical practice*. Springer Science & Business Media.

Morgan, D.J., Pineles, L., Owczarzak, J., Magder, L., Scherer, L., Brown, J.P., Pfeiffer, C., Terndrup, C., Leykum, L., Feldstein, D. and Foy, A., 2021. Accuracy of practitioner estimates of probability of diagnosis before and after testing. *JAMA Internal Medicine*, 181(6), pp.747–755.

Sox, H.C., Higgins, M.C., Owens, D.K. and Schmidler, G.S., 2024. *Medical decision making*. John Wiley & Sons.

Swets, J.A., 1988. Measuring the accuracy of diagnostic systems. *Science*, 240(4857), pp.1285–1293.

Teicher, I.R.A., Landa, B., Cohen, M., Kabnick, L.S. and Wise, L., 1983. Scoring system to aid in diagnoses of appendicitis. *Annals of Surgery*, 198(6), pp.753–759.

Whiting, P.F., Davenport, C., Jameson, C., Burke, M., Sterne, J.A., Hyde, C. and Ben-Shlomo, Y., 2015. How well do health professionals interpret diagnostic information? A systematic review. *BMJ Open*, 5(7), p.e008155.

Wilson, J. and Jungner, G., 1968. Pr and practice of screening. *WHO: Geneva*, 69(5), p.1085.

## CHAPTER 18

Prediction of 90-Day Mortality Using Machine Learning Algorithm

Ramesh K. Vishwakarma, Zillur Rahman Shabuz and Robert Cook

Learning Outcomes

Learners will understand the application of machine learning models – specifically the Cox proportional hazards model with LASSO – in predicting 90-day mortality among ICU patients. They will gain insights into handling real-world clinical data using the MIMIC-IV database and identifying key predictors, such as age, gender, admission type, and comorbidities. The chapter emphasizes the role of predictive analytics in enhancing early risk assessment, guiding interventions, and improving ICU outcomes. Students will also explore performance evaluation metrics, like the concordance index, and recognize the need for ongoing model refinement and validation across healthcare systems to ensure generalizability.

Introduction

In contemporary healthcare, mortality prediction plays a pivotal role in patient care, clinical decision-making, and resource allocation. Predicting mortality within specific timeframes, such as 90 days, involves utilizing advanced statistical methods and machine learning algorithms to forecast the likelihood of death based on various patient-related factors, disease severity markers, and treatment responses. Accurate mortality prediction is essential for optimizing patient outcomes, informing clinical interventions, and enhancing healthcare delivery.

Over the past decades, there has been a significant increase in the development and implementation of mortality prediction models across diverse clinical settings. These models aim to provide clinicians with valuable insights into patient prognosis, enabling them to identify individuals at high risk of mortality and intervene promptly to improve outcomes. Mortality prediction has become particularly relevant in intensive care units (ICUs) and critical care settings, where early identification of patients at heightened risk of death can significantly impact treatment strategies and patient outcomes.

DOI: 10.4324/9781032701004-24

Literature Review

The field of mortality prediction has witnessed remarkable advancements, driven by developments in machine learning algorithms and the growing availability of electronic health records (EHRs) and clinical data. Early studies by Hanson and Marshall (Hanson et al., 2001) highlighted the potential of artificial intelligence (AI)–based analytical algorithms in ICU settings, owing to the abundance of available data and their effectiveness in inpatient care. Subsequent research has explored a wide range of machine learning approaches, including decision trees, random forests, support vector machines, and artificial neural networks, each offering unique advantages in mortality prediction (Mokashi et al., 2024; Kuk et al., 2006, Marshall et al., 2008; Walter et al., 2012).

Studies focusing on mortality prediction within specific timeframes, such as 90 days, have provided valuable insights into prognostication across various clinical contexts. Martin et al. (Mokashi et al., 2024) demonstrated the utility of artificial neural networks in forecasting mortality following thoracic surgery and cardiac procedures, highlighting the potential of such models in risk stratification. Similarly, support vector machine models have been applied to predict mortality in post-operative patients (Gulshan et al., 2016) and to forecast mortality based on non-invasive cardiovascular spectrum analysis (Lundberg et al., 2017). Additionally, Bayesian networks, kernel methods, and variants of support vector machines with feature selection have been explored in mortality prediction studies (Molnar, 2019; Torlay et al., 2017; Lustberg et al., 2002; Goldwasser et al., 1997; Nakhoul et al., 2015; Weng et al., 2017; Wu et al., 2017; Qiu et al., 2022).

Significance of the Study

The ability to predict mortality within a 90-day timeframe using machine learning algorithms holds profound implications for clinical practice. Early identification of patients at elevated risk of death within this window enables clinicians to implement proactive interventions, tailor treatment strategies, and allocate resources effectively (Lundberg et al., 2017). By leveraging advanced predictive models, healthcare providers can optimize patient outcomes, enhance quality of care, and reduce healthcare costs associated with preventable mortality events.

Furthermore, accurate mortality prediction can facilitate end-of-life care planning, enabling patients and their families to make informed decisions about treatment options, palliative care, and advance directives (Torlay et al., 2017; Lustberg et al., 2002; Goldwasser et al., 1997). It also provides healthcare organizations with valuable insights into population health trends, enabling them to implement targeted interventions and preventive strategies to reduce mortality rates and improve overall community health.

Aim of the Study

This study aims to develop and validate a machine learning algorithm for predicting 90-day mortality in clinical settings. By leveraging a comprehensive dataset encompassing clinical, physiological, and demographic variables, we seek to construct a prediction model capable of accurately identifying individuals at heightened risk of mortality within this critical timeframe. Our ultimate goal is to improve patient outcomes, enhance clinical decision-making, and optimize resource allocation in healthcare settings.

Data and Methods

Data and Variables

We extracted data from the Medical Information Mart for Intensive Care (MIMIC)-IV database (Johnson *et al.*, 2023). MIMIC-IV collected electronic health records (EHR) of admissions between 2008 and 2019 from Beth Israel Deaconess Medical Center (BIDMC). The database is grouped into two modules, namely, *hosp* and *icu*. The hospital-wide EHR constitutes the *hosp* module, while the *icu* module contains the ICU-specific clinical information system (Mokashi *et al.*, 2024). We acquired all patients who were admitted to an ICU between 2008 and 2019. The hospital admissions identification of each patient's most recent ICU admission was used as the key for merging data from various files. Demographics information was obtained from *admissions* and *patient* files and diagnoses of disease were collected from *diagnoses_icd* and *d_icd_diagnoses* files.

The response variable of interest was the survival time of 90 days mortality from the latest hospital admission. The covariates considered were admissions type (Ambulatory observation, Direct emergency, Direct observation, Elective, Emergency unit observation, EW emergency, Observation admission, Surgical same-day admission, Urgent), marital status (Married, Divorced, Single, Widowed, Single, Missing), ethnicity (White, Asian, Black, Hispanic or Latino, Other), gender (Male, Female), age group ([18–53], [53–65], [65–77], [77–91]), and disease diagnoses. The large number (15,699) of available diagnosis codes were categorized into 13 broad categories. Finally, the data contains information about 50,904 ICU patients.

Machine Learning Algorithms for Mortality Prediction

We applied univariate analysis to describe the sample characteristics of the covariates. We also employed the Least Absolute Shrinkage and Selection Operator (LASSO) (Tibshirani, 1996) for variable selection in the Cox proportional hazards (PH) model.

Suppose T is a random variable denoting the time to death from the hospital admission and t is the specific value of T. Then the Cox PH model can be written as follows:

$$h(t, \mathbf{x}) = h_0(t) \exp\left(\sum_{j=1}^{p} \beta_j x_j \right),$$

where $h(t, \mathbf{x})$ is the hazard at the time t, given the time-independent covariate vector $\mathbf{x} = (x_1, x_2, \ldots, x_p)$, $h_0(t)$ is an unspecified baseline hazard function and $\boldsymbol{\beta} = (\beta_1, \beta_2, \ldots, \beta_p)^\top$ is the vector of regression coefficients. The parameters $\boldsymbol{\beta}$ can be estimated by maximizing the partial likelihood function.

$P_\lambda(\boldsymbol{\beta}) = \lambda \sum_{j=1}^{p} |\beta_j|$, where $\lambda \geq 0$ is a tuning parameter that can be determined separately. The LASSO penalty forces some coefficients to be exactly zero when λ is sufficiently large (Johnson *et al.*, 2023). As LASSO yields a model that contains a subset of the variables, it is easy to interpret the model. Selecting a good value of λ is critical.

The LASSO hyper-parameter, λ, controls the variable space by applying a 'shrinkage' pressure on the magnitude of the coefficients. A greater value of λ imparts a stronger extent of regularization and a greater tendency for parameter estimates to reduce to zero. The cross-validated LASSO algorithm selects two estimates for the hyper-parameter, λ (Friedman *et al.*, 2010):

1. The value of λ, which produces the optimal learning metric (i.e., the maximum cross-validated C-index), is denoted 'lambda.min' (λ_{min}).
2. The value of λ, which produces the most regularized model such that the cross-validated error is within one standard error of the minimum (i.e., the C-index of λ_{min} minus one standard error), is denoted 'lambda.1se' (λ_{1se}).

Given that $\lambda_{1se} > \lambda_{min}$, the λ_{1se} model undergoes a greater degree of 'coefficient shrinkage' and is expected to report a greater prevalence of zero-valued coefficients. Hence, the λ_{1se} model is considered a more parsimonious and conservative estimate of the underlying model. When used as a method of selecting non-zero parameters, the λ_{1se} model is expected to have a reduced Type II and an increased Type I error rate when compared to the λ_{min} model.

We applied tenfold cross-validation to select λ for which the model performs better than the other models. The commonly used goodness of fit measure, namely, the concordance index (C-index), has been used as a performance measure. Let y_i and $\hat{y}_i$ be the observed and predicted data values for the i th observation. A pair of observations is considered concordant if $(y_i > y_l, \hat{y}_i > \hat{y}_l)$ or $(y_i < y_l, \hat{y}_i < \hat{y}_l)$. The C-index is defined as the probability of agreement between the predicted and the observed data. Suppose c is the number of concordant pairs, d is the number of discordant pairs and $t_{\hat{y}}$ is the number of observations that have tied predicted scores (but not necessarily tied with observed values). Then C-index is defined as $C = \dfrac{c + t_{\hat{y}}/2}{c + d + t_{\hat{y}}}$ (Therneau, 2023). It ranges between 0 and 1. A higher C-index means better agreement among comparable pairs. Finally, we refit the model, considering all the observations using the selected value of λ.

Data management and statistical analysis have been performed in R language (R version 4.4.0). The R package 'glmnet' was employed to perform the LASSO Cox PH regression model and tenfold cross-validation.

Results

From Table 18.1, it is evident that the dataset has a diverse representation of patients across various demographic and clinical categories. The gender distribution shows a higher proportion of males (55.9%) compared to females (44.1%). In terms of age, the patients are fairly evenly distributed across the four age groups, with a slightly higher number in the older age groups, particularly those aged 65–77 (26.0%) and 77–91 (23.4%).

The majority of admissions were classified as emergency (50.5%), which is typical for ICU settings where critical and urgent care is required. Other significant admission types include observation admissions (12.7%) and surgical same-day admissions (11.3%).

Marital status data indicates that a large portion of the patients were married (45.2%), followed by single (26.8%), widowed (12.4%), and divorced (7.1%). The ethnicity distribution shows that the majority of patients were White (67.5%), with smaller

Table 18.1 Demographic and clinical characteristics of the patients

Characteristic	n (%)
Gender	
Male	28,436 (55.9)
Female	22,468 (44.1)
Age group	
(18–53)	13,113 (25.8)
(53–65)	12,646 (24.8)
(65–77)	13,248 (26.0)
(77–91)	11,897 (23.4)
Admissions type	
Ambulatory observation	16 (0.0)
Direct emergency	1,757 (3.5)
Direct observation	130 (0.3)
Elective	1,787 (3.5)
Emergency unit observation	326 (0.6)
EW emergency	25,693 (50.5)
Observation admission	6,474 (12.7)
Surgical same-day admission	5,748 (11.3)
Urgent	8,973 (17.6)
Marital status	
Married	23,009 (45.2)
Divorced	3,602 (7.1)
Single	13,656 (26.8)
Widowed	6,312 (12.4)
Missing	4,325 (8.5)
Ethnicity	
White	34,375 (67.5)
Asian	1,503 (3.0)
Black	4,655 (9.1)
Hispanic or Latino	1,710 (3.4)
Other	8,661 (17.0)

The dataset extracted from the MIMIC-IV database included 50,904 ICU admissions from 2008 to 2019. The demographic and clinical characteristics of the patients are summarized in Table 18.1.

proportions of Black (9.1%), Asian (3.0%), Hispanic or Latino (3.4%), and other ethnicities (17.0%).

Variable Selection

We employed LASSO (Least Absolute Shrinkage and Selection Operator) for variable selection in the Cox proportional hazards (PH) model. The LASSO method effectively reduced the number of variables by applying a penalty that forces some

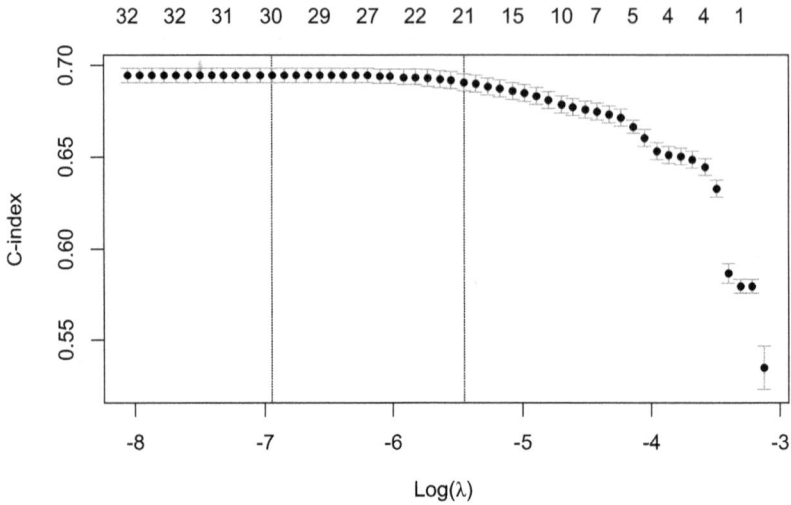

Figure 18.1 Cross-validated C-index across all folds for each λ.

coefficients to be exactly zero. This method was crucial in handling the high-dimensional data, ensuring that only the most significant predictors were included in the final model. The selected variables are listed in Table 18.2, along with their LASSO Cox PH estimates.

The left vertical line in Figure 18.1 is the minimum cross-validated error, i.e., the maximum C-index. The right vertical line is the most shrinkage model with a C-index within 1 standard deviation of the maximum.

Table 18.2 provides detailed estimates for the variables selected by the LASSO Cox PH model. Each variable's influence on the 90-day mortality prediction is shown with coefficients for both lambda.1se and lambda.min regularization parameters. The lambda.1se (standard error) parameter selects a simpler model with fewer predictors, whereas lambda.min selects a model with the minimum cross-validated error, potentially including more predictors.

Table 18.2 LASSO Cox PH estimates

Variable	lambda.1se	lambda.min
Admissions type		
Ambulatory observation	0	0
Direct emergency	0	−0.047
Direct observation	0.193	1.339
Elective	−0.712	−1.096
Emergency unit observation	0.778	1.432
EW emergency	0.237	0.263
Observation admission	−0.052	−0.119
Surgical same-day admission	−1.118	−1.508

(*Continued*)

Table 18.2 (Continued)

Variable	lambda.1se	lambda.min
Urgent	0	0.015
Marital status		
Married	0	0
Divorced	0	−0.021
Single	−0.036	−0.024
Widowed	0.037	0.07
Missing	0.39	0.432
Ethnicity		
White	0	0
Asian	0	0.128
Black	0	0.003
Hispanic or Latino	0	0
Other	0.084	0.139
Gender		
Male	0	0
Female	0.001	0.042
Age group		
(18–53)	0	0
(53–65)	0.05	0.291
(65–77)	0.324	0.545
(77–91)	0.693	0.885
Disease diagnosis		
Complications and Conditions	0	−0.033
Injury and Trauma	−0.01	−0.061
Gastrointestinal and Abdominal	−0.257	−0.334
Transplant and Organ Status	0	0.027
Chronic Diseases	0	0
Infectious Diseases	−0.019	−0.093
Personal Medical History	0	0.025
Cancer and Related Conditions	0.077	0.107
Mental Health	−0.02	−0.123
Surgical and Post-Surgical Status	0	0.041
Environmental Exposure	0.148	0.252
Noncompliance and Compliance Issues	−0.16	−0.348
Other Conditions	0	0

Model Performance

The concordance index was used as the primary performance measure to evaluate the predictive accuracy of the Cox PH model with LASSO variable selection. The concordance index for the model using lambda.1se and lambda.min was 0.691 and 0.695 (Figure 18.1), respectively. These values indicate a moderate level of predictive accuracy, suggesting that the model can distinguish between patients with different survival times to a reasonable extent.

In summary, the results highlight that the LASSO Cox PH model, applied to a comprehensive ICU dataset, can reasonably predict 90-day mortality. The selected variables and their coefficients provide insights into the factors that significantly influence patient outcomes, which can be invaluable for clinical decision-making and improving patient care in the ICU setting.

Discussion

The study aimed to develop a predictive model for 90-day mortality using machine learning techniques applied to the MIMIC-IV database. The results demonstrate that the LASSO Cox proportional hazards model effectively identified significant predictors and achieved a moderate level of predictive accuracy, as indicated by the concordance index. This discussion elaborates on the implications of these findings, the strengths and limitations of the study, and potential directions for future research.

The dataset included a diverse patient population with varying demographic and clinical characteristics. The majority of the patients were male and elderly, which is consistent with the typical ICU population (Johnson *et al.*, 2023). The high proportion of emergency admissions underscores the critical nature of the dataset (Bate *et al.*, 2024).

The LASSO variable selection process identified key predictors of 90-day mortality, including age, gender, admission type, marital status, and various disease diagnoses. Notably, older age groups and certain clinical conditions (e.g., complications, gastrointestinal and abdominal issues, and chronic diseases) were associated with higher mortality risk. These findings align with existing literature, which consistently shows that age and comorbidities are strong predictors of mortality in critically ill patients (Vincent *et al.*, 2010).

The performance metrics of the model, particularly the concordance index, indicate a moderate level of predictive accuracy. A concordance index of approximately 0.69 suggests that the model can reasonably distinguish between patients with different survival times. While this level of accuracy is not optimal, it is sufficient to provide valuable insights for clinical decision-making.

The predictive model developed in this study can serve as a useful tool for clinicians in the ICU setting. By identifying patients at higher risk of mortality, healthcare providers can prioritize resources and interventions more effectively (Lim *et al.*, 2024). For example, high-risk patients might benefit from more intensive monitoring, early interventions, or palliative care discussions. Moreover, the model can aid in informed decision-making regarding patient management and discharge planning.

The selected variables also highlight areas where targeted interventions could improve patient outcomes. For instance, addressing chronic diseases and optimizing the management of complications and gastrointestinal conditions could potentially reduce mortality rates. The findings emphasize the importance of comprehensive and individualized patient care in the ICU (Pattha Pattharanitima *et al.*, 2021).

One of the key strengths of this study is the use of the MIMIC-IV database (Johnson *et al.*, 2023), which provides a large and detailed dataset of ICU admissions. This richness allowed for robust model development and validation. Additionally, the application of LASSO for variable selection ensured that the model focused on the most significant predictors, enhancing its interpretability and clinical relevance (Friedman *et al.*, 2010).

However, several limitations should be acknowledged. First, the study relied on retrospective data, which may be subject to biases and inaccuracies in documentation. The predictive model's performance, while reasonable, indicates room for improvement, suggesting that additional variables or more sophisticated modeling techniques might enhance accuracy. The generalizability of the model is another concern, as it was developed using data from a single database. Validation with external datasets is necessary to confirm its applicability to different patient populations and healthcare settings (Bate *et al.*, 2024).

Future Research

Future research should focus on several areas to build on the findings of this study. First, external validation of the model using data from other ICU databases is crucial to assess its generalizability. Additionally, incorporating more advanced machine learning techniques, such as deep learning, could potentially improve predictive performance.

Exploring the inclusion of additional variables, particularly those related to social determinants of health and detailed clinical interventions, may enhance the model's accuracy (Pattha Pattharanitima *et al.*, 2021). Finally, integrating the predictive model into clinical workflows and assessing its impact on patient outcomes and healthcare resource utilization would provide valuable insights into its practical utility.

Conclusion

The development of a predictive model for 90-day mortality using machine learning techniques has shown promising results, with the LASSO Cox proportional hazards model identifying significant predictors and achieving moderate accuracy (Friedman *et al.*, 2010). These findings highlight the potential for such models to inform clinical decision-making and improve patient care in the ICU. However, further research is needed to validate and refine the model, ensuring its robustness and applicability across diverse healthcare settings (Komorowski *et al.*, 2018).

Discussion Questions

- How can machine learning models assist clinicians in predicting patient outcomes in the ICU?
- What are the advantages of using LASSO in variable selection within survival analysis?
- Which clinical variables were most predictive of 90-day mortality, and why might they be influential?
- What does a concordance index of 0.69 suggest about model performance, and how can it be improved?
- Lastly, what are the challenges of implementing predictive models in clinical practice, and how can they be addressed to ensure ethical, accurate, and equitable care?

References

Bate, S., Stokes, V., Greenlee, H., Goh, K.Y., Whiting, G., Kitchen, G., Martin, G.P., Parker, A.J. & Wilson, A., 2024. External validation of prognostic models in critical care: A cautionary tale from COVID-19 pneumonitis. *Critical Care Explorations*, 6(4), p.e1067.

Friedman, J.H., Hastie, T. & Tibshirani, R., 2010. Regularization paths for generalized linear models via coordinate descent. *Journal of Statistical Software*, 33, pp.1–22.

Goldwasser, P. & Feldman, J., 1997. Association of serum albumin and mortality risk. *Journal of Clinical Epidemiology, 50*, pp.693–703.

Gulshan, V., Peng, L., Coram, M., Stumpe, M.C., Wu, D., Narayanaswamy, A., Venugopalan, S., Widner, K., Madams, T., Cuadros, J. & Kim, R., 2016. Development and validation of a deep learning algorithm for the detection of diabetic retinopathy in retinal fundus photographs. *Journal of the American Medical Association, 316*, pp.2402–2410.

Hanson, W. & Marshall, E., 2001. Advanced analytics in intensive care: Unlocking the potential of AI-based algorithms. *Critical Care Medicine, 29*, pp.427–435.

Johnson, A.E., Bulgarelli, L., Shen, L., Gayles, A., Shammout, A., Horng, S., Pollard, T.J., Hao, S., Moody, B., Gow, B. & Lehman, L.W.H., 2023. MIMIC-IV, a freely accessible electronic health record dataset. *Scientific Data, 10*(1), p.1.

Komorowski, M., Celi, L.A., Badawi, O. *et al.*, 2018. The artificial intelligence clinician learns optimal treatment strategies for sepsis in intensive care. *Nature Medicine, 24*, pp.1716–1720.

Kuk, J.L., Katzmarzyk, P.T., Nichaman, M.Z., Church, T.S., Blair, S.N. & Ross, R. 2006. Visceral fat is an independent predictor of all-cause mortality in men. *Obesity, 14*, pp.336–341.

Lim, L., Gim, U., Cho, K. *et al.*, 2024. Real-time machine learning model to predict short-term mortality in critically ill patients: Development and international validation. *Critical Care, 28*, p.76

Lundberg, S.M. & Lee, S.-I., 2017. A unified approach to interpreting model predictions. *Advances in Neural Information Processing Systems*, pp.4765–4774.

Lustberg, M. & Silbergeld, E., 2002. Blood lead levels and mortality. *Archives of Internal Medicine, 162*, pp.2443–2449.

Marshall, N.S., Wong, K.K., Liu, P.Y., Cullen, S.R., Knuiman, M.W. & Grunstein, R.R. 2008. Sleep apnea as an independent risk factor for all-cause mortality: The Busselton health study. *Sleep, 31*, pp.1079–1085.

Mokashi, S. & Keane, M., 2024. The utility of machine learning for cardiology and cardiac surgery risk assessment scores. *Indian Journal of Clinical Cardiology, 5*(3), pp.258–261.

Molnar, C., 2019. *Interpretable machine learning*. Lulu.com.

Nakhoul, G.N., Huang, H., Arrigain, S., Jolly, S.E., Schold, J.D., Nally Jr, J.V. & Navaneethan, S.D., 2015. Serum potassium, end-stage renal disease, and mortality in chronic kidney disease. *American Journal of Nephrology, 41*, pp.456–463.

Pattha Pattharanitima, P., Thongprayoon, C., Kaewput, W. *et al.*, 2021. Machine learning prediction models for mortality in intensive care unit patients with lactic acidosis. *Journal of Clinical Medicine, 10*(21), p.5021.

Qiu, W., Chen, H., Dincer, A.B., Lundberg, S., Kaeberlein, M. & Lee, S.I., 2022. Interpretable machine learning prediction of all-cause mortality. *Communications Medicine, 2*(1), p.125.

Therneau, T. 2023. *A package for survival analysis in R. Vignette: Concordance*. R package version 3.5.7. https://cran.r-project.org/web/packages/survival/vignettes/concordance.pdf.

Tibshirani, R., 1996. Regression shrinkage and selection via the lasso. *Journal of the Royal Statistical Society: Series B (Methodological), 58*(1), pp.267–288.

Torlay, L., Perrone-Bertolotti, M., Thomas, E. & Baciu, M., 2017. Machine learning–xgboost analysis of language networks to classify patients with epilepsy. *Brain Informatics, 4*, pp.159–169.

Vincent, J.L. & Moreno, R., 2010. Clinical review: Scoring systems in the critically ill. *Critical Care, 14*(2), p.207.

Walter, S., Mackenbach, J., Vokó, Z., Lhachimi, S., Ikram, M.A., Uitterlinden, A.G., Newman, A.B., Murabito, J.M., Garcia, M.E., Gudnason, V. & Tanaka, T., 2012. Genetic, physiological, and lifestyle predictors of mortality in the general population. *American Journal of Public Health, 102*, pp.e3–e10.

Weng, S.F., Reps, J., Kai, J., Garibaldi, J.M. & Qureshi, N., 2017. Can machine learning improve cardiovascular risk prediction using routine clinical data? *PLoS ONE, 12*, p.e0174944.

Wu, L.W., Lin, Y.Y., Kao, T.W., Lin, C.M., Wang, C.C., Wang, G.C., Peng, T.C. & Chen, W.L., 2017. Mid-arm circumference and all-cause, cardiovascular, and cancer mortality among obese and non-obese US adults: The National Health and Nutrition Examination Survey III. *Scientific Reports, 7*, pp.1–8.

Index

Note: Page numbers in *italics* indicate a figure and page numbers in **bold** indicate a table on the corresponding page.

For Product Safety Concerns and Information please contact our EU
representative GPSR@taylorandfrancis.com
Taylor & Francis Verlag GmbH, Kaufingerstraße 24, 80331 München, Germany

www.ingramcontent.com/pod-product-compliance
Lightning Source LLC
Chambersburg PA
CBHW081050220326

41598CB00038B/7050